Dr Paula Baillie-Hamilton is a medical doctor and also holds an academic doctorate in human metabolism from the University of Oxford. She is a Visiting Fellow in Occupational and Environmental Health at Stirling University and an adviser to the Soil Association. Paula and her husband live on their family estate in Scotland with their two young sons.

The Detox Diet

*Eliminate Chemical Calories and
Restore Your Body's
Natural Slimming System*

DR PAULA BAILLIE-HAMILTON

MICHAEL JOSEPH
an imprint of
PENGUIN BOOKS

MICHAEL JOSEPH

Published by the Penguin Group
Penguin Books Ltd, 80 Strand, London WC2R 0RL, England
Penguin Putnam Inc., 375 Hudson Street, New York, New York 10014, USA
Penguin Books Australia Ltd, 250 Camberwell Road, Camberwell, Victoria 3124, Australia
Penguin Books Canada Ltd, 10 Alcorn Avenue, Toronto, Ontario, Canada M4V 3B2
Penguin Books India (P) Ltd, 11 Community Centre, Panchsheel Park, New Delhi – 110 017, India
Penguin Books (NZ) Ltd, Cnr Rosedale and Airborne Roads, Albany, Auckland, New Zealand
Penguin Books (South Africa) (Pty) Ltd, 24 Sturdee Avenue, Rosebank 2196, South Africa

Penguin Books Ltd, Registered Offices: 80 Strand, London WC2R 0RL, England

www.penguin.com

First published 2002

6

Set in 12/14.75 pt Bembo
Typeset by Rowland Phototypesetting Ltd,
Bury St Edmunds, Suffolk
Printed in Great Britain by Clays Ltd, St Ives plc

A CIP catalogue record for this book is available from the British Library

ISBN 0-718-14545-3

This book is dedicated to the many thousands of scientists worldwide whose vital individual research findings have effectively formed the groundwork from which this book has arisen.
Thank you for reporting the truth as you witnessed it, even if it turned out to be different from the 'truth' that you may have been looking for.

AN IMPORTANT NOTE: This book is not intended as a substitute for the medical recommendations of physicians or other health-care providers. Rather, it is intended to offer information to help the reader to cooperate with physicians and health professionals in a mutual quest for optimum health.

The publisher and the author are not responsible for any goods and/or services offered or referred to in this book and expressly disclaim all liability in connection with the fulfilment of orders for any such goods and/or services and for any damage, loss, or expense to person or property arising out of or relating to them.

Note on weights and measurements

The ingredients lists in the recipes are given in metric amounts (g, kg, ml), as in the majority of cookery books nowadays. Single references to weights and measurements in the text are also given in metric.

However, the height and weight charts are given in imperial measurements (in, ft, lb), as this is felt to be more easily accessible to the general reader.

Contents

Acknowledgements

No one works in isolation, and this book would never have been possible without the support and help of very many people. I want to start by thanking my entire family, beginning with my husband Mike. He has helped tremendously, not only by providing continual encouragement and suggestions, but also in providing the financial support which has allowed me free rein to follow and fully develop my ideas. Without his whole-hearted support over the last three years, this book would probably never have seen the light of day.

Likewise I am indebted to my sister Julia for her helpful review of the manuscript, as well as for her extremely constructive advice, to my parents, Pat and John, for teaching me to believe in myself, to my sister Clare for acting as a sounding board, and to my children for making everything worthwhile.

I am also more grateful than I could express to:

Fiona Gold, my editor, who expertly helped me to structure and produce my manuscript, and to her husband, Jonathon, who was one of the first to demonstrate the wonders of the programme.

Robert Kirby, my literary agent at Peters Fraser & Dunlop, who saw the promise of my work right from the very start.

Eileen Campbell, my editor at Michael Joseph/Penguin, whose clear vision and deep understanding have immeasurably enriched this project. The particularly astute Tom Weldon and of course the other members of the Michael Joseph team at Penguin Books Ltd, Lucy Chavasse, Pippa Wright, Victoria Standing, Abigail Hanna, who have been incredibly diligent and supportive, and including Kate Raffan, who has certainly proved herself as a great organizer and communicator.

Professor Kim Jobst, who gave me the support and advice I needed to follow my own intuition, and his wife, Belinda, for providing this vital connection!

Professor Sir George Radda, who gave me invaluable advice on the production of my academic paper, and his wife, Sue, for being a good friend.

Dr Basil Shepstone, from Oxford University, my first mentor, who taught me the skills necessary for conducting research as well as giving me great encouragement to continue with my future projects.

Professor Roger Watt and Professor Andrew Watterson, on behalf of and from the Occupational and Environmental Health Research Group at Stirling University, for fully supporting my research.

The staff at Callander Library, who have coped admirably in forwarding a massive number of scientific papers to me.

Elizabeth R. Nesbitt, from the United States International Trade Commission, for going beyond the call of duty by kindly photo-copying and sending me a huge amount of data from which I created several of my graphs.

Finally I am extremely grateful to all of the following: Sam Edenborough, Nicki Kennedy, Neeti Madan, Annie Lee, Professor Desmond Hammerton, Professor Vyvyan Howard, Julian Peck, Dr Gera Troisi, David Allan and Alison Craig (from PAN), Dr Philippa Darbre, Dr Graham Kemp, Francis Blake (Soil Association), Terry Spratt, Neil, Gill and Alex Baillie-Hamilton, as well as all the other people I have not mentioned who have played a role in supporting me personally or professionally in achieving my goals. Thank you all!

Introduction: Making the Discovery

I often cast my mind back to how this all began. If I concentrate hard I can just about capture a faint impression of myself emerging from the thick fog that had enveloped me following the birth of my second son – I had just snatched a free moment when he was asleep, fallen into a comfy chair and picked up a newspaper. What drives me so hard to capture that fleeting moment is that, sitting there, I stumbled across the answer to what is arguably one of the greatest unsolved mysteries in medicine today. With hindsight, I recognize that moment to be one of the most significant turning-points in my life.

You might very well wonder what on earth was in the newspaper. What caught my eye was an article about the powerful gender-bending actions of pesticides, a diverse group of highly toxic chemicals used in food production to kill all kinds of bugs. However, what really grabbed my attention was that the amount of chemicals needed to wreak such havoc with our sex hormones was not too different from the small amount of chemicals we are all exposed to in everyday life.

It just so happened that at the time I was keen to shed some weight and was finding the going pretty tough. After reading the article it struck me that if these chemicals had the power to alter our hormones so completely, then they must possess some sort of influence over our weight. I made a beeline for one of my biggest medical textbooks, thumbed anxiously through the pages, and there it was in black and white. 'Changes in sex hormones can cause weight gain.' I was hooked. Three years of uncovering revelation after revelation have resulted in this book. Never in my wildest dreams could I have imagined the sheer wealth of evidence already in the public domain, just waiting there to be found.

*

After I had made the initial connection between toxic chemicals and weight gain, there was no turning back. I can't really explain why I felt so strongly about pursuing the subject, but I felt it then just as strongly as I do now. As every day passed, it became clearer that this was no ordinary finding but a once-in-a-lifetime discovery on the scale that most people can only dream about. However, it was also becoming clear that the research necessary to prove such a finding would be fraught with difficulties.

From previous research experience, I knew that a proper investigation would take a serious amount of time and effort, as well as requiring easy access to research facilities. The problem was that, for me, life had moved on from the days when I had been working for my scientific doctorate at Christ Church, Oxford. Everything there had been set up for research, the libraries were excellent and the resources were to hand. Now I was living in a different world. After Oxford, I moved to a rural part of Scotland to become a laird's wife and the proud mother of two young boys. I was completely happy with my new life but it had become a great deal harder to do any sort of academic work.

If I wanted to consult medical or scientific papers, for example, I couldn't just stroll across the road to one of the world's biggest scientific libraries. I now had to organize a babysitter for the boys, make the three-hour return journey into Edinburgh, use the library computer to look up potential papers, spend several hours carting very heavy volumes up and down the stairs to make photocopies of the relevant pages, then rush back home again to read the material. The practical problems slowed everything down, making progress very tough.

As a result, I found myself in a difficult situation. On the one hand I was desperate to get down to some proper research; on the other I had major time constraints because of my family and where we lived. Despite the difficulties, however, I was totally gripped by the idea that I had discovered what was causing people to gain weight and by the possibility that my discovery would help millions of people. And as the evidence supporting my ideas stacked up, the more I was convinced that giving up was absolutely not an option.

★

Fortunately, this painfully slow research was soon speeded up by a visit from one of my husband's relations, Belinda Jobst. Neither Mike nor I had ever met her before, but it turned out that I had a great deal in common with her husband, Professor Kim Jobst. By a strange coincidence, he is also a medical doctor, had also gained a scientific doctorate from Oxford and had even been working in Oxford while I was there!

Yet more coincidences followed. He too was very interested in pesticide-free foods and alternative forms of medicine, in fact he is the editor-in-chief of the *Journal of Alternative and Complementary Medicine*. So I had now come across an expert in the right area, with a similar background to my own in orthodox medicine and science.

The meeting had come at just the right time: I was already feeling the need to talk to someone else about this discovery. Every piece of evidence I had found over the previous months pointed to the conclusion that toxic chemicals were making us fatter. But I recognized that I had been working pretty much in isolation for a long time and I really needed to hear from someone else that I was on the right track. So one day I told him about my ideas and waited with bated breath to see what he would say. He paused, then smiled and said, 'Paula, you have got to write a book about this.' This was just the tonic that I needed: there would be no stopping me now!

Hot on the tracks of this encouraging response came the news that it was now possible to access all the scientific information that I needed from the Internet. The National Libraries of America had started to provide free Internet access to Medline, a database of all the medical research papers published worldwide. This was the breakthrough that I needed. Instead of going to Edinburgh, I could now access all the information I needed on my computer at home. My research really took off, as I now had easy access to all the hundreds of thousands of scientific studies that had been published over the past forty years. To everyone at the National Libraries of America – I love you all!

The astonishing fruits of my research, set out in this book, will at last expose the full story behind the tide of excess weight engulfing

approximately 30 million UK citizens, and an overall total of
1.2 billion people worldwide.[1] By being led through what has
effectively been the last three years of my life, you will discover the
primary causes of weight gain and the previously undisclosed key
to permanent weight loss in the twenty-first century.

To help guide you through this book, I have divided it into four
parts. Part One, Our Polluted Bodies, examines the reasons why
we are having such a problem with our weight today. Although
these initial chapters can in places be quite detailed, they set the
scene for the rest of the book. These are full of vital slimming
information and advice, making essential reading for all those who
want to understand the problem more fully.

Part Two identifies which are the most fattening chemicals in
our lives, where in our food and environment they are found and
how to avoid them. The advice given here should in its own right
promote significant weight loss without involving any form of food
deprivation – truly effortless weight loss.

Part Three contains vital information on how to safely remove
the large quantities of existing fattening chemicals or *Chemical
Calories* in our bodies. This speeds up the weight loss process and
is ideal for those who want to lose weight more quickly.

Finally, Part Four tells you how to maintain and enhance your
new slimmer figure. It also contains valuable information on some
of the many health benefits available to you if you follow this
programme.

So if you want to know how you can be part of this major new
discovery – which will revolutionize the way that we should all
now set about losing excess weight – read on. This book will help
you, possibly for the first time, to achieve your dream of permanent
weight loss, improved body shape, and glowing health, virtually
effortlessly.

The programme has already helped many people to lose weight
– let it help you too. You will be totally amazed by the results. Say
farewell to your excess fat and hello to a new slimmer, fitter and
healthier you.

PART ONE

Our Polluted Bodies

1. The Fat Epidemic
Why are We Eating Less but Still Getting Fatter?

Human beings have unravelled the mysteries of the chromosome, split the atom, walked on the moon and even taken photographs of the most distant stars in the Universe, yet until now we have had no idea what is causing so many of us to become uncomfortably overweight or even dangerously fat. Indeed, many doctors have publicly admitted defeat, effectively raising the white flag in the battle of the bulge.[1]

The situation has become so bad that leading doctors have suggested that much of the world is in the grip of a full-blown fatness epidemic. William Dietz, the director of nutrition at the Center for Disease Control, certainly pulled no punches when he said in 1999: 'This is an epidemic in the US, the likes of which we have not had before in chronic disease.'[2] Another leading scientist has even gone so far as to say that if the fat epidemic is not checked, almost all Americans will be overweight within a few generations.[3]

What makes the situation even worse is that our children appear to be increasingly at risk. A staggering 25 per cent of Canadian children are now overweight.[4] In addition, excess weight seems to be becoming a problem at an increasingly young age. This has set loud alarm bells ringing, since it is well known that overweight children are far more likely to stay overweight throughout their adult lives.

As for adults, we already know that the depressing trend for adults is to get heavier as they get older. Current estimates suggest that the average woman gains 450g each year and the average man gains 225g.[5]

It's not too difficult to believe these frightening figures – just take a look around and you can see for yourself. More people are now overweight than ever before. Even seats in public places are no longer wide enough and are having to be replaced.

OUR BODY SHAPE IS CHANGING TOO

But it doesn't stop at our weight: it is increasingly apparent that even our basic body shape seems to be changing. Women are gaining more weight around the abdomen and hips and are also developing bigger busts.[6] Men are becoming more rotund, particularly around the waist. These relentless increases in weight and ballooning in shape have been so dramatic that the standard clothing sizes used for the last fifty years have had to be scrapped and completely revamped.[7]

An experienced underwear fitter I met recently confirmed this. She told me that when she started her career forty years ago, a DD bra fitting was extremely uncommon and an E fitting simply didn't exist. Now DD and E fittings are among the most common bra sizes she sells!

DIETING SIMPLY DOESN'T WORK!

Somewhat incomprehensibly, our battle with our weight seems to grow and grow in spite of our best efforts to hold back the tide. It has been estimated that at any one time over half the adult female population in the US is actively dieting.[8] And it is not only those who are overweight who feel the need to keep their weight from rising: many people who are considered to be of normal weight are also dieting – for example, one study showed that over 33 per cent of adolescent normal-weight girls were on a diet at any one time.[9]

Yet the harder we try, the less effective our efforts seem to be. Surely, if traditional dieting methods really worked, the fat epidemic should have been stamped out long ago? Granted, in the short term, many people do lose weight through sticking to a particular diet or regime. But the overwhelming evidence is that they will regain all the weight lost, and then some more, as soon as they return to 'normal life'.[10]

However, that's by no means the end of the bad news. For when you diet, the proportion of lean muscular tissue you possess dramatically falls while the proportion of your body fat greatly increases, producing a disastrous effect on your overall body shape.[11] Then when you regain the weight you have lost the body gains fat in preference to lean muscle, so you end up with a greater proportion of body fat than when you first started.

For many people, therefore, their final reward for all those weeks or months of deprivation and exertion is that they are likely to end up being heavier, fatter and more out of shape than they would have been if they had put on more weight just by over-eating! To add insult to injury, by the time you are driven to try the next new diet, your excess weight will be that much harder to shift.

So not only do diets not work, but there is increasing evidence that they are actually making us fatter!

BEING OVERWEIGHT DESTROYS SELF-ESTEEM

The harsh reality is that as long as there is widespread prejudice against being overweight, most people will ignore all the above evidence and keep on trying diet after diet to try to reach their ideal body weight. The motivation to be slim is extremely powerful and should never be under-estimated.

Magazines, film and television all promote images of people who are unrealistically skinny. But because of their powerful influence on our society, the message taken on board by most people is that this is the shape people have to be if they want to be considered attractive or be loved.

The flip side of this message is considerably more negative, with fatter people being labelled as either greedy or lazy. Since over-indulgence and laziness are signs of weakness in our society, being seriously overweight is considered a massive social stigma, a self-inflicted and ugly problem, gaining very little sympathy or understanding.

Like it or not, appearance plays a hugely important part in how we relate to others and how they react to us. Society treats overweight people very differently from their slimmer counterparts. Overweight children often bear the brunt of teasing in the classroom and can become withdrawn, developing fewer social skills. With adults the effects are subtler, such as not being selected for a job or having more difficulty in finding a partner. This can cause people to remove themselves from many situations, particularly high-profile or intimate situations where they would be visible or exposed.

While many of us would just like to lose a few pounds to reach our ideal weight, for others being overweight can take a huge personal toll on our lives, driving us to seek ever more desperate ways of losing that unwanted fat. Indeed, many people would do virtually anything to achieve their goal, such as putting themselves through major operations and treatments, with the accompanying pain and danger, in an attempt to become slimmer.

PUBLIC HEALTH ENEMY NUMBER ONE

But it's not just our appearance that is at stake. Life-threatening illnesses such as heart disease, diabetes, cancer and strokes are all closely linked to being overweight and they are all on the increase. Excessive weight is swiftly developing into public health enemy number one, not just because of the problems it causes in its own right but because of all the other illnesses that accompany it.[12]

Yet being overweight in itself is not the only factor behind the higher rates of illness suffered by overweight people. Research has shown that people whose weight 'yo-yos' from one extreme to the other can have up to double the death rate from all forms of illness (particularly diabetes and heart disease) compared to those whose weight remains stable.[13] So if people try to tackle their weight and health problems by traditional dieting methods, they can unwittingly be putting their own health at risk.

Before I leave this serious subject, there is one more aspect to the fat epidemic, one that sends shivers down the spines of hospital administrators and politicians. It is the cost to the nation of treating overweight and fat-related problems. In the UK this cost is currently estimated at over 3 billion dollars every year and in the US at a massive 68 billion.[14] And, as the years go on, these figures keep on growing. So to have any chance of dealing with the rising tide of illness, governments are now being forced to become more and more involved with the issues, treating the fat epidemic as a national health problem as well as a personal challenge for millions of people.

Unfortunately, the authorities are currently helpless: until they understand the cause of excessive weight gain they can offer us no new answers. Their best recommendation is that we should eat less and exercise more. Well, what do they think the majority of us have been trying to do all these years?

THE FAT EPIDEMIC IS A VERY RECENT PHENOMENON

Why are we still getting fatter? With untold sums being spent every year on trying to lose weight, the last thing we want to hear is that there is no cure. Despite increased awareness, eating less, buying low-calorie foods, booming membership of fitness clubs, we are becoming fatter than ever. What on earth is going on?

To understand the situation we need to look back to the time before our weight started to be such a huge problem. Take a look at Fig. 1, which tracks weight gain throughout the last half-century. You can see that the increase in the number of overweight people was initially very slow and consistent in the 60s and 70s, but that suddenly in the 80s and 90s the numbers simply rocketed.[15] This graph reveals that we are not just dealing with a gradual trickle of cases but are in the grip of a totally new phenomenon.

To understand still more about our current predicament we now need to look back to our dieting past, to get more of a feel for what factors could be behind the present problem.

A BRIEF HISTORY OF DIETING

The next time you see an old black and white film, or flick through old photos in your family album, count how many people are over-weight. There will be a few, certainly, but the problem was on a

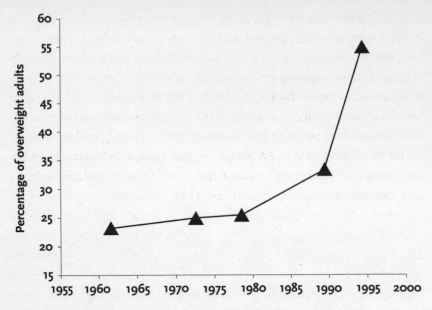

Figure 1. The percentage of overweight US adults over recent years.

much smaller scale than it is today. In truth, dieting as we recognize it today didn't even exist until about midway through the twentieth century. Before then excess weight had been treated by fasting, or other methods such as nibbling on soap or taking laxatives.

All this changed with the conception of the food restriction 'diet' by Drs Johnston and Newburgh in the 1930s at the University of Michigan in the United States. Their theory was simple and is well known by most people today. If a person consumes fewer calories than his or her body burns, then the body will burn its fat stores to make up the energy deficit. This simplistic theory has provided the basis for most of the thousands of diet books written since then, which basically differ from each other only by fiddling about with the proportions of fats, carbohydrates and proteins that they allow.

As the number of overweight people continued to increase through the 40s and 50s, more people started asking for expert help. It seemed as if the natural checks and balances that had served us for centuries didn't work any more.

One of the first diet 'bibles' was *The Slimming Business*, written by the nutritionist Professor John Yudkin and published in 1958. He recommended a diet very low in carbohydrates, with higher levels of fat-rich foods, which is actually very similar to the low-carbohydrate diets popular today. Very low-carbohydrate diets were found to induce an abnormal metabolic state known as ketosis,[16] as well as mood changes, carbohydrate cravings and irritability. Even if dieters were prepared to risk these side-effects, low-carbohydrate eating also caused the body to accumulate fat more quickly when people came off the diet.

In the 70s, very low-calorie diets or 'crash diets' came into fashion. Powdered protein drinks were promoted as a 'scientifically balanced' replacement for two or three meals every day, encouraging dieters to stick to around 1,000 calories a day. This form of dieting soon fell from favour because it made people lose both muscle and fat, the drinks tasted pretty revolting and it did not change long-term eating habits. So any weight lost was regained very quickly.

Possibly the best-selling diet book ever written was *The Complete Scarsdale Medical Diet*, by Dr Herman Tarnower, published in 1978.[17] It was the first diet I ever went on, and my lasting memories of it are painful to say the least. Fundamentally it was a high-protein low-carbohydrate diet, and it did help me lose weight, albeit temporarily. However, the gastric side-effects from eating vast quantities of onions, carrots, cabbage and tomatoes, which were often the only foods allowed to be eaten freely, were unreal.

It was followed in the 80s by Judy Mazel's glitzy *Beverly Hills Diet*, which was based on the food-combining theory of eating proteins and carbohydrates separately. Because of its nickname, 'the diarrhoea diet', I decided not to use this diet to remove the pounds I had regained following the Scarsdale Diet. I was most definitely not going to do anything which upset my gut in any way again!

The 90s were hit by Barry Sears's very fashionable *Enter the Zone*, which recommends a low-carbohydrate and high-protein intake.[18] Recently, more books promoting low-carbohydrate eating have been released, most notably Dr R. Atkins's *New Diet Revolution*.[19]

These are a variation on the earlier diet books of the 50s, so fashion appears to have come round full circle.

Yet despite the attractiveness of the concept, to date no studies exist to support the idea that a simple calorie-cutting diet is effective for long-term weight loss. It now seems pretty clear that no amount of fiddling with proportions of food alone can result in a permanent solution.

SOLVING THE GREATEST
TWENTY-FIRST-CENTURY MYSTERY

You could choose almost anyone at random from a crowd and they would be able to quote the popular wisdom that we are getting fatter because we are eating more food, eating more fat, eating too much processed food, exercising less, living less active lives, and watching too much television.

Prominent scientists refer to this as the gluttony or sloth theory.[20] They say that if our food intake is more than the amount of food we use up by exercising, then we will gain weight. This clearly implies that people become fat through their own fault alone, either by eating too much or by being lazy. But is it really true that we are becoming greedy and lazy?

It is true that our diet has changed dramatically over the last seventy or eighty years. Foods have become increasingly processed and 'convenient'. Our intake of fat and sugary carbohydrates has increased while that of unrefined fruit, vegetables and starchy carbohydrates has fallen, making a larger proportion of the foods we eat more calorific.[21] However, it is also the case that (contrary to popular opinion) we are actually eating much less food than we did at the turn of the century.[22]

Regarding physical activity, there is also controversy. It is easy to assume that we are exercising less due to the increase in car ownership, invention of the television and the decrease in manual labour. However, the amount of exercise that we take can only drop by a limited amount, since most of us do not stay in bed all day.[23]

Interestingly, the first major national health survey carried out in the UK, in 1992, by Allied Dunbar, investigating physical fitness, actually found a rapid growth of leisure-time sports and little evidence of a dramatic fall in the amount of exercise people took. Indeed, they reported that increasing numbers of people of all ages were taking part in regular physical exercise.[24] So while the level of exercise may have decreased a little, it has certainly not dropped to the level needed to explain the current fat epidemic.

Just looking at the facts, the equation doesn't seem to add up to the enormous problem that we have today. If we are not eating vastly more or exercising dramatically less, how can we still be putting on weight like there is no tomorrow? There is one possible answer which could explain these findings, but its implications are very serious indeed. It is possible that our bodies are losing their natural ability to regulate their own weight.

WHAT COULD CAUSE SUCH A DRAMATIC CHANGE?

The ability to control body weight is one of the most fundamental and highly developed of all our bodily functions. It has evolved over many hundreds of thousands of years, allowing our bodies to adapt and survive through different environmental stresses such as famine and drought as well as times of plenty.[25]

For many of our ancestors, size was literally a matter of life or death. If you were too fat it reduced your ability to hunt effectively or flee from the occasional sabre-toothed wildcat which came your way. If too thin, you could perish. Survival of the fittest ensured that those who could adapt to different situations would be the winners.

If something is indeed poisoning our weight-control mechanisms, then until it is identified no amount of dieting will ever make us lose weight. So what could be causing it?

Well, we need to go back to the basics of whether a problem is inherited or acquired. The time needed for a change in our genetic make-up big enough to have brought about this fat epidemic is thousands of years. Since it has occurred over a couple of decades, this cause can effectively be ruled out. So the potential cause can be narrowed down to changes in our environment.

Could there be a way in which our environment has significantly changed over the past century? And could this change have caused a fundamental difference to the way our weight-control systems work?

Unfortunately the answer is yes. During this century we have been exposed to substances that have been shown to cause profound damage to all the systems involved in weight control. These substances are used on a vast scale and cause damage at the levels at which they are currently found in the environment.[26] Their use has been so insidious that we have hardly noticed. Their manufacture has grown from nothing to a multibillion-pound-a-year industry worldwide.[27] Considered essential by most that use them, these substances have changed the practice of farming and industry to such an extent that life without them now is almost unthinkable. Yet they have only been around for a very short time.

What are they?

Man-made chemicals.

2. The Synthetic Revolution
How Toxic Chemicals Have Invaded Our Bodies

In this chapter you will discover how the production of man-made or synthetic chemicals has, in some way, touched everybody's lives. Since their first creation, over 150 years ago, these substances have been produced in massive quantities and appear to have the ability to contaminate and damage both wildlife and humans. Yet most people, and indeed the majority of doctors, seem to know next to nothing about what is going on in their environment and indeed, more specifically, underneath their very own skin.

In trying to explain the sheer enormity of the problem we all now face from this chemical onslaught, we need to know a bit more about the current size of the problem, the ways in which these chemicals compromise our health, what sorts of substances are involved and just why they cause such extreme havoc to our well-being.

I can fully appreciate that much of the information in this chapter may be worrying. But you have got to realize that by understanding the issues, you will be one short step away from dealing with them. Don't become too alarmed, since the rest of the book will contain the ground rules for simple ways to adapt your body to deal effectively with the new polluted environment that we now find ourselves in.

By following the advice contained in this book, you will get all the relevant know-how you need, not only to survive in the twenty-first century, but to positively thrive!

FROM NO EXPOSURE TO OVER-EXPOSURE

The creation and widespread use of toxic synthetic chemicals in the late twentieth century has permanently changed the face of our planet. As a result, every single region of the planet has been permanently contaminated with a cocktail of toxins. Whether you go to the North Pole or to the desert, these toxins can now be found everywhere.[1]

Don't make the mistake of thinking that the only people at risk are those who are exposed to them at work, for in this man-made polluted environment in which we all now live, every last one of us is bombarded on a daily basis by massive amounts of these chemicals. OK, admittedly few people deliberately set out to expose themselves to these toxins, but the simple act of eating certain contaminated foods or using certain 'treated' products could be putting you at risk without you even realizing it.

And don't think that just because you can't see them, they are not there. After all, the many hundreds of billions of kilograms of these synthetic chemicals produced every single year have to go somewhere!

We end up eating these chemicals in our foods as pesticides, preservatives, additives, pollutants and contaminants from food containers. We drink them in tap water, which contains chemicals leached from contaminated soils, environmental pollutants and even chemicals added deliberately. We absorb them though our skin from cosmetics, toiletries, treated wood, sprayed plants, treated areas of public parks, golf courses and swimming-pools. We even inhale them in air contaminated with solvents, car fumes, industrial waste and environmental pollutants. As you can see, there are very few places left to hide.

THE EXTENT TO WHICH WE ARE NOW CONTAMINATED

It has been calculated that one new industrial chemical enters industrial use every twenty minutes, and many hundreds of thousands of them are already out there.[2] As a result, the average person living in the developed world is now contaminated with up to 500 industrial toxins, few of which have been properly tested for harmful effects.[3]

One government study, which measured levels of pesticides in animal fat, also tested biopsies of human fat for some of the most poisonous and persistent toxins – organochlorines. The results were shocking. Using the results provided in this study, I calculated that human fat contained not just double or triple the level of organochlorines commonly found in animal fat (in this case beef suet), but on average approximately 500 times the total amount of organochlorines found in UK animal fat.[4]

The stark truth is, we are all so polluted that if we were cannibals our meat would most certainly be unfit for human consumption!

THE IMPLICATIONS FOR OUR CHILDREN

One of the really desperate consequences of this extreme level of bodily contamination is that chemicals appear to be affecting our children before they are even born. Newborn babies have already been affected by the chemicals in their mother's bodies;[5] even their father's sperm at conception may have been damaged by chemicals.[6]

In an unexpected twist, one of the few effective ways of ridding our body of significant amounts of the most persistent and harmful chemicals is by having a baby, as chemicals are passed, in a form of toxic inheritance, from the mother into the baby's blood. Following delivery, much larger doses are passed on in the mother's milk. As many of the most persistent and toxic of these chemicals tend to accumulate over the years, by the time most women have babies their breast milk can be loaded with a highly toxic chemical cocktail.[7]

Just consider this. The average woman's body is now so polluted that the breast milk she lovingly feeds her baby can easily contain many times the level of toxic synthetic chemicals she has in her blood at the time.[8] This is because many of the chemicals are extremely fat-soluble, and as breast milk has a high fat content, they tend to accumulate there.

If you turn again to recent government data and compare the levels of contamination in breast milk with the milk that we pile into our trolleys at the supermarket, breast milk can contain over 100 times the level of toxic organochlorines pollutants commonly found in cows' milk.[9]

So it is hardly surprising that in many countries the contaminants found in breast milk are way over the recommended 'safe' limits set by the World Health Organization (WHO) for toxic chemicals in milk for adult consumption, let alone those for babies.[10]

MY OWN PERSONAL DILEMMA

I remember vividly the moment I heard the first suggestion about the toxicity of human breast milk. I had just had my second baby, and after feeding him myself for a few months I had switched him on to formula milk. Around this time there had been a scare in the press about chemical contaminants (polychlorinated biphenyls or PCBs) found in formula baby milk, which were linked to 'gender-bending' effects (abnormalities in sexual development).

As I had never heard of these chemicals and, judging by the initial newspaper articles, few other people had too, I was very concerned that I was contaminating my baby with scary toxins. But at least I felt relieved that I had been breast-feeding him for quite a long time prior to starting him on formula milk. My relief, however, lasted only until the next day, when I read a report that the levels of chemicals in breast milk were in fact far more toxic than the levels found in formula milk.

At that point my blood turned cold. My previous satisfaction at making the considerable effort required to breastfeed my baby quickly evaporated. Had I unwittingly been poisoning my own son?

But despite this extremely unwelcome news the report had unexpectedly served a very useful purpose. By dramatically raising my curiosity about these toxic substances in food, it effectively set the scene for my discovery about toxic chemicals and weight gain. It also prompted me to think about discovering ways in which this problem could be dealt with. As you can well imagine, there is no greater spur than direct personal interest, and by this point I was already fired up and very keen to find out ways in which I could reverse some of the damage I might unwittingly have done.

Although I definitely do not want in any way to discourage

women from breastfeeding, I would strongly suggest that they need to do it in a way that reduces the risk to their babies, as this is now possible. I will be addressing this topic again in Chapter 20.

THE GROWING LINK BETWEEN CHEMICALS AND DISEASE

As every year passes it becomes more and more apparent that the introduction of these highly toxic chemicals into our lives has resulted in setting off a disease time bomb. It now seems that a staggeringly large number of the most common diseases of the developed world are related to or can be triggered by these toxins. This list includes most kinds of cancer, hormonal disorders, low energy levels, chronic fatigue syndrome, sexual problems, immune disorders and heart disease.[11]

The consequences for future generations, exposed to higher and higher levels of toxic chemicals, are dire. Our children are actually far more vulnerable than we are, because their chemical detox-ification systems have not yet fully developed and their immature body systems are much more susceptible to chemical damage.[12] Because of this increased vulnerability, synthetic chemicals are thought to play a role in a whole range of childhood disorders such as learning difficulties, attention deficit disorder, autism, dyslexia, diabetes, cancer, eczema, asthma – the list goes on and on.[13]

SO WHAT ARE THESE CHEMICALS?

The chemicals that appear to be causing all these problems can basically be divided into two main groups: toxic heavy metals and synthetic chemicals.

Toxic heavy metals include substances such as lead, cadmium, mercury and manganese and they have been around as long as we have, since they are part of our natural world. The problem is that, due to the explosive increase in manufacturing, we are now exposed to levels far higher than our bodies were ever designed to withstand. As a result, these unnaturally high levels have been found to cause a whole range of health problems, such as impaired intelligence and permanent nerve damage, as well as triggering a number of other diseases.[14]

Synthetic chemicals are definitely not natural, since they are all manufactured in chemical laboratories. Because of the massive quantities produced, along with their widespread use and potential for excessive toxicity, they appear to be the main troublemakers. In addition, unlike the heavy metals, which we have developed some mechanisms for dealing with over the years, we simply have no way of dealing with many of these chemicals. Many of them just end up accumulating in our bodies.

SYNTHETIC CHEMICALS

Synthetic chemicals are extremely big business. Production in the United States alone in 1994 was worth a staggering 101 billion dollars, and Fig. 2 shows the phenomenal increase in production of these substances throughout the twentieth century.[15]

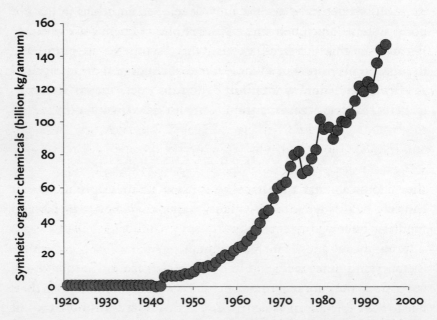

Figure 2. The annual US production of synthetic chemicals in the twentieth century.

We use synthetic chemicals in pesticides, plastics, solvents, dyes, medicines, industrial chemicals, rubber, food preservatives and many other products. As more and more uses for new chemicals keep on being found, the quantities produced keep on rising. This has seriously affected the markets for more traditional materials, which as a direct result are becoming less and less popular. Think about it: when was the last time you bought supermarket milk in a glass bottle?

WHY DO WE USE SYNTHETIC CHEMICALS?

To get to the bottom of why synthetic chemicals are so widely used in preference to naturally occurring substances, we need to know a bit more about them and what makes them so popular with manufacturers.

It may surprise some, but most synthetic chemicals are actually derived from natural substances, usually either crude oil or coal, which themselves are the products of organisms that lived many thousands of years ago. During the industrial revolution in the nineteenth century we discovered how to convert crude oil and coal into synthetic chemicals by subjecting them to extreme temperatures, among other methods. What happens is that the molecules of the natural oils or coal tar are manipulated and rearranged into an entirely new structure that simply does not occur in nature.

With this new structure often comes a whole new set of properties, such as increased stability, increased longevity, high toxicity and reduced biodegradability. These new qualities are the reasons why synthetic substances are so widely used, as in many cases they can offer clear advantages over more natural materials.[16] For instance, why buy wooden window frames that need to be painted regularly when you could buy lower maintenance plastic ones instead?

As a result, since we first discovered these man-made substances, research has been intense to discover new compounds that possess even more 'beneficial' qualities. And so hundreds of thousands of synthetic chemicals have now been created, each with its own particular properties.

Chemicals that are extremely stable can be used as fire-retardants or insulators. Chemicals that powerfully manipulate our bodily functions tend to be used as medicines, for both humans and animals, or as pesticides to kill insects as well as many other forms of life. Chemicals that possess strong colours are used as pigments or food colourings; chemicals that add malleability are used to make plastics flexible.

UNNATURAL PROPERTIES CREATE NEW PROBLEMS

As the raw ingredients of synthetic chemicals (oil and coal) are the products of fossilized plants and animals, these new synthetic substances are therefore made up from the same molecules that were found in once-living creatures. This makes the new chemicals similar enough to natural materials to be recognized by our bodies. However, their new properties (increased stability, different structures and so on) make them act in a completely unnatural way. This is in fact the very heart of the problem.

On the one hand, this similarity to naturally produced substances allows them to be assimilated into many of our body's natural processes, including all the systems essential in supporting animal life.[17] In other words, synthetic chemicals can mimic natural substances and can fool the body into carrying out certain functions, and so be very useful, for example, as medicines.

On the other hand, because of their different shapes and increased stability, they do not react in the same way as natural substances, which tend to break down or are switched off after having completed their work. As a result, many synthetic compounds do not break down or get 'switched off' after performing their function.[18] Instead they can keep on falsely stimulating or disrupting our bodies twenty-four hours a day, seven days a week.

This low-grade but continual long-term damage to many of our body's systems is precisely why they appear to pose such a major problem to our health.

WE ARE NOT DESIGNED TO COPE WITH
SYNTHETIC CHEMICALS

Before we can start to deal with the multitude of problems caused by chemicals we need to appreciate why these chemicals are causing so much chaos.

Over millions of years, our bodies have developed very sophisticated detoxification systems to rid themselves of most naturally produced toxins on a day-to-day basis – there are plenty of different natural toxins in our environment, such as certain fungi and bacteria. The problem is that these new artificial compounds have structures which are totally alien to our highly developed detoxification systems, as our bodies have never previously been confronted with them. As a result, our waste-disposal systems can manage to process some of these 'alien' chemicals but often fail miserably in dealing with others. This results in a build-up of certain toxic chemicals in our body.[19]

In effect, most of the chemicals that we cannot eliminate end up being stored in our adipose tissue (body fat) due to their high fat-solubility. Contrary to popular belief, however, once in the fat stores they are not effectively stored out of harm's way, because once there they just set to work in damaging our fat metabolism.[20]

If there were some way in which we could break down many of these chemicals into more harmless products they would not be so dangerous. But because some are so untouchable, our bodies cannot get rid of them and so they keep on accumulating throughout our lives.[21] It is this inability to remove many of these toxic substances which has made us into one of the most contaminated species on the face of this planet.

WE NEED TO ADAPT TO SURVIVE

It is also becoming clearer that people whose systems are better able to deal with these chemicals are far less prone to chemical-related problems than others.[22] Darwinian theories hold true here. Those who are better able to adjust to their new environmental conditions will pull through, in the survival of the fittest. So what makes some people better able to process these chemicals than others?

Well, the first important factor is the current state of nutrition. The additional work caused by our bodies' efforts in processing these new chemicals has resulted in a 'devitaminizing effect'. In other words, we are now using up certain of our vitamin supplies more rapidly than we have probably ever done in our history. So the presence of these chemicals has had the effect of considerably increasing our requirement not only for these vitamins but for all the other nutrients which are vital in processing these toxic substances.[23] Thus to all intents and purposes the presence of artificial chemicals has permanently increased our overall nutritional needs. Those people who have a better level of nutrition will possess a greater ability to process these chemicals compared to those with less good diets.

But it is not just the state of nutrition which determines the individual's ability to deal with these chemicals – a whole range of other factors, such as genetic predisposition, age,[24] level of exposure and even dieting history,[25] have their own influences.

The bottom line is that the more able a person is to rid their body of these chemicals, the less susceptible they will be to piling on the kilos, as well as being less vulnerable to a whole range of chemical-related illnesses. The key is to discover how to adapt to our new environment. That is the essence of this book.

HOW DO THESE CHEMICALS ENTER OUR BODIES?

So how do these chemicals actually enter our bodies? Well, the main way is in our food and drink, but they are also readily absorbed through the skin and breathed in through the lungs.

Rather than discussing this now, I will limit the discussion in the rest of this chapter to explaining the main ways in which our intake of chemicals has increased via our food.

THE ORIGINS OF 'CONVENTIONAL' FARMING IN THE
TWENTIETH CENTURY

After the creation of synthetic chemicals at the end of the nineteenth century, scientists found that certain compounds possessed a deadly ability to interfere with many of the vital processes essential for life – so much so that even the tiniest amounts of these substances could kill virtually any life form.

This was a gift to the authorities, who realized and developed the potential for chemical warfare. But after the Second World War was over, they needed to find other uses for these substances, which they were now producing in ever-increasing quantities. It was then that these deadly chemicals started to be used as pesticides in the farming community.

It soon became clear that these new pesticides were just as good at killing insects as they had been at killing humans. So it made good economic sense to farmers to use them in reducing the pest damage done to their crops. In fact these 'wonder' chemicals were initially so effective that, before long, chemical pest-control had spread throughout the international farming community with breathtaking speed, changing the way we farmed beyond all recognition. This new way is now known as conventional farming.

CHEMICALS ARE POISONING OUR FOODS

As a result of this fundamental change to the way we now farm, most of the food we eat today has been sprayed with all kinds of highly toxic chemicals, designed to kill insects (insecticides), fungus (fungicides), bacteria (antibacterials), animals (rodenticides) and weeds (herbicides). Collectively these are all known as pesticides. After your food is harvested, it may be sprayed again to prevent it going bad in storage. And before it is packaged, it may be treated with yet more chemicals.

Apples and pears are commonly sprayed with pesticides an average of twenty-one times while they are growing and during packing.[26] Even processed foods commonly have chemicals deliberately added to them, just to increase their shelf life. This has resulted in approximately one third of the foods we eat having some amount of detectable deliberately added pesticide still on them.[27]

This is a totally unnatural state of affairs. Never before has food contained these destructive toxins, all of which have been designed to kill. By carrying on in this way we are effectively poisoning our food supplies and with them ourselves.

But because of the widespread contamination of our environment, our food is contaminated not only by the pesticides that are deliberately added to it, but also by a whole raft of industrial waste products which are present in the air, water and soil. And I'm afraid it doesn't even stop there. Food packaging, which is mostly plastic, can add even more chemicals wherever it is in contact with food. Many of the chemicals in plastics are highly fat-soluble and rapidly leach into fatty foods, particularly dairy produce or fatty meats. So by the time your food gets to you, not only will it contain the ingredients listed on the label, but the chances are it will contain an awful lot more.

Now that I have set the scene by introducing you to the many problems that exposure to these chemicals has created, it is time to give you what you really want to know. So sit back, turn the page, and you will discover for yourself the startling evidence supporting my discovery that these toxic chemicals appear to be making us all fatter.

3. Chemicals Make You Fat
The Medical Evidence

When I started researching this book, never in a million years did I expect to find the overwhelming evidence that I've now uncovered. The solution to the puzzle of why we are all becoming fatter is under our very noses. It lurks in every bite of food we eat, in every sip of liquid we drink and in the very air we breathe. Now the time has come for the evidence to be pieced together. I think the easiest way to explain it is to use a simple financial example.

CHEMICALS CAUSE WEIGHT GAIN

Imagine a beef farmer, who raises cattle and sells them for slaughter. One of his major outgoings will be animal feed and his profit will be linked to the final weight of the cattle. The more it costs him to feed the cattle, the less profit he will make. If he had a magic 'fattening' pill his cows would eat less food and put on more weight, so he would make more money. It is therefore not surprising to learn that farmers have actually been using powerful fattening synthetic chemicals to force animal weight gain for a long time. For example, since 1976, the increasing use of growth-promoting feed additives, selective breeding and high-protein diets has reduced the amount of feed needed for broiler chickens to reach 2kg by almost 40 per cent.[1]

The way that most of these chemicals act is to greatly improve food efficiency: in other words, they alter the animals' metabolism so that less food goes much further. Animals that eat these chemicals in their feed end up gaining more weight than untreated animals, even when the untreated animals are eating *more* food.[2] It makes total economic sense.

More animal weight for less food. Food bills are reduced, and the income increases since the farmer will get a better price at market. And after the animals are sold, guess what? We eat them, chemicals and all.

SYNTHETIC CHEMICALS ARE MAKING US FAT

Our metabolism appears to be affected by a massive range of synthetic chemicals in a very similar way – with the 'fattening' effect intended for animals in all probability working on us too.

Different synthetic chemicals achieve this in one or more ways in humans and other mammals. First they appear to damage the appetite 'switch', so that more food is eaten than is generally needed.[3] Another way is by reducing the amount of food the body needs by damaging the ability to burn off food and so making the food that is eaten go further.[4] But possibly the most important way is by seemingly preventing the body burning up existing fat stores.[5]

So in effect, many synthetic chemicals appear to possess the potential to poison critical parts of our weight-control system,

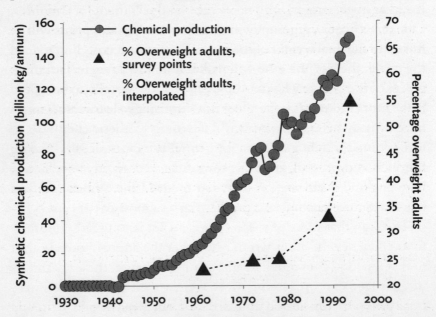

Figure 3. The increase in number of overweight US adults and the increase in the US production of synthetic chemicals in the twentieth century.

effectively putting it out of action. What's worse, unless properly tackled, the effect could be cumulative or even synergistic, dooming us to become fatter and fatter as long as we keep exposing our bodies to these chemicals.

At this point I think it would be very useful to look at how the timescale of the fat epidemic relates to the increased production of synthetic chemicals. Fig. 3 shows the relationship between the rising production of synthetic chemicals in America and the rise in the percentage of US adults who are overweight.[6]

You can see for yourself that the explosion in production of synthetic chemicals precedes an equally dramatic recent rise in the number of people who are becoming overweight. The very speed of the recent marked increases in overweight people indicates that changes in the environment are far more likely to be the source of the problem than genetic changes, which would take much longer to occur. This timescale would also fit with chemicals being the cause of the fat epidemic.

Although the graph in itself does not prove that the two are linked, it certainly gives an indication that this suggestion is plausible. The added fact that synthetic chemicals are actually known to cause weight gain just adds more weight to my ideas.

So, considering the ever-increasing amounts of these chemicals that we are being exposed to in our lives, is it surprising that it has been said that excessive weight gain is becoming a normal response to the American environment?[7]

This would also explain why simple food-restriction dieting simply does not work over the long term, as it totally fails to deal with removing fattening chemicals from our lives. Their removal is a vital part of tackling the problem.

SO WHERE IS THE PROOF THAT THESE CHEMICALS CAN MAKE US FAT?

In making the revolutionary claim that our exposure to synthetic chemicals is at the heart of the current fat epidemic, it is vital to be able to back the statement up. So when I started my investigations,

I spent many months scouring medical and scientific libraries up and down the land, gathering together hundreds of academic papers which could help me get a grip on what was happening.

This is where my medical and scientific background really kicked in, as my specialist knowledge enabled me to ask the right questions and get the right answers. But it was only towards the end of this lengthy but thorough process that the full picture gradually but spectacularly fell into place.

These papers revealed how growth promoters, pesticides,[8] plastics,[9] toxic chemicals[10] and a whole range of the most common environmental pollutants about us[11] produce fattening effects in animals and humans. In plain English, I discovered that these chemicals appear to be making us fat.

The sheer number of fattening chemicals in our environment meant that it took me over a year to get all my evidence together. Every step of the way I kept making new discoveries that confirmed my initial suspicions. Time and time again, when I learned about a different group of pesticides or environmental pollutant, I would soon discover that they too could cause weight gain.

Remarkably, the evidence was already there in a very large number of scientific papers and studies, but no one had put the whole picture together. In fact, after a few months I realized that the commonly used chemicals that *didn't* cause weight gain were extremely few and far between.

IF IT'S POISONOUS, IT SHOULD CAUSE WEIGHT LOSS, NOT GAIN!

So, you may well ask, if all the evidence is already there, why has it taken so long to come to light? Until very recently, scientists have believed that because pesticides and other synthetic chemicals are toxic, the only possible effect on weight could be one of weight loss.[12] I suppose this prejudice was not so surprising – large doses of chemicals are indeed extremely toxic and will tend to cause those affected to be very unwell, and if you are feeling dreadful your appetite is not going to be up to very much.

What I have uncovered is that this weight-gain effect is found at the other end of the exposure spectrum, where the person or animal is exposed to extremely low doses of chemicals. At these low levels the weight-control systems are still damaged but the person or animal doesn't actually feel ill and stop eating.

The main problem I had in finding my evidence directly resulted from this prejudice, because any study designed to assess the toxicity of a chemical, but which found weight gain rather than weight loss, tended to ignore the finding as irrelevant to the study or even tried to explain it away. I even found one report, investigating the toxicity of plastics, which actually apologized for finding weight gain, as it was not at all what the scientists had hoped for![13] This particular study showed a remarkable weight-gain effect, with no sign of weight loss at all, but just to show to the world they had tried to find a weight loss they stated: 'Ideally in these studies the top dose should cause some measure of general toxicity *such as a small decrease in weight gain* to ensure that the dose is high enough to produce effects'!

More recently, scientists have accepted that chemicals *can* cause weight gain,[14] but because of the difficulty of retrieving much of this 'hidden' evidence from the past, the fuller picture has simply not been seen until now. Because weight gains were not reported in the summaries of many earlier scientific papers, there is currently no way of discovering whether a study showed a weight-gain effect or not by searching modern scientific databases, as these only contain information extracted from the summaries.

It was because I was so convinced that a weight-gain effect was happening that I spent a huge amount of time ordering up batches of research reports on spec, in the hope that a few of them would reveal these weight-gain effects. Typically one study out of every ten of the papers I had ordered had used doses low enough to reveal this weight-gain effect. Subsequently every time I found one of these precious papers showing that yet another major group of chemicals produced weight gain, I was absolutely elated!

These numerous small but highly significant discoveries over time were essential in strengthening my ideas and acted to spur me on to uncover the whole picture. The more I delved into the subject the more extensive and conclusive the evidence became. Reflecting back on the situation, if I had simply accepted the easily accessible summaries at face value and not actually spent months retrieving and reading the full original papers, this book would never have been written.

THE CHEMICALS WHICH MAKE YOU FAT ARE ALL AROUND US

With hundreds of thousands of synthetic chemicals already out there, and with a new substance being introduced into industrial usage every twenty minutes, I needed some way to simplify my research. So, rather than looking at each chemical individually, which would have been virtually impossible, I grouped the chemicals together according to their structure. This approach soon proved invaluable, as it opened my eyes to the discovery that one type of chemical can actually have lots of different uses.

This became more and more apparent as I went through each one of the dozens of different synthetic chemicals found as pesticide residues in food. It rapidly became clear that not only were these chemicals used for the purpose of killing a huge variety of different forms of life, but the same chemicals or very similar ones were also being used to promote growth in animals,[15] associated with weight gain in humans,[16] and were even regularly used as medicines to treat a whole range of human illnesses.[17]

But it didn't stop there: I also discovered that the same or similar chemicals were also widely used in a huge range of cosmetics, toiletries and other household products. In other words we were being exposed to these fattening chemicals in a whole variety of different ways.

So what are these chemicals? Well, there is a whole range of chemicals which cause weight gain, including pesticides, medicines, heavy metals,[18] plastics,[19] solvents, environmental pollutants, fire-retardants,[20] and many other substances. Because of the sheer number of chemicals I have found with fattening effects, it would be far too confusing to deal with all of them at once. So I have decided to highlight just those chemicals which are actually used to promote fattening in animals.

Following this, I will expose some of the human evidence which shows that chemically induced weight gain can be deliberately induced on occasions, but is more commonly an unwanted side-effect of many synthetic medications. After that I will explain how certain persistent chemicals are already present in some of us at levels which appear to be making us fatter.

THE ANIMAL GROWTH-PROMOTERS

When I found the first paper showing that one of the most commonly detected pesticides in our food was actually used as a growth-promoter to fatten up animals, I knew I was on to a winner. It's one matter to find that chemicals cause a fattening effect in animals but quite another to discover that they have been deliberately used for this purpose in real life. Suddenly the whole thing turned from a hypothesis into reality. The extensive group of substances that I am about to describe proves, I believe, beyond reasonable doubt that chemicals can make you fat, because they have been used for precisely this purpose for many years.

Although some of these growth-promoters are now banned from this particular use, we are still being exposed to them, both as pesticides in our food and in many other products commonly used around the home and in our environment. As a result, the following information is highly relevant to our lives. So which are the worst offenders and where else can these substances be found?

ORGANOPHOSPHATES: The organophosphates are particularly good examples of 'fattening' synthetic chemicals. After being created, they were used in the gas chambers at Auschwitz as nerve gas. Later it was discovered that as well as being highly toxic to humans, they were also very effective at killing insects. This discovery led to their extensive use on food crops and now they are some of the most common pesticides found in our soft fruit and vegetables.

However, what really struck me about organophosphates was that this same group of chemicals had a further commercial use: to fatten up livestock! Although many studies had shown that organophosphates possessed a marked fattening effect, to discover that they were actually used for this purpose really drove it home. What made it even worse was that the same type of chemical used to fatten up cattle (at very low doses) was also found on our food (again in very low doses) because of its use as a crop insecticide. It could even be found in many other products, for example flea powders and household fly spray.[21]

So how does this group of chemicals promote fattening? Well, at low doses organophosphates appear to fatten up cows by severely reducing their ability to use up existing fat stores. As the animals' fat-burning abilities slow right down, they gain weight more quickly, since they just can't burn off body fat as well as they previously could. Their food needs also fall, as less food appears to go further. Though the use of organophosphates as growth promoters has now been banned, they are still one of the commonest pesticides used in many of our foods. They are also commonly used in the manufacture of rubber and plastics, in gasoline as additives and in lubricating oils.

It really doesn't matter how you are exposed, whether it is from a can of fly spray or from pesticide residues in food, once they get into your body the chances are they will proceed to damage your weight-control systems, making it just that little bit harder to lose weight in the future.

While I am on the subject of organophosphates, I must mention their toxic effects on the nerves and muscles (remember, they were originally developed as nerve gas). When I was working as a hospital doctor there was an incident that really shocked me at the time and to this day I can remember it quite clearly. We got a call about a person who had deliberately swallowed a teaspoon of household pesticide. We had no idea what chemicals were in the poison, and just had to wait until the ambulance appeared.

Virtually the first thing the patient did after being wheeled into casualty was to stop breathing. This was followed by continual violent convulsions, and it took a whole team of us several hours to stabilize the patient in intensive care. When coming round a few days later, the patient's muscles were extremely weak, to such an extent that the head could hardly be lifted from the pillow. It turned out that organophosphate was the main active ingredient in the pesticide.

It is this extreme damage to the muscles that I want to highlight here. As well as having the ability to reduce and slow down fat metabolism, organophosphates are extremely damaging to the ability to exercise. They can permanently damage nerves,[22] break down the structure of muscle fibres, reduce the ability to produce energy to power exercise and, to cap it all, reduce the desire to exercise.[23] This powerful ability to lower exercise levels makes organophosphates even better growth-promoters, as exposed animals that exercise less will use up fewer calories. Remember that the next time you think about wielding a can of fly spray.

CARBAMATES: Carbamates are some of the most widely used chemicals in agriculture because they are generally reckoned to be among the least toxic of the pesticides. In addition to being common insecticides for crops such as tobacco and cotton, and their frequent use in the treatment of wood infestations, they are also found in large quantities in an extensive range of foods, including potatoes, peanuts and citrus fruit, along with many other fruit and vegetables, because of their use as fungicides (when they are more commonly known as bisthiocarbamates). Because fungicides tend to be added to food *after* it has been harvested and before it is put in storage, there is no opportunity for it to be washed off by the rain. As a result, carbamates can often be found in relatively high levels in food.

As well as being commonly used as pesticides, carbamates possess extremely powerful fattening abilities which, in combination with their antibacterial properties, have resulted in their widespread use in animal husbandry. The main way in which they are thought to cause fattening is by reducing the overall metabolic rate, in essence making less food go further.[24] In addition they, like the organophosphates, can also lower the overall level of physical activity.[25]

The irony is that most people eating fruit and vegetables treated with these chemicals would think they had chosen low-fat healthy foods to help them keep their weight down!

THYROID DRUGS: Some of the most critical hormones our bodies use to burn off excess weight are the thyroid hormones. So it is not surprising that several chemicals designed to suppress the production of this potent fat-burning hormone have been used as growth-promoters because of their ability to make animals pile on the fat.[26] Although all these thyroid-hormone-suppressing or 'anti-thyroid' compounds are now banned for this use, similar compounds are still being commonly found on our foods as pesticides.

We definitely know that they also cause weight gain in humans, as these anti-thyroid substances are commonly used in humans to suppress overactive thyroid disease,[27] and if too large a dose is given, it causes excess weight gain.

However, it gets worse: I have found that not only do a couple of chemicals possess these anti-thyroid actions, but a very large number of synthetic chemicals used on our foods and in our environment appear to damage the thyroid to different degrees.[28] So the more synthetic chemicals we are exposed to, the more our thyroid hormones are damaged and the fatter we will become.

STEROIDS: Many people already know that certain steroids used in medicine can pile on the pounds. They include those that act on the sex hormones, such as the contraceptive pill. They also include steroids prescribed to prevent an asthma attack and some steroids used in cancer therapy. Side-effects can make a patient blow up like a balloon and stimulate a ravenous appetite, particularly for carbohydrates.[29] So it is hardly surprising to learn that steroids have been used to fatten up animals for many years. In fact, some steroids were so good at increasing levels of body fat that when oestrogens were given to broiler chickens, they caused such an increase in body fat that the practice had to be stopped. The meat was just too fatty to sell, and the high levels of fat deposited in the main blood vessels threatened the animals' lives.[30]

More recently, because of food safety concerns, the use of steroids has been banned in animal farming across Europe, although they are still widely used in the United States.

You don't even have to be exposed to the steroids themselves to be affected, as a whole range of synthetic chemicals to which we are all commonly exposed can alter our natural levels of steroid hormones to induce the same fattening effects.[31]

The really scary thing about these steroids is that if they are given to pregnant animals the offspring not only weigh more, but they also have higher weight gains all through their lives due to increased appetite and improved feed efficiency.[32] This suggests that our children are potentially at risk of obesity in later life if their mothers are exposed during pregnancy to large amounts of steroids or any of the synthetic chemicals that mimic their effects. This may help to explain the increasing weight problems now found in children.

ANTIBIOTICS: Antibiotics tend to have a more positive image because of their ability to clear up infections and kill germs. So when I found that antibiotics were commonly used to fatten animals, I assumed it was because they killed nasty bugs that made the animals lose weight through illness. What I didn't know then, but have discovered since, is that antibiotics will treat infections if given in high doses, but not at the minute doses at which they are given to animals. At these lower levels they actually lack the ability to kill bacteria. However, they are present at a level which can promote animal weight gain.[33] Again, these chemicals appear to promote weight gain by damaging the weight-control hormones and metabolism in such a way that weight gain results. Is this beginning to sound familiar?

The scale at which these antibiotics are used in animals is stunning. They account for over half of the antibacterial drugs manufactured in the United States and in the UK, and the vast majority of all forms of livestock will be exposed to antibacterial growth-promoters at some stage of their lives. Residues from antibiotics are found in meat from treated animals, so you will be taking them too and more often than you think. And although many antibiotics are naturally derived substances, an awful lot more are synthetic chemicals with the ability to fatten.[34]

But don't let this put you off taking a course of antibiotics if you need them. They can be life-saving, and the short, high-dose courses prescribed by doctors should not have a weight-gain effect.

So, to round up, all these chemicals are in the food chain today and have been there for a long time. Not only do they cause increased weight gain but many have actually been formulated for the purpose. Considering our constant exposure to all these substances, just think what effect they're having on us. Is it any wonder we are in the grip of a fat epidemic?

THE HUMAN GROWTH-PROMOTERS

While the fact that synthetic chemicals make animals fat is of vital importance, the ultimate proof that these chemicals can make us fat is that doctors use them in hospital conditions for that very purpose.[35] It is obvious that if a drug is used deliberately to cause weight gain under medical supervision, a similar chemical will produce a similar effect if you are exposed to it from another source without realizing it.

I think that if people were more widely aware of the fact that, through pesticides in their food and pollutants in their close environment, they are being exposed to chemicals which are similar to those used by doctors to fatten up patients, they wouldn't be too happy. So what are these substances and how are we exposed to them?

There are quite a few medical conditions that cause people to lose too much weight. Anorexia is one obvious example. In the past, a large number of different 'fattening' drugs have been used in an attempt to promote weight gain. Although this way of treating anorexia has been frowned upon recently, many drugs did appear to produce positive weight gain.[36]

One of these substances is known as sulpiride. This chemical works by attacking and lowering the levels of our most powerful natural slimming hormones, our catecholamines. Indeed it is so powerfully fattening that if animals are exposed to it they become obese within a short time. It is also a very commonly used antipsychotic medicine in psychiatry, which not so surprisingly causes great problems with unwanted weight gain during treatment. Because of these powerful fattening 'side-effects' and the ability to stabilize mental conditions, it has been used to promote weight gain in anorexics.[37]

But we don't have to be on medication to get a dose of these chemicals, because we are exposed to a whole range of other catecholamine-attacking chemicals with actions very similar to sulpiride in our foods, again in the form of pesticide residues.

Elderly people can often suffer from a dramatic drop in weight due to loss of appetite. Drugs that have been used successfully to bring their weight back up again include corticosteroids and megestrol.[38] These and similar drugs were found to cause excessive weight gain when used to treat patients with breast and prostate cancer. Again, these substances are closely related to and have similar actions to certain pesticides used in our food.

A third group of people – cancer patients – are regularly treated with drugs to counteract the loss of appetite caused by cancer therapy. I have found a study that tested the ability of a bisthiocarbamate (see page 33) to prevent the normal dramatic fall in weight after toxic cancer therapy. In fact, it was so effective that it even produced mild weight gain.[39] The exact same chemical is one of the commonest anti-fungal pesticides used in food production, and is present in many fresh fruits and vegetables.

WEIGHT GAIN AS A KNOWN SIDE-EFFECT

The other main way to show that synthetic chemicals cause a fattening effect in humans is to look at the wealth of studies on the side-effects of different medications. Everyone at some time in his or her life has known or heard of people who have had weight problems caused by a prescribed medication. The pill is one, steroids are another. In fact, a very large number of medications made up of synthetic chemicals can upset your metabolism, including some antihistamines, anti-sickness medications, a whole range of cardio-vascular drugs, antifungals, certain antibiotics, and drugs to treat disorders of the nervous system.[40] Many of these, in particular the long-term medications, in trying to treat your illness can also appear to make you gain weight.

You will be horrified to find that you don't have to be on medication to be exposed to these compounds. Once again, very similar chemicals are found as pesticides in our foods or pollutants in our environment.

But please understand, I'm not suggesting for one moment that you should stop taking medication if you are ill. The point I am making in all this is that there is proof in abundance that synthetic chemicals have the ability to make us fat, and that we are being exposed to similar substances in our food and many non-food products which could be making us fatter, but without our knowledge or consent.

THE ORGANOCHLORINES YOU HAVE ACCUMULATED THROUGHOUT YOUR LIFE ARE MAKING YOU FAT

So now we know that there are a huge number of chemicals in our diet and environment which can cause weight gain. But how do we know that they are present at a level that will make us fat? Experts have estimated that each of us has on average approximately 300–500 industrial chemicals in our bodies, but it would be impractical and far too expensive to measure all of these routinely.[41]

The strongest evidence to show that we are contaminated with certain chemicals, at levels which appear to be making us fat, comes mainly from a group of extremely toxic pesticides and environmental pollutants more commonly known as organochlorines.

Of the synthetic chemicals that we are now exposed to, organochlorines are possibly the most fattening of all. This is largely due to their ability to cause continual damage to our weight-control systems, in combination with our relative inability to process them or get rid of them from our bodies.

Better-known members of this group are the extremely poisonous insecticides DDT and lindane, as well as a very common group of environmental pollutants known as polychlorinated biphenyls (PCBs). PCBs were once very widely produced and were used as fire-retardants and insulating substances, but they have now been banned because of their extreme toxicity and longevity.

Despite many, but certainly not all, organochlorines having been banned for many years, they are still present in our bodies at levels far above those needed to damage our hormones, as unfortunately they tend to persist in our tissues for many decades.[42] They are also highly fat-soluble and tend to concentrate in fatty tissues. Because of these characteristics they are now present in most life forms, including us. Since our bodies are virtually unable to break them up and kick them out, as the years go by our stockpile of them just keeps on increasing.[43]

DDT, one of the most fattening of all the organochlorines, is one which has actually been banned for several decades in most developed countries but is still commonly found in people's bodies. Low levels of DDT have been shown to be powerful inducers of weight gain in animals.[44]

Lindane is also extremely fattening and has been shown to promote obesity in animals.[45] Despite being banned from use in the UK only fairly recently, it is still legal in other countries, where it is freely available in flea powder, anti-nit shampoo and insecticides, and can be found on many grassy areas that have to look pretty, such as golf courses. It is also present in much of our food, particularly animal products and chocolate.

Yet another member of this fattening group is the pesticide hexachlorobenzene (HCB). Unlike DDT and lindane it is still commonly used in the UK, as a fungicide on wheat and other foods. This organochlorine was found to possess such extreme fattening effects that in one animal study, when the food intake was cut by 50 per cent, animals treated with HCB still managed to gain more weight than the untreated animals did on full rations![46]

Now this is where it gets kind of up close and personal. I have compared the levels of these organochlorines already present in our bodies with the levels which have been shown to cause weight gain in animals and they are frighteningly similar. This suggests that our bodies are probably already being exposed to high enough levels of these organochlorines to make us gain weight. As most people get contaminated with these chemicals from food, could it be possible that people who eat food which contains more of these chemicals will become more contaminated and so gain more weight?

Despite the relative scarcity of scientific studies comparing organochlorine contamination and body weight, I managed to hit the jackpot with the few that I did uncover. These findings suggest that far from being just a hypothesis, this link between bodily contamination and excess weight appears to be very real.

As with many of the previous studies, despite revealing evidence suggesting that the greater the contamination by organochlorines the greater the body weight, this vital connection was far from understood by the scientists performing the study – probably because they were not looking for it.

MEDICAL STUDIES LINK CURRENT LEVELS OF CONTAMINATION TO INCREASED BODY WEIGHT

A study carried out in Long Island, USA, looked at a number of ordinary women who did not have any reason to be exposed to dangerous chemicals at work or at home, or to eat foods from a known contaminated source. It revealed that those with higher levels of organochlorines in their bodies (measured in fat stores and circulating in their blood) generally had a higher body mass index (BMI) – in other words, they were fatter than those who were less contaminated. By the way, the BMI is just a way of comparing your weight with your height to assess the level of fatness. Anyway, the study concluded that the accumulation of these contaminants over time was mainly from the types of food these women ate.[47]

Several other studies provided further evidence that people who eat certain more contaminated foods were likely to be fatter. One study examined the effect of eating fish from the Great Lakes of America, which are known to be relatively polluted with organochlorines (DDT and PCBs). It looked at fishermen who ate the salmon and trout that they caught from the lakes (as commercial fishing is banned, these were sport fishermen). Compared to the fishermen who didn't eat the fish they caught, the fish-eaters had higher levels of PCBs and DDT, as well as the heavy metals cadmium and lead. Significantly, they were also fatter.[48]

OUR CHILDREN ARE AFFECTED TOO

In looking for these studies I stumbled upon something exceedingly worrying. Not only were higher levels of organochlorines linked to excess weight in adults, but it also seemed that they could cause the same fattening effect in our young. A further study was made up of mothers who had eaten large amounts of salmon (12kg or more over the last six years) caught from Green Bay, Wisconsin. The mothers who had eaten more fish were found to be more contaminated with PCBs but, more worryingly, they gave birth to significantly larger babies.[49]

So, you say, what is the problem? – a bigger baby is healthy. While bigger babies may indeed be healthy, increased birth weight can also be an indication that the weight-control mechanisms have been damaged even before birth.

It gets worse: another group of fish-eating mothers, this time from Lake Ontario, showed that mothers who had eaten relatively large amounts of fish (high in PCBs) not only gave birth to slightly bigger babies (an average increase of 100g) but they themselves were on average 4.7kg heavier than the non-fish-eating mothers.[50]

What's more, the heavier babies appeared to have a marked degree of damage to the nervous system. They had abnormal reflexes, less mature autonomic response and less attention to visual and auditory stimuli – it may not surprise you that organochlorines can also cause these signs of nerve damage in babies.[51] So not only does it seem that by eating more contaminated foods we could effectively be programming our children to be fat, but it also appears that in fact we could also unwittingly be making them unwell.

So, to round up, we now have real evidence to suggest that the level of contamination of the food that we eat appears to affect our overall body weight. This is actually very positive, because if we can identify the foods which are more contaminated and therefore 'fattening' we are well on the way to reducing our exposure to them in our diet.

SO WHY AREN'T WE ALL FAT?

If we gain weight by absorbing dangerous chemicals, and if these chemicals are all around us, then why aren't we all fat? We know from personal experience that many slim people eat sprayed and treated foods. The answer is that we are all made differently. Some of us are born with systems that can cope with these chemicals better than others. Those of us with sensitive systems are affected more, resulting in more weight gain. Even people with high resistance suffer from the build-up of chemicals over time. They damage the body's chemistry little by little until its defence mechanisms are strained to breaking point. At this point we start putting on weight.

Despite all this gloom and doom, there is a whole lot of good news about this discovery. At last we appear to know what is making us fat, so for the first time we can start addressing the problem. If we know how our bodies control our weight then we are brought one step closer to understanding how chemicals can disrupt this system and, for the first time in our lives, we will be able to tackle the problem head on.

Fortunately, the vast majority of the damage done by these chemicals is not permanent, and if you follow the advice given in the rest of this book you will find out how to lose weight in such a way that it is extremely likely to stay off for good.

In the next chapter I will introduce the idea that we all have a highly developed weight-control system, explain the way it works, and tell you what you need to do to maximize your ability to lose weight permanently.

Please believe this – it is never too late to start. The fattening effects of chemicals really can be reversed. The secret of how to do it is here in these pages, so keep reading!

4. Your Natural *Slimming System*

All About Your Highly Evolved Weight-control System

This chapter is a vital one, because it lays the foundations for a fuller understanding of how chemicals can actually make us fat. Since you can only deal with a problem once you know what the problem is, the following pages will give you a unique insight into how the body controls its weight.

It cannot be denied that this is one of the more in–depth chapters, designed to give you a basic and thorough understanding of a whole range of essential dieting issues such as:

- What our natural *Slimming System* is and why it is so important.
- Why we have powerful food cravings and how to minimize them.
- How our body shape is controlled.
- Why dieting as we know it simply doesn't work.
- Why some people are more likely to gain weight than others.
- Why it can be extremely hard for some to lose excess body fat.
- The importance of the *Slimming System* in long-term weight control.
- Simple ways in which the *Slimming System* can be enhanced.

The chapter is packed with stacks of vital slimming information and advice to help you to maximize your weight loss. The bottom line is that by understanding how your body controls its weight you will be able to see how this whole self-regulatory process has gone wrong. From there you will be able to work with your body, rather than against it, in order to put things right.

WE ALL HAVE A NATURAL *SLIMMING SYSTEM*

In the battle of the bulge our body has developed an extremely powerful weapon which if it is working well can keep excess fat firmly at bay, but if not can result in us putting on weight. For want of a convenient term I have dubbed this natural weight-loss mechanism our *Slimming System*.

Our *Slimming System* covers a whole network of body systems, such as appetite, metabolism, hormone levels, fat-burning, body heat, exercise and more, which work together to maintain our ideal weight. Most experts agree that we all have an ideal weight and that our bodies will try to maintain it come famine or times of plenty by altering different parts of these weight-control mechanisms. As most of these adjustments take place without us even knowing, we actually have much less direct control over our weight than we might imagine.

Just as our bodies have homeostatic mechanisms to maintain body temperature at a certain level, our weight is also controlled by homeostatic mechanisms to maintain a largely predetermined weight 'set-point'. This is the weight at which the body will try to remain through thick and thin.[1] In fact it can only be altered and set at a higher body weight if the underlying mechanisms get damaged.[2]

The fact that the average woman eats over 20 tonnes of food between the ages of twenty-five and sixty-five and yet tends to gain only a fraction of this weight in kilograms over these years shows that the mechanisms used to maintain the set-point are extremely accurate. If it is protected and well cared for, the ability to control our own weight can actually be a natural *Slimming System*.

WHY WE NEED AN EFFICIENT *SLIMMING SYSTEM*

A person who has an efficient *Slimming System* will find it very easy to maintain their body weight despite eating lots of food. I think we all know people like that, who can eat and eat yet not gain any extra weight. On the other hand, people with a less effective *Slimming System* will lack the same ability to burn off excess calories. So, unhappily for them, less food will go much further.

But the natural *Slimming System* doesn't just control weight, it also determines our body shape. The amount of muscle we have, whether we have a flat belly or a pot belly, slim hips or full hips, all this is determined by our natural *Slimming System*. So we can see that our *Slimming System* plays a key role in determining not only our weight but also our shape.

The problem at the heart of the fat epidemic is that most people's *Slimming Systems* appear to be constantly under-achieving. This is because they are under attack from toxic chemicals and are lacking the nutrients they need in order to work properly.

The good news is that by reducing our exposure to the most damaging or 'fattening' of these chemicals and by increasing our intake of 'slimming' nutrients, it suddenly becomes possible to revitalize our *Slimming System*. Once this happens, it can then start working properly to actively reduce our weight. But before we can find out the best way to repair our *Slimming System*, we need to know more about what exactly it is and how it works.

WHAT MAKES UP OUR *SLIMMING SYSTEM*

The body's personal *Slimming System* is largely made up of the following four parts:

1. A control centre (in the brain).
2. A large number of different 'slimming' hormones.
3. An intact body structure.
4. A good supply of nutrients.

These four parts of the *Slimming System* are highly interlinked, with changes in one affecting all the others. Together they form a sort of dynamic body metabolism. A problem in any one of these areas could seriously reduce our overall ability to lose weight.

On the other hand, when these four parts are working well

together they alter our appetite, energy levels and metabolism in such a way that our weight is kept low with virtually no conscious effort on our part. Let's find out more about these four key areas.

1. CONTROL CENTRE: The brain is where all weight-control really happens. Messages about how much fat is stored around the body are relayed from the brain around the body by hormones, which then feed information back to the brain. This information is processed in the control centre, known as the hypothalamus, which is deep inside the brain and acts as the body's pilot.[3] If the brain thinks the fat stores are too large, it will send directions for the body to burn the excess off. If the brain thinks there is not enough fat stored, it will send signals to drive you to find something to eat. At all times, the constant aim is to keep your body at its predetermined weight set-point.

But it works both ways, as the set-point is itself determined by the efficiency of the whole *Slimming System*. So if the system has all the nutrients it needs to function properly and is intact and working well, the set-point will be at a low level and the person will be lean. If, however, the system is not working smoothly and there are shortages of nutrients or damaged body organs, the set-point will be higher, resulting in a fatter body.

For example, if the hypothalamus is injured, huge fluctuations in weight can occur as people lose their natural ability to control their appetite. This can get so extreme that people who have tumours in the hypothalamus area can, if untreated, actually die from overeating.

2. HORMONES: If our brain is the most important part of our *Slimming System*, our hormones must come a close second. Hormones are natural chemical molecules acting as internal messengers. They carry information and instructions around the body, enabling one part to talk to another. Although only minuscule amounts of hormones are produced, they control virtually all the body's functions, including food intake, ability to exercise, metabolism,

maintaining body heat, growing, reproduction and, of course, controlling size, weight, shape and how much fat we store.[4]

All the major hormones, for example the catecholamines, thyroid hormone, insulin, growth hormone, steroids, leptin and the sex hormones (oestrogens and testosterone), play a vital role in our *Slimming System*. Out of all these hormones, the catecholamines, more commonly known as our 'fight or flight' hormones, are possibly the most important 'slimming' hormones because of their prime role in enhancing fat-burning.[5] They are produced by the nerve cells of the sympathetic nervous system (SNS), the part of the brain that coordinates the burning and storing of fat. As well as being produced in the brain, they are also produced from certain nerve endings throughout the rest of the body. As you will discover, they play a vital role in explaining the weight problems we are now facing.

3. INTACT BODY STRUCTURE: An intact and efficient body structure is essential in allowing all these vital processes to take place. For example, to burn up foods by exercising we need our muscles to be working properly. And for our muscles to work, our nerves must be intact so that they can stimulate the relevant muscles!

4. NUTRIENTS: Last, but by no means least, our natural *Slimming System* needs a whole range of different nutrients such as vitamins, minerals, carbohydrates, proteins and essential fatty acids. These nutrients power, accelerate and facilitate the millions of individual reactions taking place in the body and so govern the overall speed of metabolism. The faster our metabolism is, the more fat we will use up. So you can see that an efficient metabolism is vital in order to keep in shape.

Now we will move on to discover the ways in which our *Slimming System* works to alter our appetite, the amount of exercise we do and even our metabolism to maintain our weight at its optimum weight set-point.

APPETITE AND YOUR *SLIMMING SYSTEM*: ARE YOU
REALLY IN CHARGE OF HOW MUCH YOU EAT?

Of all the messages controlled by your *Slimming System*, the one you will be most aware of is your appetite. You may think that you are in control of how much you eat, but in reality your hormones call all the shots. They manipulate your appetite according to what they perceive your present needs to be.

In fact, your hormones can even dictate the type of food you choose to eat, the amount you eat, and when you eat throughout the day. Different hormones stimulate an appetite for different foods, and as their levels change throughout the day they will drive you to seek out whatever your body needs at any particular time.[6] So when you open the fridge door and decide what to eat next, you are not making an impartial choice. Your hand will be guided by the hormones running through your brain, telling you what your *Slimming System* wants.

For example, have you ever wondered why carbohydrates, such as toast, cereals and fruit, are among the most commonly eaten foods for breakfast? Well, this is because your body needs readily available energy to get it powered up after the night's fast. As carbohydrates are the foods most easily converted into energy, the body produces large amounts of steroid hormones first thing in the morning to increase the appetite for carbohydrates.

It is a simple way of making sure that you make the right food choices. The carbohydrates will kick-start your body into action and replenish the small existing carbohydrate stores in the muscles and liver which are essential for ensuring you have lots of energy all day long.

Later in the day, once your body gets going, your appetite for other food groups such as fats and proteins will increase. This is achieved by a changing balance in a whole number of different hormones.

WHAT DRIVES US TO EAT MORE FAT?

Our appetite for fat, on the other hand, is largely driven by the *absence* of hormones, specifically catecholamines. People fortunate enough to produce large amounts of catecholamines will tend to be lean and eat less fatty foods, because catecholamines suppress appetite in general and the desire for fatty foods in particular. They are known as the 'fight or flight' hormones because they are released in stressful situations – and as you can imagine, eating is the last thing you want to do if being chased by a bull!

Catecholamines work by increasing activity in the sympathetic nervous system (SNS), and any increase in SNS activity will automatically suppress the appetite. High levels of catecholamines also cause people to eat less fat. So a person with an active SNS tends to be driven to eat not only less food – but also less fatty food.

The effect is so powerful that for many years now the most effective slimming-pills have mimicked the appetite-suppressing effects of catecholamines. There are two main types of these appetite-suppressants. The early type caused the release of a natural catecholamine, dopamine, from its stores in the brain. These drugs were widely known as amphetamines and are rarely used now because of their potential for abuse. Their place has been taken by a group of similar drugs with fewer side-effects.

THE SHEER POWER OF HUNGER

This tendency to seek out specific foods to supply a particular nutrient is especially marked in pregnancy and is known as pica. It can cause a very powerful urge to eat, for example, raw meat or apples. The body will do all it can to persuade the pregnant woman to seek out foods with high levels of whatever nutrient it needs.

The same kind of thing happens in pre-menstrual women. The body needs more of a certain protein and, as large amounts of this substance (phenylethylamine) are found in chocolate, the brain produces a craving for chocolate.[7]

Since our bodies keep adjusting our appetite according to our needs, it makes extreme dieting (and in particular restrictive single-food diets) very difficult to follow. Your brain will deliberately do its very best to make you break the diet, increasing your appetite sharply to send you off in search of food.

Constant hunger pangs and food cravings are very uncomfortable to ignore – because your body has been designed to give in to them! This obviously makes trying to control your weight simply by eating less very difficult to do, as you end up fighting your own drives and needs.[8] This is why very restrictive diets are exceedingly uncomfortable and usually fail.

HOW BODY SHAPE IS CONTROLLED BY THE *SLIMMING SYSTEM*

Not only does the *Slimming System* control weight, it also controls our basic body shape. Several of the 'slimming hormones' also play a major role here, but two of the most important ones are the male and female sex hormones.

The male sex hormone, testosterone, builds muscle and burns fat, causing men to be generally leaner and more muscular than women. A reduction in the levels of testosterone as men get older creates a tendency for muscles to shrink and fat to gather particularly around the abdominal area; in other words it is largely responsible for a paunch.[9]

The female sex hormones, oestrogens, encourage fat storage, particularly in the breasts, thighs and buttocks. This is most obvious during puberty, when rising levels of female sex hormones create the curvy outline we normally associate with women. It also explains why women tend to store more body fat than men – and why women on the pill can sometimes gain weight.

EXERCISE AND THE *SLIMMING SYSTEM*

Exercise is a vitally important tool in maintaining our weight. It is also one of the few ways in which you can positively reduce your weight set-point and improve your body shape.[10]

This is not just because exercise burns off lots of calories, but because when you exercise you will actually increase your body's production of certain vital 'slimming' hormones.[11] This hormonal effect lasts way beyond short-term calorie-burning – as after good spells of exercise these slimming effects can extend for several days or even weeks.

Once again, you might think that the amount of exercise you take is totally voluntary. In fact, your level of spontaneous activity is strongly controlled by your hormones and depends on an intact body structure and all the necessary nutrients that generate energy to power the muscles.

We all differ in our natural activity levels, even from birth. Some babies are far more active than others and will tend to grow up to be the type of people who seem to have endless energy, take part in more strenuous activities and are constantly on the go.[12] These fortunate people are far less likely to have a weight problem than those born with a lower energy drive, who tend to take less exercise, tire more easily and have to make more of a conscious effort to take exercise.

So what determines our energy drive? Well – in a nutshell – our hormones do. Hormones affect both long-term and short-term aspects of muscle metabolism; they stimulate growth, maintain muscle volume, increase energy levels in muscle and alter our metabolism to make available the foods necessary for sufficient levels of energy production.

Though a wide range of hormones may play a role in controlling the amount of exercise we take, the catecholamines play the leading role. So you can see why they make such good slimming aids. They can reduce your appetite but they can also increase your energy levels,[13] so you feel like taking more exercise in all aspects of your life.

Catecholamines not only increase your conscious activity, such as walking, but they also increase the amount of involuntary fidgeting movements you make.[14] Although you may not be so aware of them, these fidgeting actions can burn up quite a significant amount of energy and can play an important part in allowing your *Slimming System* to do its job.

WHAT REDUCES OUR ABILITY TO EXERCISE?

Although we inherit much of our body chemistry, which largely determines how active we are, several other factors also affect the amount of energy we produce. They include metabolic disorders, hormone imbalances and even a lack of essential nutrients in the food that we eat.

Most people don't appreciate how our hormones stimulate the will to exercise until they have a hormone deficiency or imbalance. A feeling of tiredness or lack of energy is one of the commonest symptoms of hormone problems and is also commonly found in people with vitamin or mineral deficiencies.

By the same token, damage to any part of the body structure involved in exercise, from the nerves stimulating the muscles through to damaged muscle fibres, will prevent us burning off calories through exercise. As the body uses up approximately 25 per cent of the energy derived from food in exercise, a reduced ability to exercise resulting from damage or illness would most definitely affect the overall balance – increasing the chances of weight gain.

WHY OUR ENERGY LEVELS CAN FALL DRAMATICALLY WHEN DIETING

Just as your body alters your appetite to adapt to changing circumstances, so your body is also able to alter its energy levels to control the amount of exercise you take.

Fluctuating energy levels are particularly noticeable if you cut your food right back in an attempt to lose weight. Because of the shortage of nutrients, rather than 'wasting' them on powering non-essential exercise the body will redirect them to power its most important life-support systems.

The resulting feeling of tiredness and lack of energy is therefore a natural defence mechanism to prevent you doing too much in these conditions – your body effectively compensates by dropping your energy levels so that you take less exercise. It will also cut your level of involuntary movement (fidgeting) in order to make further energy savings.

This helps to explain why crash dieting rarely works, as the body instinctively tries to protect itself from a sudden weight loss by dramatically reducing the desire to exercise. And, if you force yourself to take strenuous exercise on a limited food intake, for the remainder of the day your body will tend to reduce the amount of energy you spend on non-essential tasks by dramatically reducing your energy levels – making you feel tired and forcing you to rest.

Weight-control mechanisms also kick in if you try to lose weight by simply increasing your levels of exercise. For example if you spend thirty minutes every day doing vigorous aerobics, the extra exercise will definitely help you lose lots of excess fat and develop more body muscle, but you will not burn off 12 kg of body fat after a year, which is the fat equivalent of the total number of calories used up from the aerobic exercises. This is because your natural weight-control mechanisms actively compensate to some extent for this higher activity level.

By the same token, if you change from a very active job to a less active one your appetite will reduce to compensate.[15] This ability to compensate is known as your dynamic metabolism.

YOUR METABOLISM AND THE *SLIMMING SYSTEM*

Fig. 4 shows how the body uses up the energy we get from the foods we eat.[16] You can see that exercise uses up only a quarter of your daily intake of food, while another quarter is burned off by hormones such as catecholamines. But clearly the biggest energy user of all is the body's basic metabolism. Since our metabolism is such a major player in weight control, it is important to understand what it is and how it works.

Metabolism is a convenient term to cover the billions of reactions taking place in our bodies to convert food to fat or energy. On average, just keeping your vital functions running accounts for about half of the energy you burn off every day. The speed of your

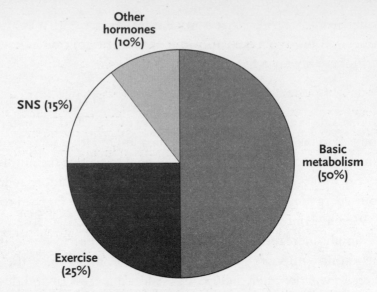

Figure 4. The relative importance of different systems in using up energy.

metabolism, or your metabolic rate, can vary quite a lot from person to person.[17] Two people can be exactly the same size and have the same amounts of muscle and fat, yet the person with the faster metabolism can burn up more calories than the other. This means that the person with the slower metabolism has to eat less food than the person with the faster metabolism just to stay at the same weight.

What determines whether you are a faster or slower fat-burner? Well, surprise, surprise – your hormones do. Hormones, or the lack of them, strongly influence the speed of your metabolism. For example, an excess of thyroid hormone can actually double your metabolic rate, resulting in weight loss, whereas a deficiency can reduce it by more than half, causing weight gain.

So the overall speed or efficiency at which our hormones are working will play a very important role in determining where our weight set-point will be fixed.

WHAT UNDERLIES AN EFFICIENT
FAT-BURNING METABOLISM

Your hormones have a natural rhythm that helps to order the metabolic reactions in a way that maximizes the efficiency of the entire process. A deficiency in one particular hormone or nutrient can disrupt the overall rhythm, thereby reducing the efficiency of the reactions.

In order to keep these processes working to full capacity we need to ensure that we feed our metabolism with all the essential nutrients it needs to work, as well as providing it with enough vitamins and minerals to act as catalysts for all the millions of reactions taking place.

I'll go into much more detail about nutrients and supplements to power your metabolism in Chapter 13: Repair and Revitalize Your Natural *Slimming System*. For now, the important thing is to realize that a good metabolic rate is vital if you want to keep your weight down.

HOW WE BURN OFF EXCESS FAT STORES

The hormones that control metabolism are also in control of the rate at which fat is burned up, and the most important hormones in this process are, once again, the catecholamines. They are vital to our ability to burn off body fat stores – without them we simply could not break down fat.

Another way in which our body burns up large amounts of energy is in controlling our body temperature. The heat-producing process known as thermogenesis is designed to keep us warm if the temperature drops – but it also helps the body to burn off excess food by raising the overall body temperature to a higher level than normal.[18] In this way, excess food or body fat stores can be converted into heat which can then be easily dispersed.

Carbohydrates in particular are good at increasing heat production. This helps to explain why you will get a warm feeling after eating foods rich in carbohydrates. Their ability to release catecholamines into the body ensures that excess carbohydrates are burned off and not stored as fats.

In fact, one of the main thrusts in the development of new slimming drugs is to find a way of enhancing thermogenesis so that more food and excess body fat can be burned off as heat. The sad thing is that if your *Slimming System* was working well this would all be done by your body automatically and there would be absolutely no need for these drugs.

WHAT HAPPENS TO OUR METABOLISM WHEN WE DIET?

Traditional methods of dieting depend on the idea that a certain amount of food has a fixed calorific value and by cutting your food intake you will lose weight. However, the body's dynamic metabolism means that if you cut your intake of calories, your body will respond to this pretty quickly, by slowing down the rate at which you burn off food as heat. In this way your body can make internal energy savings. This has the effect of making less food go further.

This is a basic survival mechanism that protects (among others) pregnant or lactating women in poorer countries. Rather than starve the baby of food, the mother's body will shut down any waste of food energy. This mechanism is so powerful that even mothers with physically demanding jobs can produce adequate amounts of breast milk to feed their babies with.[19]

Ideally, if your *Slimming System* is working well, the reverse will happen if you over-eat. The rate at which your body produces heat should increase until you burn all the excess food off.

This dynamic metabolism explains why dieting by food-restriction alone will never work in the long term. The body will strive to return to its set-point not just when you are dieting but also after you stop. Dieting alone simply cannot alter the weight set-point and only makes the body more efficient with the food it has got.

So, while you can lose weight in the short term, when you stop dieting your body will do all it can to compensate for the food shortage and you will end up weighing at least as much as you did before you started.

I think by now it should be absolutely clear that you will never be able to lose weight by following traditional dieting methods alone. The experience of the past fifty years or more backs this up completely. With such a large chunk of the population dieting at any one time, if traditional diets really worked there would actually be few fat people left!

OVERWEIGHT PEOPLE HAVE LESS EFFECTIVE METABOLISMS

It will come as no surprise to any of you who are actually eating less than your slimmer friends that overweight people appear to have less efficient metabolisms. The same amount of food that will maintain the weight of slimmer people can make overweight people fatter. What's more unfair is that overweight people also appear to use up proportionately less energy in carrying out a whole range of different body functions.

Studies have shown that in overweight people there is a basic malfunctioning in the most important part of the body's *Slimming System* – the sympathetic nervous system (SNS).[20] If a person has an underactive SNS, their appetite will tend to be greater, particularly for fatty foods, since they produce fewer fat-burning catecholamines. The amount of energy they appear to burn up to heat the body is likely to be lower.[21] They even seem to use up less energy than a naturally slimmer person would use if they took the same amount of exercise.[22]

This obviously creates an energy imbalance, as the numbers of calories taken in are far greater than those which are being used up. These excess calories may then be stored as fat deposits.

OVERWEIGHT PEOPLE ARE ALSO LESS ABLE TO USE UP THEIR EXISTING FAT STORES

But the problem doesn't stop there, because the SNS needs to be functioning properly for fats to be released from adipose tissue. As the SNS is less active, the total rate at which fat can be used up from these stores could plummet.

So, with less fat readily available to burn, overweight people tend to produce less heat after eating a meal or if the surroundings get colder. Since they cannot raise their body temperature as much as lean people, they use up less excess body fat and end up getting colder and fatter. So despite the ever-increasing stores of fat being there, they simply cannot actively mobilize them and use them up.

The bad news is that even if they do lose weight temporarily by traditional food-restriction diets, they will still have an underactive SNS, so the struggle to keep excess weight off will continue throughout their lives.

Now don't despair at this point. There *is* a way to boost your *Slimming System* and SNS to a new level of improved functioning which will lower your weight set-point, and therefore your body weight too.

Many of the toxic chemicals we are regularly exposed to damage not only the *Slimming System* but also specifically target the SNS.[23] This damage could result in increasing the overall weight set-point. By reducing our exposure to these chemicals, the *Slimming System* can be revived and allowed to function properly again.

OVERWEIGHT PEOPLE ARE LOW IN CERTAIN VITAMINS AND MINERALS

There is one more vitally important difference between overweight and lean people: overweight people tend to be markedly deficient in certain vitamins and minerals compared to the non-overweight. Just because you are getting enough calories in your diet, it doesn't automatically mean that you are getting enough vitamins and minerals. On the contrary, the fatter you are, the more deficient you are likely to be.[24]

So it will hardly come as a surprise that the vitamins and nutrients that overweight people lack are the same ones that play vital roles in maximizing the ability to burn off fat.[25] This shortfall in vital nutrients not only reduces your ability to lose weight, but it starts a vicious circle, making your whole system less efficient.

I know that if I forget to take my vitamins for more than one day then by the second evening I can really feel tiredness coming on. To me, this is a sign that my metabolism hasn't got what it needs to produce enough energy to power my body fully. If being tired makes you exercise less, then you have little chance of burning off excess food.

WHICH NUTRIENTS SEEM TO BE MISSING?

So which vitamins and minerals are we talking about? Well, in all the studies I have read, the ones cropping up again and again are vitamins A, B, C, and E and the minerals zinc and magnesium. In fact, studies have shown that the fatter a person becomes the more likely it is that they will be deficient in vitamins A, C and E and several of the B group vitamins.

In a study of very overweight women, 58 per cent were deficient in vitamin C, but among women of average weight the deficiency level was a very low 3 per cent.[26] In another study, which looked at overweight boys, the levels of vitamins A and E in their blood were 50 per cent lower than those found in normal-weight boys.[27]

The evidence that these vitamins play a crucial part in our *Slimming System* was supported by yet another study, which actually found that if obese non-dieting women were given 1 gram of vitamin C three times a day for a period of six weeks, they lost 2.5kg without even trying to diet.[28]

This is potentially very good news, because it suggests that, for whatever reason, overweight people tend to be extremely deficient in certain nutrients which are vital to the smooth running of their *Slimming Systems*. It opens up the possibility that one of the reasons overweight people *are* overweight is because they lack the appropriate nutrients to bring about weight loss, either because they use up nutrients faster than the average person, or because their diet is particularly lacking in them, or a combination of both factors.

This problem is actually much more common than you might suspect. The number of people worldwide thought to be deficient in at least one vitamin or mineral has been estimated at a stunning 2–3.5 billion – many of these being people who are overweight.[29] By taking the appropriate vitamin supplements, you allow the *Slimming System* to function properly, perhaps for the first time ever, and so get to work in burning off excess weight and keeping it off.

It also appears that deficiencies in certain vitamins and minerals could be partly responsible for altering your body shape. The evidence is strongest for vitamin E. For example, a study by Ohrvall in 1993 found that the lower the level of vitamin E in the blood, the greater the abdominal measurement.[30]

Another study looked at Indian men with abdominal obesity. It found that the more abdominal fat they had, the lower their blood levels of vitamin E, vitamin C, magnesium and zinc would be.[31] Again this is actually marvellous news, as it is relatively easy to remedy vitamin and mineral deficiencies by taking the right balance of supplements.

To optimize your *Slimming System* it is now clear that you need to give your body all the nutrients it needs to work to its maximum ability (see Chapter 15).

USE YOUR NATURAL *SLIMMING SYSTEM*

The aim of this chapter has been to show you that will-power alone is not your greatest asset in losing weight. Your greatest asset is, in fact, a healthy and efficient *Slimming System* – as any attempt to lose weight by just reducing the amount of food you eat will be countered by the body doing all it can to fight the change. It will increase your appetite, reduce the amount of exercise you do and even reduce the rate at which you burn off calories. Your body will maintain its existing food stores as if its life depended on it – millions of years ago it probably did!

The only effective way forward for those who want to lose weight permanently is to get your body to work with you in losing weight rather than fighting against you all the way.

The next chapter will explain how chemicals have poisoned the body's natural *Slimming System*. This totally new and ground-breaking information has never previously been published in a book and is set to take the dieting world by storm. By understanding just how these chemicals damage us, we move one step closer not only to preventing any further damage but also to restoring our *Slimming System* to its former glory.

5. How Chemicals Make You Fat
Why Dieting without Detox Will Always Fail

You may not have realized it, but there is a war going on inside your body. As you read this, synthetic chemicals are currently engaged in an increasingly one-sided battle against your natural *Slimming System*. Judging by the number of overweight people, the chemicals appear to be winning hands down.

The evidence that many of these highly toxic substances have the ability to destroy our natural weight-control systems is overwhelming. What's more, it seems that this is happening at our current exposure levels. In order to win the battle against chemicals, and win it we most definitely can, we need to raise our defences and fortify our shields. This, in a nutshell, is what this chapter is all about.

It will tell you how toxic chemicals are able to attack every single major part of our *Slimming System*, how the subsequent damage can make us fat, the ways in which chemicals can alter our body shape, how traditional methods of dieting can make us fatter, and, last but not least, how the fundamental way in which we diet has to change in order to adapt to the new environment we find ourselves living in.

Like the previous chapter it will be more detailed than the rest of the book, but the proof of the pudding is in the eating, so to speak, and I think that after you have read it you will understand why I have spent so much time clarifying these issues.

So take heart: weight gain is not simply down to weak willpower, greed and laziness. Most of it is due to your body's inability to deal with toxins in your food and environment. And once you understand exactly what is happening, you will be well on your way towards dealing with the problem. Please believe me when I say that there is light at the end of the tunnel, because by reading this book you will be brought yet another step closer to achieving the body of your dreams. Go on – you're worth it!

WHAT MAKES OUR *SLIMMING SYSTEM* ONE OF THE FIRST SYSTEMS 'HIT' BY THESE WELL-ARMED INVADERS?

Toxic chemicals are well-known for their ability to damage a whole number of body systems. However, there are certain reasons why our *Slimming System* is probably more susceptible to chemical damage than the rest of our other body systems.

The most important tissues making up our *Slimming System*, for example, our brain, glands and body fat, tend to have a high fat content and a relatively good blood supply. Unfortunately, for the following reasons, tissues which have these characteristics tend to be more vulnerable to chemical damage. The first problem relates to the fact that many of the more toxic synthetic chemicals are extremely fat-soluble. So when they are released into the blood they make a beeline for the fattier parts of the body. Due to their high fat content, the most central parts of the *Slimming System* present an easy target for these chemicals.

Second, as the brain and our hormone-secreting glands have some of the highest blood supplies of all the existing organs in our body, they end up being exposed to the highest amounts of blood-borne toxins.[1]

As a result, the most toxic and persistent synthetic chemicals tend to concentrate in the most sensitive and vulnerable parts of our *Slimming System*. So it comes as no surprise that out of all the systems in our body, our *Slimming System* will be among the first in the firing line to be damaged by chemicals.

OK, now we know what makes our *Slimming System* particularly vulnerable to injury, we need to move on to discover exactly what type of damage takes place. Let's return to the four main parts of our *Slimming System* and see how this fattening effect is brought about in each individual situation.

BRAIN AND NERVE DAMAGE

The brain controls everything about who we are and what we do. No exception is made when it comes to body weight and eating, as the brain governs all our eating behaviour, appetite and metabolism. On top of this it also controls the body's weight 'set-point'.

Unfortunately, the brain is exquisitely sensitive to damage from all kinds of chemical toxins, not only because of its high fat content and excellent blood supply, but also because it appears to be less able than most parts of the body to deal with certain chemical toxins.[2] In addition, unlike most other tissue, most brain cells once poisoned cannot regenerate themselves.

Here is an example of how our brain is put at risk by these chemicals. One of the features which make certain synthetic chemicals 'good' pesticides is their ability to act as nerve agents, paralysing the functioning of certain parts of the brain.[3] The probability is high that many of the pesticides in our food will act in a similar sort of way on us to the way they do on insects. To put it brutally, many of the chemicals deliberately added to our food could therefore be acting as small doses of nerve agent on our brains. How does that grab you?

HORMONES, THE FAT CONTROLLERS

In recent times the media have publicized a whole range of synthetic chemicals thought to have powerful hormone-altering properties, with 'gender-bending' effects. Gender-bending is just a phrase to describe unexpected changes in sexual behaviour.

Although gender-bending in particular has caught the public imagination, this is not the only problem resulting from hormonal damage; if truth be known, the whole range of hormones involved in weight control can essentially be altered to promote excessive weight gain.

When I was in the midst of my research, it didn't take long before I realized that virtually every one of the pesticides found in our foods – in addition to the majority of the other synthetic chemicals I was investigating – appeared to have a significant effect on at least one of the major weight-controlling hormones.

More specifically, the trend was that these chemicals tended to increase the levels of fattening hormones such as insulin and steroids,[4] while reducing the levels of slimming hormones such as thyroid hormone, sex hormones, growth hormone and catecholamines.[5]

OUR NATURAL 'SLIMMING' HORMONES, CATECHOLAMINES, ARE PARTICULARLY TARGETED

Out of all the hormones affected by chemicals, it appeared to me during the course of my research that those which seemed to come most frequently under attack were our most valuable group of slimming hormones, the catecholamines. Not only was a powerful catecholamine-lowering effect evident in animals, but it was also frequently found in humans.

For example, one study of workers in a pesticide factory manufacturing organochlorines, organophosphates and carbamates revealed that the workers themselves produced at least 40 per cent fewer 'slimming' catecholamines in their blood than the average person.[6]

This may in part be explained by the fact that the adrenal gland, which is responsible for producing a large amount of 'slimming' catecholamines, has been described as being the gland most susceptible to chemical-induced toxicities.[7] With fewer catecholamines being produced, is it any wonder that we are losing the ability to stay slim?

BODY STRUCTURE

To burn off excess food, the basic fabric of your whole body needs to be in good shape. The problem is that many chemicals can directly injure much of our body's basic structure. As many of these chemicals can also inhibit the overall amount of body protein created, the overall structural damage is magnified.

As protein-rich structures make up much of our body structure and in particular much of the fabric of our *Slimming System* (specifi-cally in the form of hormones, enzymes, mitochondria and muscles), chemical damage has a significant knock-on effect on the entire efficiency of our *Slimming System*.

To give you an example of this happening, sheep farmers who dip their sheep in organophosphate sheep dips to kill the parasites were found to have smaller calf muscles than quarry workers who do a similar amount of work, but have no contact with organophos-phates.[8] This well-documented muscle-shrinking effect is thought to be caused in the following way. First the nerves that stimulate the muscles are damaged or destroyed, so that the muscle they would normally stimulate ends up just wasting away. Second, the muscle fibres themselves can be directly damaged by these chemicals, as well as the energy-producing mitochondria which exist within the muscle. This promotes muscle shrinkage and a lower level of energy production.[9]

In addition to shrinking muscles the level of stamina falls, as muscles become fatigued more quickly. This is a direct result of a slow-down in energy production, such that the supply can no longer meet the demands. This is why the commonest symptoms of chemical toxicity are weak muscles and general fatigue.[10] You can imagine that if you don't feel like exercising, you are far less likely to burn off excess body fat.

If marked, this muscle toxicity can make you feel so tired that you don't want to get out of bed, let alone go for a walk, and here I speak from personal experience. In my case, though, this chemically induced muscle poisoning was due to dieting, and I will tell you all about that dreadful but thankfully temporary experience later, in Chapter 14.

SYNTHETIC CHEMICALS ARE DEPLETING YOUR BODY OF ITS 'SLIMMING' NUTRIENTS

To ensure the smooth running of the body's natural *Slimming System*, we need to provide it with all the fuel it needs and cannot manufacture itself, such as vitamins, minerals, proteins and certain essential fats. A shortage of any one of these vital nutrients may result in the overall efficiency of your entire *Slimming System* plummeting.

Synthetic chemicals have had a major destructive role even here. It seems that not only can they interfere with the way that our bodies absorb nutrients from foods, but they can directly destroy some of the more delicate nutrients, prevent the production of other essential nutrients, increase the rate at which the body uses various nutrients and even increase the rate at which the body excretes nutrients.[11]

So the overall effect is to promote in our bodies a form of chemically induced nutrient deficiency. This deficiency involves all the previously mentioned nutrients, but perhaps the most affected of all are the antioxidants, namely vitamins C and E. This is because when toxic chemicals damage our tissues, the body needs to repair the harm caused by the subsequent blast of free radicals released. As the body soaks up free radicals with antioxidants, this could explain why our need for these particular vitamins seems to have sky-rocketed.[12]

The knock-on effect to us is that these chemicals appear to deprive our *Slimming System* of a whole range of nutrients essential for its smooth functioning. And if the *Slimming System* cannot work to its full capacity, the chances are we will end up gaining weight.

OUR NEED FOR CERTAIN NUTRIENTS HAS BEEN PERMANENTLY INCREASED

Because of the increasing presence of synthetic chemicals in our bodies and lives, our need for certain nutrients has increased to a greater level than it has probably ever been. We now appear to need far higher doses of certain nutrients than the recommended daily dosages commonly laid down as guidelines, because these values were simply not created with chemical damage in mind.

Regrettably our nutrient intake from food has in all likelihood dropped to an all-time low. To aggravate an already bad situation, we are now eating a fraction of the nutrients that we once did thousands of years ago. The problem is that even by eating the perfect diet of nutrient-rich foods, our need for certain vitamins has increased so much that we will never be able to get the levels we need from our food alone – even with the best will in the world.[13]

Fortunately, this situation can be fully dealt with. By taking the right supplements you can give the body the nutrients it needs to power its vital systems as well as its *Slimming System*, and in so doing, help combat any potential damage by chemicals. The recommended doses of nutrients are given in Chapter 15.

HOW CHEMICALS CAN INCREASE YOUR APPETITE

As we have seen in the previous chapter, hormones control our appetite. So it is not surprising to discover that hormone-damaging toxic chemicals can also have a powerful influence on our appetite.[14]

What tends to happen is that chemicals can disturb the usually tight balance between the amount of food that we eat and the amount of food that we actually require. The overall effect will be an increased appetite which can drive us to eat more than our body actually needs.

This appetite-enhancing effect is one of the more important ways that synthetic chemicals can work in promoting animal growth and is a major reason for the effectiveness of many chemicals which have been used to fatten up humans. It also contributes to why certain medications such as steroids and antihistamines appear to have powerful fattening side-effects.[15] Ask anyone on even a short course of steroids and they will tell you how their cravings for carbohydrates escalate.

However, not only is our overall level of appetite affected, but the hormones damaged are those which control our appetite for fatty and sugary foods – such as the catecholamines and steroids – so if the level of these hormones is altered, our desire for these foods can increase. Perhaps this explains the popularity of fast foods, since they meet the criteria of increased fats and sugars perfectly. Unless we can fight our body's natural urges every day, chemical damage could make us eat more than we need. And I don't imagine for one second that you need me to tell you that this will ultimately make us fatter.

CHEMICAL DAMAGE AND A REDUCED ABILITY TO EXERCISE

Yet again, synthetic chemical interference appears to severely affect all aspects of our ability to exercise, making our get-up-and-go simply push off. I must admit that when I started researching into the effects these chemicals have on our ability to exercise, I never anticipated finding such wide-ranging and damaging results, as all aspects of muscle function seem to be touched.

As well as shrinking the muscles, which reduces strength and stamina, they also reduce our energy drive. And at this point the catecholamines come into the equation again. As well as controlling our appetite, they also effectively 'set' our energy levels and our desire to exercise. Consequently any fall in catecholamine levels, such as the reductions produced by an extremely large number of synthetic chemicals, will not only reduce the amount of voluntary exercise we feel like taking, but will also probably lessen the involuntary movements that we usually don't even notice.[16] The overall effect is rather like a chemical cosh.

Adding further insult to injury, chemically damaged muscles will probably be less able to burn up energy than non-damaged muscles.[17] This will reduce the ability to burn up calories even further. This damage to our ability to exercise will have a serious effect on our overall weight, as exercise is one of the main ways in which our bodies burn off excess calories.

Again, don't despair as you read this. It is possible to regain your natural energy drive, even if it is currently low. By following the instructions in this book you can overcome this chemical damage to improve not only your natural energy levels, but also your level of fitness – just keep reading and soon all will be revealed!

HOW CHEMICAL DAMAGE AFFECTS METABOLISM

The last major part of our *Slimming System* to be considered is our metabolism. As our basic metabolism is by far the biggest user of energy, any damage to our metabolism, however small, can have very serious weight implications.

Once again, synthetic chemicals can damage virtually all aspects of our metabolism. By lowering the amount of hormones that speed up metabolism and by reducing the availability of a whole range of essential nutrients – by using them up to rid the body of these new chemicals – they can effectively slow down the rate of energy production.[18] This ability to reduce energy expenditure means they make great animal fatteners, since less food goes further. But on the other hand it can devastate our ability to lose weight or to stay slim.

Added to this, as if we needed more bad news, our ability to use up certain foods, for example carbohydrates, also appears to be impaired by certain chemicals.[19] This could be one of the reasons why a diet high in carbohydrates leads so easily to weight gain.

But, despite this apparent slow-down, we still need a certain amount of carbohydrates in our diet because they powerfully rev up our metabolism by stimulating the production of catecholamines. They are also essential for our ability to detoxify chemicals.[20] So carbohydrates in moderation, rather than cutting them out completely, seems to be the answer.

CHEMICALS PREVENT US FROM USING UP OUR
FAT STORES

But it is not only carbohydrates which are affected. Synthetic chemicals specifically appear to reduce our ability to burn up our existing fat stores.[21] This is probably done in two main ways: first by lowering our ability to generate body heat,[22] and second by reducing the levels of hormones essential for releasing body fats from storage.[23]

Chemical damage appears to make people less able to raise their body temperature – particularly marked when surrounding temperatures fall. This can be seen in people who are severely damaged by chemicals, as they tend to have a lower than average body temperature.[24] So if they produce less heat they end up using less energy.

The reason for this inability to convert existing fat stores into heat is that the hormones which are essential in mobilizing fats, namely catecholamines, have been severely lowered. Because of this, our fat stores cannot be exploited fully to produce heat energy or indeed energy for any other reason.

So, once our fat is in storage, it becomes very difficult to shift, creating ever increasing amounts of fat stores that our bodies simply cannot use up.

Weight control, then, is not just a matter of regulating what we eat and how much we exercise, but involves a huge diversity of systems, which can all be damaged by chemicals. You can see for yourself that the weight you are depends far less on your will-power than on the state of your *Slimming System*.

NOT JUST HEAVIER, BUT FATTER TOO

Yet more bad news: not only do toxic chemicals appear to make us heavier, but it seems that some of these chemicals could also make us fatter. As the kilos pile up, certain chemicals tend to increase the proportion of body fat while simultaneously lowering the proportion of body muscle.[25] The overall result is a fatter, less shapely body.

And it doesn't stop there: these changes could have a knock-on effect on our skin too. As there is a certain amount of muscle in skin, any subsequent reduction in the amount of muscle will affect the firmness of the skin, making it softer and flabbier.

In addition to worsening the condition and appearance of our skin, this could also increase our amount of cellulite. This is because the packages of fat stored under the skin will be held in less firmly and will be more visible if the skin is thinner.

WHY CERTAIN FAMILIES SEEM TO HAVE MORE WEIGHT PROBLEMS THAN OTHERS

You might ask, since we are all exposed to these chemicals, why aren't we all fat? After all, most slim people eat contaminated foods and live in the same environment. The answer is related to the overall amount of pollutants that we are exposed to and to our nutritional status, as well as to our individual ability to deal with toxins.

For years, the view was that people were stuck with the particular balance of hormones that they were born with. The ability to inherit 'overweight' genes was thought to explain why the problem of excess weight tended to run in families and left people believing that there was absolutely nothing they could do about their weight if they inherited these genes.

Now it is clear that our body chemistry can be totally altered by toxic chemicals. So perhaps what these families have really inherited is a vulnerability to toxic chemical damage. We already know that there is a huge genetically based variation in our ability to detoxify certain chemicals.[26] For instance, some racial groups cannot metabolize alcohol as well as others.

In addition to explaining why some racial groups seem to be vastly more susceptible to weight gain than others, this raises the possibility that people from fatter families could now become thinner by reducing their exposure to toxic chemicals and by eliminating their body stores of fattening chemicals.

WHY IS THE EPIDEMIC GROWING SO FAST?

If you turn back to Fig. 1 on page 8 you will see that this fat epidemic is a relatively recent problem. The big question is: why is the epidemic growing at such a pace?

The most obvious reason by far is the ever-increasing levels of chemicals to which we are now exposed. However, before we can deal with the problem effectively, a full understanding of the potential reasons is essential.

By looking at the broader picture, several other likely reasons emerge. These include the early age at which our children are being exposed to chemicals, the increasing chemical stores we gather throughout our lives, our worsening nutrition and lastly our increased tendency to diet.

ARE OUR CHILDREN BEING PROGRAMMED TO BE FAT?

As previously explained, children are far more sensitive than adults to the potential damage that chemicals can cause. In fact, they appear to be most vulnerable to damage while still in the womb.[27] So, if they are exposed to chemicals at certain critical stages, their *Slimming Systems* can be permanently affected. To illustrate this, tests have shown that pregnant animals treated with certain synthetic growth-promoters produce offspring that are not just heavier at birth but also weigh more throughout their lives.[28]

Now if we take a closer look at the average weight of our newborn babies, it seems that the average birth-weight has been increasing over recent years.[29] In addition, children seem to be becoming overweight at an ever younger age, with the problem for some children starting almost from birth.[30] Childhood obesity is now at the highest level that it has ever been, and there is every sign that the situation is getting worse. So early exposure to chemicals may be an important factor in causing the recent fat epidemic.

WHY WE ARE BECOMING INCREASINGLY FATTER AS WE GET OLDER

It is not only children who are getting fatter – we adults are gaining weight throughout our lives at a greater speed than ever before. This increasing tendency to gain weight as we get older can largely be put down to several different factors.

First, throughout our lives our body load of chemicals tends to increase. The greater the build-up, the more disrupted the *Slimming System* will be. Second, these increased levels of chemicals will most probably result in a greater level of existing *Slimming System* damage. And last, the body's detoxification system also tends to become less effective as we get older.[31]

All these factors tend to reduce the effectiveness of our *Slimming System*, making future weight gain almost inevitable.

HOW OUR INCREASINGLY PROCESSED FOODS AND NUTRIENT-POOR DIETS ARE MAKING US FATTER

Given the quantity of toxic chemicals in our food and environment and the way they increase our need for nutrients, it has been said that even the best-balanced diet could not contain all the nutrients we now need without some form of supplementation.[32]

Food-processing, storage and conventional farming techniques have all done their bit to reduce the quality of protein, vitamins and minerals now present in our food. Add to this the fact that an extremely large percentage of the population is now actively dieting, and this reduces the chances of getting sufficient nutrients from food even further.

So on the one hand our need for nutrients has actually grown but on the other our *Slimming Systems* are being increasingly starved of the nutrients they need. Not surprisingly, the consequences of this increasing nutrient imbalance are now clearly evident in our escalating weight problem.

HOW CONVENTIONAL DIETING CAN ACTUALLY MAKE US FATTER

While you may think you are doing the right thing by going on a conventional diet, you could actually make the problem worse. This is because when you diet, your body will have to burn up more fat to power its systems.

You might think that was a good thing, and it probably was hundreds of years ago. However, your fat stores now contain a large amount of accumulated toxic chemicals, which are mobilized into your system in a big whoosh as soon as you start burning off your fat.[33] Once set free in your body, these toxins will redistribute themselves and cause havoc in the most vulnerable parts of your *Slimming System*.

Added to this is the problem of insufficient nutrients, as by restricting your intake of food you will have fewer nutrients to repair the damage.

So every time you go on a diet without protecting your body against the release of stored toxins and chemicals, you will be effectively damaging your *Slimming System*. This is most probably why people who lose weight quickly seem to put back the weight they have lost, plus a bit extra. This can also explain why the next time you try to diet, it seems even harder, because in truth it really will be.

Yet if done in the right way, you can use food-restriction dieting to lose weight. However, here the whole method has to be changed. Rather than using food-restriction alone, the emphasis is on detox-ification and on protecting your natural *Slimming System*. The up-side is potentially fantastic though, for if done properly, not only can detox dieting accelerate your eventual weight loss but it can also lower your body weight set-point.

SO HOW DO YOU KNOW IF YOUR *SLIMMING SYSTEM* IS DAMAGED?

There has been a lot of talk about what causes damage to the *Slimming System*, but how do we actually know if our *Slimming System* is damaged or not?

Well, the biggest and most obvious sign that your *Slimming System* is flagging is if you are already overweight. Another sign is that of easy weight gain, especially if it seems a daily struggle to keep your weight down.

Other relevant clues include a great desire to eat fatty and sugary foods, a tendency to feel the cold, and a changing body shape, for example a pot-belly or proportionally bigger hips and thighs.

If you have to make continual efforts to restrict the amount of food you eat, or to exercise regularly to maintain a stable weight, the chances are that your *Slimming System* is not working as well as it should. These signs also indicate that the *Slimming System* is now in need of urgent attention.

THE NEW WAY WE NEED TO LOSE WEIGHT

We must realize that to lose weight in our new chemically contaminated environment, we have to adapt the way we diet to the new situation we find ourselves in. Thus, today, dieting should always take place hand in hand with detoxification. In fact dieting without detox is not just ineffective but potentially dangerous.[34]

The benefits of combining diet and detox include permanent weight loss but also a whole raft of other health benefits, because by removing the toxic chemicals that make you fat, you will also do away with the ones that appear to make you ill.

So now we know how chemicals damage our natural *Slimming System*. The next step is to find out which are the worst offenders. As it is clearly no longer possible to remove all synthetic chemicals from our lives, we need to devise a plan to reduce our exposure to the most fattening of these chemicals as well as finding ways of increasing their removal from our bodies.

In this way not only can we prevent future damage to our *Slimming System* but we can also boost its effectiveness to a degree that we may never have experienced before.

So I now have the pleasure of introducing Part Two, which will start you on your way to lasting slimness. By learning which chemicals are the most fattening, what they are used for and where they tend to be found, you will be well on your way to discovering the real secret of how to lose weight in the twenty-first century.

PART TWO
Chemical Calories

6. All About *Chemical Calories*

The Dieter's No. 1 Enemy

This chapter presents some of the most innovative material in the book. For the first time ever, the doors have been thrown wide open to a completely new way for us to identify the most fattening chemicals in the food chain and the environment – singling them out from the hundreds of thousands of others that are less fattening so that we can avoid them.

Sadly, we have to accept that to cut out all synthetic chemicals from our lives would be virtually impossible. The prospect would be daunting, the cost astronomical, and in many cases the appropriate chemical-free substitutes would simply not be available. But while total exclusion is out of the question, we can all be far more selective.

Cutting out the most fattening chemicals first will enable us to make an enormous difference with comparatively little effort. And as we begin to see the weight loss benefits for ourselves, we can take a more informed view about limiting the chemicals in our food as well as considering how far to go in removing potentially fattening products from our homes. In the longer term we can also make educated decisions about how to choose less fattening products or materials when the time comes to replace existing items. So how can all this be achieved?

Well, there is a key and the key is the *Chemical Calorie*.

THE ORIGINS OF THE *CHEMICAL CALORIE*

The idea of the *Chemical Calorie* was first conceived a few months after my initial discovery that chemicals could make us fatter. By then I had already come across a very large number of chemicals that produced fattening effects – but it was becoming clearer by the day that the ability to fatten varied greatly between these different chemicals.

As there were so many different types of these substances, it became more and more evident that I had to find some way to rank them according to their 'fattening' ability. This kind of ranking system would really enable people to tackle the problem head on, since by knowing which were the worst offenders, the foods or places in which they were found could be avoided.

It was while I was turning all this over in my mind that I decided to take a break with my young sons – so I took them to their favourite play area. As they were romping around, I found myself toying with several different words on a piece of scrap paper. Initially I got nowhere and stopped to take a break, bought myself and my boys a drink, then after a while returned to take a second look at what I had been doing. Then it happened.

The words 'chemical' and 'calorie' placed accidentally side by side, suddenly leapt out at me. Eureka! I had inadvertently written down the name of a totally new unit, which would provide a revolutionary way of measuring the fattening ability of the chemicals in virtually every conceivable type of food and household product.

At that moment the *Chemical Calorie* was born.

CHEMICAL CALORIES V. TRADITIONAL CALORIES

Chemical Calories are very different from calories in the traditional sense. Conventional calories are simply units of energy. As your body is able to convert food into energy, food too can be described as having a certain calorific value. So the more conventional calories in a food, the more energy the food will produce – this is why fats possess more calories than carbohydrates, as the body can extract more energy from fats. So how do *Chemical Calories* work by comparison?

Chemical Calories produce their fattening effect in an entirely different way. Unlike foods, these toxic chemicals have no inherent energy value. They contain no conventional calories as such. So how can they make us fat?

What they do have is an ability to slow down and disrupt the efficiency of our *Slimming System*. If our *Slimming System* is less able to work, our body will become less able to convert foods into energy. So the 'left-over' foods, which the body is now unable to convert into useful energy, end up being stored as fat.

Effectively, then, the fattening ability of a chemical can be measured by the degree of damage caused to the *Slimming System* – and it is this damage which is measured in units of *Chemical Calories*. As a result, the chemicals which produce more damage to the *Slimming System* will generally contain more *Chemical Calories* than those which bring about less damage.

CHEMICAL CALORIES IN FOODS

If a food is high in *Chemical Calories* it means that the chemicals found in that food are likely to be particularly damaging to the *Slimming System*. So if your body is exposed to lots of these fattening chemicals in a meal, and if you already have quite a few of these fattening chemicals stored in your body, the most likely effect will be to reduce your overall ability to convert the food you have just eaten into usable energy.

Thus, after eating a meal, your body will possibly not be able to use up the food you have just eaten as well as it would have done in the absence of these chemicals – because of the damage to your natural self-regulating systems. Any excess food will then tend to end up adding to our existing food stores. So, in effect, much of our extra fat stores may well be created as a direct result of chemical damage to the *Slimming System*.

The overall effect of these chemicals is probably to fool your body into thinking that it has eaten more calories than you really have, effectively 'upsizing' your meal for you. It's a bit like eating a two-course meal – with your body thinking you have eaten three courses, or had an extra helping of mayonnaise.

In this way, chemicals could 'add' more calories to a meal without you ever having had the pleasure of eating them. The more *Chemical Calories* you are exposed to, the greater the mismatch may be between what you eat and how much of it you can use up. And the greater the disparity, the more food you will end up storing as fat.

So the reason why *Chemical Calories* are fattening is because they actually seem to reduce your food requirements – not because they add to your food in terms of quantity, or nutrition. This could help explain how we are all eating less, yet still getting fatter.

FINDING *CHEMICAL CALORIE* VALUES FOR
DIFFERENT FOODS

Just as a kilo of butter has more conventional calories than a kilo of rice, a fixed amount of one chemical could make you much fatter than the same amount of another chemical, if it possesses more *Chemical Calories*.

As a result, foods that contain large amounts of these chemicals that I have assessed to be particularly fattening will be rated very high in *Chemical Calories* – so if you want to lose weight, these are the foods to avoid. Foods that contain lower amounts of the less damaging chemicals will have a medium or low *Chemical Calorie* rating.

In effect, some chemicals possess the fattening abilities of full-fat cheese while with others it will be like eating an extra grated carrot.

So you can see that the key to identifying which foods are the most fattening comes from the work done in trying to quantify the fattening ability of chemicals. By working out the extent to which a chemical is likely to damage our *Slimming System*, we can estimate its fattening ability, and work out the *Chemical Calorie* rating for many types of chemicals, and the food that contains them.

This is actually how the *Chemical Calorie* food charts in Chapter 18 were created. These totally revolutionary food charts will give us an idea of which foods are more likely to contain the chemicals which make us fatter. Now I will tell you how this major step forward was actually achieved.

IDENTIFYING THE MOST FATTENING CHEMICALS

There are currently hundreds of thousands of different chemicals in use. As it would be virtually impossible to analyse them all separately, the first thing I did was divide them up into groups that shared similar features – for example, all the different types of organophosphate pesticides were analysed together.

Once I had established the main chemical groups involved, I turned my attention to identifying the most important parts of the *Slimming System*. I found that these included the major hormones involved in weight control; fat, protein, carbohydrate and energy metabolism; and the ability to exercise.[1]

Using information gleaned from thousands of scientific papers, I then scored each group of chemicals according to the degree and extent to which they appeared to cause damage to each individual part of our *Slimming System*.

Lastly, the overall total figure was multiplied by a figure relating to the time taken for the chemical to be excreted from our bodies. The final figure obtained from these calculations was the actual *Chemical Calorie* rating.

Despite being estimates, my *Chemical Calorie* ratings appeared to correlate remarkably well with each chemical's ability to fatten. Virtually all the chemicals with low *Chemical Calorie* ratings tended not to be strongly associated with weight gain, while those with high or very high ratings appeared to actively cause weight gain. The higher the *Chemical Calorie* rating, the stronger the fattening effect seemed to be.

Of course it would have been better to try to measure this effect in the laboratory, but to obtain such information would have involved many years of research and been extremely costly. Even then, we would still be left with the potential problem of working out how all these chemicals react with each other to possibly magnify their fattening effects. Until someone can directly measure these effects, these estimated ratings provide a unique way for us to determine where the most fattening chemicals can be found in our food and environment right now, instead of in ten or twenty years' time.

At this point, it's time that you were introduced to the groups of chemicals which appear to be causing the most trouble with our weight.

THE *CHEMICAL CALORIE* 'HIT LIST'

Based on the above estimates, I have found the most fattening groups of chemicals to be as follows:

1st place	Organochlorine pesticides (DDT, lindane, etc.)
2nd place	Organochlorine (PCBs) and organobromine (PBBs and PBDEs) industrial pollutants
3rd place	Heavy metals (e.g. cadmium)
4th place (joint)	Other pesticides (organophosphates, carbamates, etc.)
4th place (joint)	Plastics (plasticizers, PVC, styrenes)
6th place	Solvents (e.g. trichloroethylene – TCE)

Now you may recognize some of the names of these chemicals, not only because I may have previously mentioned them, but because they include substances which are extremely widely used.

As time goes on we will be cross-checking these results, so the actual rankings may change somewhat as we do further research – but we've done more than enough research already to know that these groups of chemicals will remain among the worst offenders.

The good news is that by having this ranking, not only do we now know which substances to avoid, but it now becomes possible to create ways to specifically target their removal from our bodies. So let's find out more about these chemicals on our hit list.

ORGANOHALOGENS (ORGANOCHLORINES AND ORGANOBROMINES)

I have previously introduced the best-known examples of this group of chemicals, the organochlorines, in Chapter 3, but you can see that they need to be described further because of their top ranking and widespread presence.

In the earlier part of the twentieth century organochlorines were used very extensively as pesticides. Though the use of some of this group has largely been stopped in developed countries, they are still found virtually everywhere – in our bodies, in our food and in the environment – because of their sheer stability.

Just because some organochlorines have been banned, it doesn't mean that we are not still being exposed to them. Some countries still produce 'banned' organochlorine pesticides in large quantities, shipping them overseas where they can easily be used on food crops. We may then get them 'returned' in imported foodstuffs. Our local foods are still being treated with other pesticides from this group, and all the time yet more organochlorine pesticides enter the food chain through environmental contamination. The relevant message is that despite their production being gradually reduced, they are still very much out there and will be for many future generations.

Since organochlorine pesticides appear to be the most powerfully fattening chemicals around us, I believe their avoidance and elimination from our bodies to be essential for achieving permanent weight loss.

The second most fattening chemicals are extremely common, not just in food, but in water and in the air around us. They are known as polychlorinated biphenyls, or PCBs. Because of their extreme stability, PCBs used to be popular as electrical insulators. Since being banned (because of their extreme persistence) they have become some of the most common environmental pollutants and contaminate a whole range of foods.[2]

The polybrominated biphenyls (PBBs) and polybrominated diphenyl ethers (PBDEs) are similar compounds which share a high degree of structural similarity with PCBs and DDT, so are extremely stable as well as being potentially highly toxic.[3] They have been used to lower the flammability of an extensive range of products. In fact it is illegal for certain goods – upholstered furniture for example – not to be treated with flame-retardants! Despite environmental concerns about their use, as yet they have not been banned.

OTHER FATTENING CHEMICALS

As you can see from the 'hit list', there are many other types of chemicals which appear to possess a powerful fattening effect. Starting with the heavy metals, cadmium in particular is high in *Chemical Calories*. Although the fattening effect of this group in general does not appear to be as marked as the organochlorines, they still rank very highly because of their extreme persistence – once we have absorbed heavy metals, they tend to remain in our bodies for many years.[4]

Next come a large number of pesticides commonly used on our foods, such as organophosphates and carbamates. The fact that many of these chemicals have also been used as growth-promoters testifies to their weight-enhancing potential (see Chapter 3).

Plastics also appear to contain a large amount of *Chemical Calories*, in particular the plasticizer chemicals (used to give plastics their flexibility) and the styrenes (as in polystyrene).[5] Although you don't deliberately set out to eat them, by eating foods which have been packaged in plastics you will effectively consume all the chemicals which have migrated from the packaging into the packaged food or drink.

Finally there is a whole range of solvents, such as trichloroethylene (TCE), the dry-cleaning solvent, and those used widely in industry and in paints, glues and cleaning fluids, which possess moderate amounts of *Chemical Calories*.[6]

I have found that the longer these chemicals remain in the body, the bigger the potential problem they tend to cause. So the chemicals which last for years, rather than days and weeks, will possess far more *Chemical Calories* than those less persistent substances. However, as we tend to be exposed to much larger daily amounts of the latter substances, such as solvents and plastics, which are less long-lived in our bodies, they can still cause a significant problem.

If you want to know more about these substances, what they are used for and where they are found, see Appendix A on page 337.

DETERMINING THE *CHEMICAL CALORIE* CONTENT OF FOODS

One of my main aims in working out the *Chemical Calorie* ratings of chemicals was to discover which foods made us fat by virtue of their chemical content. I admit that a mixture of personal and public interest was there right from the start – after all, who wants to unknowingly eat foods which could be making them fatter? So much effort is put in by people to cut out conventional calories from their diet, so why should potentially fattening chemicals be treated any differently?

In order to work out the *Chemical Calorie* content of a food, we need to know two things. First, the *Chemical Calorie* rating for all the individual chemicals detected in the food; second, the levels at which these chemicals are present. As national food agencies conduct regular tests to measure the levels of pesticide residues on commonly used foods,[7] it should be relatively easy to use this data to work out the overall *Chemical Calorie* content of a food or drink – and this is exactly what I have done.

The *Chemical Calorie* value of a food can then be reached by multiplying the *Chemical Calorie* rating for each particular chemical by the amount of that chemical detected in the food tested. If there are multiple chemicals present, then the *Chemical Calorie* value of the food is the sum of these values. And there you have it!

CHEMICAL CALORIE CHARTS

I can tell you when I first worked out the *Chemical Calorie* content of a whole range of foods, no one was more interested in the outcome of these calculations than me. And when I saw the results,

I started to see some of our everyday foods in a completely new light. It was quite frankly shocking – many of the foods which we have been told for years are extremely healthy revealed themselves as anything but!

Now the aim of these charts is not to stop people eating these foods completely, but to reduce their exposure to the most contaminated versions of them or to find ways of preparing them in order to make them less fattening.

The charts in Chapter 18 will, I hope, help you towards that goal. They reveal which foods are low, medium, and high in *Chemical Calories*, and the data is presented in a similar way to ordinary calorie charts. Better still, most of the foods that you would typically find in ordinary calorie charts are also listed – including a wide range of meat and meat products, dairy products, fish and shellfish, fruit, vegetables, grain products, oils and fats, herbs and spices and processed foods.

This information will be particularly welcome, as food labels are not yet required by law to give any information about pesticides and other such chemicals used during production and packaging – at present it is simply impossible to assess how contaminated your food will be just from reading the wrapper.

Hopefully, my user-friendly *Chemical Calorie* charts will help change all that. They will let you see at a glance how foods vary in their *Chemical Calorie* levels. Use this as a guide to help you discover which foods are likely to be the most contaminated, which tend to be the safest, when it is necessary to buy organic (foods produced with a minimal use of artificial chemicals) and when it is not.

Although most organic foods are low in *Chemical Calories*, you will still need to watch out for the few which can be relatively contaminated from environmental pollutants, such as certain fish and animal products.

The good news is that you can now lose weight just by choosing the less contaminated food option. No deprivation is required. Painless dieting, after all these years of suffering from hunger and repetitive meals – what could be better than that!

CHEMICAL CALORIES IN NON-FOOD PRODUCTS

Once you have mastered the way to avoid *Chemical Calories* in food, you may find yourself looking around to discover other ways in which we are exposed to *Chemical Calories* – once absorbed into your body it doesn't matter if a fattening chemical is from a food or cosmetic, it will still potentially interfere with your *Slimming System*. But unlike the *Chemical Calories* that we absorb from our food, the levels of *Chemical Calories* that enter our bodies from non-food products are much harder to measure.

When we eat food, we absorb most of the *Chemical Calories* it contains – so effectively we know exactly how many *Chemical Calories* we are being exposed to. But when we absorb *Chemical Calories* from the environment, we breathe them into our lungs and absorb them through our skin. Because these modes of absorption are less easily measured, it is more difficult to estimate precisely the amounts of *Chemical Calories* we take in from non-food products.

However, it is possible to get an idea of the level of *Chemical Calories* in specific materials such as paint, carpet or cosmetics by looking to see what the product is made of. This, in combination with the way the product is used, enables us to determine which non-food products are more likely to expose us to higher levels of *Chemical Calories* than others.

USING THE *CHEMICAL CALORIE* TO REACH YOUR TARGET WEIGHT

The discovery of the *Chemical Calorie* has enabled us to target the problem of fattening chemicals with far greater accuracy than has ever previously been possible. It now enables us to have much more control over our exposure to toxic chemicals, as well as arming us with enough information to eliminate what appear to be the worst culprits from our diet and surroundings.

So now you know the theory, it's time to be introduced to the findings. The following chapters will explain why some foods contain more *Chemical Calories* than others – including the top twelve, or 'dirty dozen', most 'fattening' foods I have found so far, based or the reports published by the UK Government's Ministry of Agriculture, Fisheries and Food (MAFF), now known as the Department for Environment, Food and Rural Affairs or DEFRA.

Because a significant part of our exposure to *Chemical Calories* is from non-food sources, Chapters 11 and 12 will expose all the areas around the home, office and garden where high levels of *Chemical Calories* can be found – making it easier to adopt the lifestyle changes necessary to cut your overall exposure dramatically.

Although the rest of this section will go into great detail about where you will be exposed to *Chemical Calories* in every aspect of your lives, you need to bear in mind that most of us are exposed to the largest amounts of these substances from our foods. So if you are keen to get on to the diet itself, you can skip the non-food-related chapters and come back to them later. In addition, you should realize that you can achieve significant amounts of weight loss just by cutting down on *Chemical Calories* in your food and by taking the right supplements.

So don't feel overwhelmed by the rest of the information found in this section. Just pace yourself and understand that you don't have to follow all the advice given. Just do what you can when you can. The reason I have gone into so much detail about where *Chemical Calories* are found in non-food products is to save people from coming back after they have successfully lowered their dietary intake of *Chemical Calories* and then asking, What can I do now?

So whether you follow some or all the recommendations I have given you, all the advice that follows will be of immense value to any dieter, since it provides a relatively easy way to help you lose weight which doesn't involve any food deprivation or discomfort. Not only will cutting down on *Chemical Calories* help you to lose weight and stay slim for life, but it will also help lift the toxic burden off your body and boost your health for years to come. Now that's certainly worth striving for!

7. What Makes Lettuce More 'Fattening' Than Avocado?

Which Foods are Highest in *Chemical Calories*?

It used to be so much easier to work out which foods were fattening and which were not. We were told that if we counted the conventional calorie content of foods and did not exceed recommended figures, we could control our weight. In fact, that's what we're still told.

We see calorie counts on chocolate bars and yogurt pots. We see calorie counts at the top of recipes. We see calorie counts in countless magazines. We are bombarded with the words 'low-calorie' and 'low-fat' on 'diet' food packaging and advertising. Calories are everywhere! They are so ingrained in the western culture that it is understandably difficult for somebody brought up in this environment to accept that there might be another way of thinking – much less to actually believe it. But look at the facts presented here and come to your own conclusions. And then try it out.

I clearly remember, when I was a teenager, studying calorie charts with my friends probably more intensely than we studied most other subjects. At that time I could quite easily quote to the last digit the precise calorific value of a whole range of different foods. Now the rules have changed – chemical contamination has made some 'low-calorie' foods remarkably fattening. We urgently need to find out how the new rules work. And fortunately help is at hand.

You will find the information in this chapter totally liberating. It will allow you for the first time to make more informed choices about how to choose foods low in *Chemical Calories*. After telling you how foods come to be so contaminated, it will then reveal the top twelve most contaminated foodstuffs – the 'dirty dozen' on the

Chemical Calorie scale of most fattening foods. Following this, it will go through all the major food groups identifying why some foods are higher in *Chemical Calories* than others, exposing the worst offenders and explaining what makes them apparently so bad.

Armed with this information, with the advice on how to lower your intake of *Chemical Calories* given in the next two chapters, and lastly with the full *Chemical Calorie* charts in Chapter 18, you will be completely capable of dramatically reducing your exposure to *Chemical Calories* from food.

While I accept that all this might take a bit of getting used to, the good news is that for the first time ever you now have the 'know-how' to help you on your way to achieve safe and permanent weight loss. Now that's something really positive.

SO HOW CAN LETTUCE BE MORE FATTENING THAN AVOCADO?

Take a look at any calorie chart and you will discover that lettuce is extremely low in conventional calories while avocados are very high. Even to suggest that the reverse is true seems to go against absolutely everything that we have been taught.

So what does make lettuce more fattening than avocado? The answer is very simple. Lettuce has far more *Chemical Calories* than avocado. This is because it is a relatively fragile food crop that tends to be sprayed repeatedly with 'fattening' pesticides and preservatives to keep it looking fresh and crisp on the shelf.

On the other hand, the avocado is a much more robust crop that needs hardly any active intervention at all. As a result, it is much lower in *Chemical Calories*. So from the *Chemical Calorie* viewpoint, lettuce becomes more fattening than avocado.

FOOD IS THE MAJOR SOURCE OF CHEMICAL CONTAMINATION

For the majority of people, who do not come into contact with large amounts of chemicals at work, food will be their main source of chemical exposure – since most *Chemical Calories* creep into your body unseen on the food that you eat. And once they are inside your gut, your body is forced to deal with them, either by storing them or by breaking them down, if indeed it can.

We have already seen that weight can be affected in people who make the 'mistake' of eating modest amounts of even one type of highly contaminated food. If you go back to some of the studies quoted in Chapter 3, you will see that they show that just by eating average amounts of contaminated fish, ordinary people can actually become fatter. If just one type of food can be found to have such a significant effect, you can imagine the effect that all the other types of polluted foods could be having on our weight.

To lose weight we need to know which out of all the multitude of foods available are the most fattening, so that we can cut them out of our diet – substituting them with safer and less fattening foods.

Of course, you will still need to pay attention to the types of food you eat – a diet of organic crisps, chocolate and fatty foods is not going to help you lose much weight at all. The answer lies in a balanced diet, containing all the nutrients that the body needs to fully power its *Slimming System*.

WHERE THE CHEMICALS IN OUR FOODS COME FROM

How do chemicals actually get into the food that we eat? It would be relatively easy if all the chemicals in our food were from deliberately added chemicals such as pesticides or preservatives. However, life is never that simple. In real life chemicals can enter our food in a variety of different ways:

- Pesticides, additives, preservatives or colourants are deliberately sprayed on to or added to food crops.
- Farm animals are treated with drugs or hormones and have antibiotics added to their feed.
- Food crops or animals are affected by environmental pollution.
- Chemicals leach out into foods from packaging materials.

Despite the variety of ways in which chemicals enter foods, government agencies tend mainly to test and monitor the levels of food contamination caused by pesticides. While there are occasional studies which look at contamination from packaging or from environmental pollutants, they are usually relatively small or funded privately. As a result, the levels of pesticides in foods offer virtually the only official large-scale information on food contamination generally available. Because of the availability of this information, in combination with their extensive testing in this area, I have based all the following figures on this pesticide information alone.

While this will give you an excellent guideline to the potential level of *Chemical Calories* from pesticides in a product, it will not be able to give you the total figure. However, to help you make a more accurate assessment, I will also provide you with loads of relevant advice, which will help you limit your exposure from all forms of food-borne *Chemical Calories*. Don't worry, once you know what to look for it will become quite easy to spot the potential problem areas.

THE DIRTY DOZEN

Now we have arrived at the nitty gritty – which of all our foods are the most contaminated with *Chemical Calories*? I have created the list below from the reports published by the UK Government's Ministry of Agriculture, Fisheries and Food (MAFF), now the Department for Environment, Food and Rural Affairs (DEFRA).[1]

In order to work out the *Chemical Calorie* content of all the following foods, I have used four years of pesticide residue testing data (1995 to 1998) published by MAFF. Although the reports track food for sale in the UK, you will see that many of the items are imported from other countries. At the No. 1 spot, as you can see, eels are according to my calculations the most contaminated food *Chemical-Calorie*-wise, with the others following in descending order.

1. Eels (UK)
2. Fish oils (Canada)
3. Lamb (New Zealand)
4. Oranges (Spain + others)
5. Mint leaves (no country listed)
6. Cocoa butter (used in chocolate) (no country listed)
7. Dill (no country listed)
8. Salmon (farmed, UK)
9. Sugar snap peas (Kenya)
10. Geese (France)
11. Winter lettuce (UK)
12. Trout (farmed, UK)

Rather than explain each result individually, it will be easier to go through all the major food groups, starting with those containing foods with the highest levels of *Chemical Calories*. For each group I'll explain how the foods come to be contaminated and suggest particular foods in each group that are also likely to be particularly high or indeed low in *Chemical Calories*.

This explanation is probably more important than the table above, as the exact rankings of different foods are bound to change as we do more and more research – but the general rules and guidelines below will remain valid even if particular foods climb up or fall down in the rankings as we get to understand more about *Chemical Calories*.

FISH AND SHELLFISH

Fish appears four times in the dirty dozen, and this in itself should provide a severe warning about including a lot of fish in your diet. This will probably come as a shock to many, since fish are generally regarded as a healthy low-fat food.

The main problem at the heart of this issue is the large-scale contamination of our lakes and oceans with organochlorines (such as DDT). These toxic and extremely persistent chemicals have invaded every environment on the face of the earth through their ability to evaporate into the air, circulate in the atmosphere and be carried back down to the ground in rain, resulting in the pollution of most water sources.

Since these chemicals are extremely fat-soluble, they are easily absorbed across the surface of fish gills and thereby enter the fish. They will also cling to particles in the water which are then eaten by fish.[2] Those fish may well carry the chemical in their bodies for good. The problem with eels, which as you can see have come straight in at the No. 1 spot, is that they are great scavengers, and voraciously eat the rubbish and detritus which settles and accumulates on the sea floor or on river beds. Unfortunately, much of this waste originates from living creatures, which over the years have been building up their own levels of personal contaminants that remain locked in the animal after its demise. Thus the diet eels tend to eat will be potentially more polluted and has resulted in them being awarded this dubious honour.

Before you sigh with relief, since the chances that you eat eels are relatively slim, eels are not the only water-living victims of a contaminated food source. As we see from the dirty dozen, salmon and trout are also laden with *Chemical Calories*. Low levels of water-borne fat-loving chemicals move from the water into micro-scopic plants and animals (known as plankton) which are eaten in vast quantities by fish like salmon and trout, resulting in significant accumulation of these chemicals in their tissues. Trout and especially salmon have very fatty meat, which means that compared with other species, their tissues are ideal sinks for fat-loving chemicals. Carnivorous predators like tuna, salmon and trout eat large quantities of small fish, thus further scaling up the levels of contamination (a process called biomagnification), since none of the species involved is capable of breaking down and eliminating these persistent chemicals.

Rather than fish itself, it is fish oils which have come in at the No. 2 spot. This is because the most persistent *Chemical Calories* will tend to accumulate in fatty tissues. As a result, it is the fish oils which will tend to contain the highest levels of these pollutants, and cause them to rank so highly in the above list.

Farmed salmon and trout may also be treated with many other chemicals, added to the water and foodstuffs to treat infections. This is why farmed salmon and trout also rank in the dirty dozen.[3]

The really scary thing is that eels, fish oils, salmon and trout earned their rankings based on the figures for pesticides alone. In reality, fish may also be polluted with large doses of the environmental pollutants PCBs, dioxins and heavy metals, all of which are extremely high in *Chemical Calories*. If the environmental pollutants and heavy metals had also been tested by MAFF, the additional *Chemical Calorie* value might have pushed certain types of fish right off the charts.

But if you are a fish-lover, don't become too despondent. There is some good news, since non-carnivorous fish, which includes most types of fish with white flesh such as cod, tends to be much less polluted. This is because these fish feed lower in the food chain, on plankton which are less contaminated. In addition they also have a much lower fat content, and so have much less of a build-up of fat-loving pollutants. So white fish is much more likely to possess considerably lower levels of *Chemical Calories*. Shellfish also seem to be less contaminated with pesticides and so appear in my charts to be relatively low in *Chemical Calories*. But due to the fact that they often contain relatively high levels of heavy metals and other chemical contaminants, they may in the future be found to contain higher levels of *Chemical Calories* than these pesticide charts initially suggest.

MEATS AND POULTRY

Meats vary far more in their *Chemical Calorie* content than most other types of food. This is because animals are exposed to a larger number of potential sources of contamination. Animals are affected not only by the environment they have grown up in, but also by the food they have been fed, as well as the other chemicals they have been directly 'treated' with.

These highly variable factors can mean that some meats, such as lamb, tested from one source high in *Chemical Calories*, whereas the same type of meat originating from another source may be low in *Chemical Calories*. But fortunately many of these differences can be dealt with if the source of the contamination is located and removed.

For example, for several years a number of rabbits from China were found to have higher levels of the organochlorines pesticide lindane. However, when this problem was addressed, the chemical was found to originate from a contaminated food source. And once the contaminated food source was stopped, the problem effectively ended.

The proportion of fat in meat also appears to have some relationship to the overall *Chemical Calorie* loading. This is because most animals tend to store chemicals that they cannot metabolize in their body fat. Meats low in fat tend to be lower in *Chemical Calories* – chicken, venison and turkey are good examples. A high-fat meat such as goose is much more likely to be high in *Chemical Calories*.

Another thing to bear in mind is that some animals, particularly those farmed intensively, may have been treated with growth-promoters. Unfortunately MAFF did not publish their test for growth-promoters/antibiotics in the published figures I used to produce these charts.

However, a report by Richard Young and Alison Craig, recently published by the Soil Association, shows that a significant number of chicken samples – chicken livers, muscle and eggs – contained very high levels of toxic synthetic antibiotics, reported to be dangerous to human health.[4]

This could definitely influence the overall levels of *Chemical Calories* not just in chickens and eggs, but in meat from any animal reared intensively. To keep the chances of contamination down I would recommend buying either organically produced meats or meats produced using less intensive farming methods.

In this as well as in other areas, as more information keeps coming to light and as agricultural and industrial practices change, there will be a continual need to keep the charts fully up to date using the latest information, and I fully intend to do this. So you must expect the estimated levels of *Chemical Calories* in different products to vary, sometimes substantially, from year to year.

FRUIT

The main source of contamination for fruit is from pesticides that are deliberately added during the growing process or to prolong life in storage. As growers in similar climates across the world tend to use similar types of pesticides on similar food crops, there is relatively little difference between, say, strawberries produced in the UK and those produced in another country. So the country in which the fruit was produced tends to become less critical.[5]

For example, apple growers in the US will use the same chemicals in roughly the same amounts as apple growers in the UK. The only major difference arises when growers in countries with less stringent regulations occasionally use cheaper but also potentially more fattening chemicals, which are banned in other countries.

Oranges rank fourth in the 'dirty dozen' and are regularly the most contaminated fruits in our supermarkets. Out of all the samples MAFF tested, those grown in Spain had the largest number of different chemicals found on them, but oranges from other countries – Israel, Argentina, Cyprus, South Africa, Morocco, Uruguay, Turkey and Sicily – all had detectable levels of pesticides too.

This is because growers everywhere can use large amounts of pesticides to kill pests which attack crops of oranges. In addition, fungicides are applied liberally to the outside of the orange (sometimes in a wax coating) to stop them going off in storage.

Few consumers realize that wax coatings used for all kinds of fruit can contain several fattening chemicals. Lemons, apples, cantaloupes, peppers, passion fruit, grapefruit, melons and tomatoes are potentially coated with extra pesticides as a result of being waxed.

It has to be said at this point that although oranges rank very highly, most of the chemicals detected stay on the peel. People do not usually eat the peel, unless they are using it in cooking, and the inner part is generally far less contaminated.[6]

Fragile crops such as soft fruit (strawberries, raspberries and peaches) also tend to be sprayed more heavily, as fruit gets a better price when it has an unblemished exterior. This explains why apples and pears can be very heavily sprayed and also why oranges that are intended for marmalade tend to be much lower in *Chemical Calories* than those sent to the supermarket. Marmalade oranges simply don't need to look good, since they will be mashed up anyway, so it appears that growers spray them less.

Testing also shows that plums, pineapples, rhubarb and some dried fruits (figs and dates) are usually sprayed less than other fruits, so they are also likely to be lower in *Chemical Calories*.

HERBS AND SPICES

This was the category that surprised me the most, probably because I hadn't really thought of herbs and spices as containing any sort of calorific value. But it soon became apparent that some herbs can contain very high levels of *Chemical Calories*. In fact the sheer number and high level of pesticides found on a couple of herbs sent me straight to my kitchen to throw the relevant stocks away.

This extensive spraying of herbs is probably due to their fragility and tendency to go off quickly. Mint was the worst offender, in both fresh and dried form, followed by dill, parsley, coriander and rosemary.

The levels of *Chemical Calories* in spices were actually pleasantly lower than I had expected. Admittedly, due to the small amounts of herbs and spices we use, they will cause less of an impact on our overall exposure compared to other foods, but even so, if there is a readily available safer alternative for the more treated ones, I would much rather use it.

PROCESSED FOODS

This group is a mixed bag of different foods, from chocolate to coleslaw. Government agencies test very few processed foods, so it is difficult to estimate *Chemical Calorie* content for many standard supermarket products. However, from the information available on a limited range of foods, the highest scorer in the *Chemical Calorie* ratings is chocolate.

Yes, I'm sorry, but it's true. The organochlorine pesticide lindane appears to be widely used in the production of cocoa beans, so most products containing chocolate have more than their fair share of *Chemical Calories*. In fact cocoa butter ranks sixth in the dirty dozen.

VEGETABLES

Once again, the main source of contamination for vegetables is the deliberate spraying of pesticides at different stages of the growing and storing process.

As with fruit, the factors that control how often a vegetable crop is sprayed with chemicals (and how high it will be in *Chemical Calories*) are down to the fragility of the crop during growth and storage, whether it is a cash crop or not, and how important it is for the vegetable to look good. The more fragile or easily damaged the crop tends to be, the more chemicals will be used to prevent it being damaged while it is being grown and to stop it going mouldy in storage.

One of the most heavily used insecticides and fungicides for vegetables worldwide also happens to act as a growth-promoter (organophosphates),[7] so it is not too surprising that a large number of vegetables are significantly high in *Chemical Calories*. If it is important for a vegetable to be free from blemishes, or if it is essential as a cash crop, then the chances are that it will be treated even more intensively.

Lettuce grown in the UK, in particular lettuce produced in winter, comes eleventh on the list. Lettuce tends to be treated with a whole range of chemicals wherever it is grown and whatever time of year. But in general the use of these chemicals increases over the winter because of the colder and damper conditions, which favour the growth of fungi. The average Briton eats over 3kg of leafy salad a year and the average American eats over 5kg a year,[8] so this one food alone can seriously add to our intake of *Chemical Calories*. Other salad vegetables such as celery, baby vegetables and peppers also contain significant amounts of *Chemical Calories*, potentially making these apparently healthy foods quite fattening!

DAIRY AND EGG PRODUCTS

Dairy products rank just after meat and fish because of their levels of highly fattening organochlorines. While it is true that dairy and egg products contain much lower levels than those found in fish, for example, western diets contain a lot of dairy products, making them a significant source of chemical contamination.

The average American consumes over 13 kg of cheese (excluding cottage cheese) a year. Add to this the average consumption of milk, cream, ice cream, eggs, butter and yoghurt, and you have a large dietary source of *Chemical Calories*.

Dairy foods tend to be so vulnerable to contamination because one of the few ways in which animals can rid themselves of persistent chemicals is by expelling them in their milk, or by having offspring. Chickens and other farmed birds can also offload their persistent chemicals or indeed any other chemical they are exposed to, in their eggs.

As most of the *Chemical Calories* tend to be stored in fats,[9] the highest levels will tend to be found in cheese, butter, egg yolks and cream. Consequently, dairy products that are lower in fats also tend to be lower in *Chemical Calories*, for example skimmed or semi-skimmed milk, low-fat yoghurt and cottage cheese.

FATS, OILS AND SHORTENINGS

From looking at the previous sections, you can see that the way *Chemical Calories* get into food varies slightly between animals and plants. In animal fats and shortenings, the most important source of *Chemical Calories* is from environmental exposure and the extent to which the animal's food supplies are contaminated. As this level can vary greatly, it can make the overall amount of *Chemical Calories* in animal-derived fats relatively difficult to predict and potentially more risky.

In plant-based oils, the major source of contamination tends to be from deliberately added pesticides, such as those sprayed on vegetable oil crops. Interestingly, in most cases these vegetable crops tend to contain levels of *Chemical Calories* similar to animal fat sources such as lard.

BEVERAGES

Drinks such as coffee and wine are on the whole relatively low in *Chemical Calories*, though tea can be moderately contaminated. Yes, I can hear a collective sigh of relief from all you coffee and wine lovers out there. Again, grapes grown for wine are destined to be mashed and do not need to look pretty. So it may follow that they are not treated with the chemicals designed to preserve their looks.

The only other problem seems to come from beer. Although no samples of beer were tested by MAFF in any of the four years of reports published, they did test samples of the hops which are used for making beer. Unfortunately these revealed themselves to be very highly contaminated, so much so that if they were a food they would have been ranked fourth in the above charts! So while I haven't included beer in the *Chemical Calorie* food charts, as it wasn't actually tested (see Chapter 18), it might be sensible to consider drinking the organic version if given the choice.

GRAIN PRODUCTS

The average Briton consumes over 50kg of bread each year and 80kg of cereals, so any contamination of grain products will make a huge impact based on quantity alone.

Grain is routinely sprayed with chemicals that speed up and slow down the growth of crops. During the growth cycle it is extensively sprayed with potentially fattening insecticides, then after it has been harvested and put in storage it is sprayed with even more insecticide to prevent infestations. It is also relatively common for organophosphates, in the form of a fine powder, to be mixed into piles of grain and then not removed at a later date.

From my findings, oats are the crop most likely to be contaminated with *Chemical Calories*, followed by wheat. Corn (maize), barley and rice seem to contain the lowest levels. Wholemeal flour tends to have twice as many residues as processed white flour, with the highest levels of *Chemical Calories* being found in bran, since the residues cling to the outside of the grains. As a general rule, the more processed the grains are, the lower they are in *Chemical Calories* – but also the lower they will be in nutritional value.

NUTS, SEEDS AND PULSES

Although nuts, seeds and pulses have been known to contain residues of organochlorines in the past, virtually all the nuts, pulses, lentils, beans and seeds tested by MAFF (with the exception of cocoa beans) were extremely low in *Chemical Calories*.

This is excellent news, as these foods are naturally rich in 'slimming' nutrients such as vitamins, minerals, proteins and essential fats, while lacking the higher levels of *Chemical Calories* found in animal produce.

SUGARS, PRESERVES AND HONEY

Only a few of these foods were tested, and the level of *Chemical Calories* was very low.

TRADITIONAL DIETING IS BAD FOR YOU!

Chemical Calorie ratings clearly show that many of the foods traditionally associated with dieting – salad vegetables, fruit and fish – are likely to be very heavily contaminated with chemicals. So by eating a much larger proportion of these foods in your diet, you would in all probability be exposing yourself to higher levels of *Chemical Calories* than you would when not actively dieting, defeating the whole purpose of trying to lose weight!

Another more sinister possibility also emerges. The so-called 'safe doses' of pesticides in a typical daily diet could easily be exceeded by dieters because of their tendency to eat more of these relatively heavily contaminated foods. In that case, not only will dieters be more likely to become fatter in the long term, but their risks of getting chemically related diseases could also increase. This could help to explain why people whose weight fluctuates frequently are at a much greater risk of getting a whole range of different illnesses.

By now you will have realized that many of the foods you have previously eaten, in addition to any previous dieting attempts, may actually be the source of your continual struggle with your weight. But don't despair – it really is possible to repair the damage from the past as well as reducing your risk of future weight gain.

The next chapter will tell you how to reduce your exposure to *Chemical Calories* while still eating the foods that you love. What better way could there be to lose weight for good!

8. Don't Panic, Go Organic

Getting the Most Benefit from Organic Foods

At this point you are probably reeling from the news that many of the foods you have been eating in order to lose weight in the past could have been having quite the opposite effect. You just have to be philosophical about this, and accept that what is past is past – but think of it this way, at least you now appreciate this and can start doing something positive about it.

Your goal should now be to eat the foods which contain the lowest possible levels of *Chemical Calories*, without overdosing on conventional calories. Not only will they help you to lower your weight but they will also help improve your figure. While it is totally possible to dramatically cut your intake of *Chemical Calories* on a diet based on conventionally grown foods, the easiest way of achieving this is by eating more organically.

This chapter will explain what it means to be organic, how to recognize organic foods and where to buy them. It will also tell you why organic foods are generally much lower in *Chemical Calories* than 'conventionally' grown foods and why they really do taste far better – in other words, why in my opinion they rank among the best slimming foods you can now eat!

SO WHAT ARE ORGANIC FOODS?

Organic foods are simply foods which as far as possible are produced naturally, with a minimum level, if any, of synthetic pesticides, antibiotics, growth hormone or fertilizers – pretty much like all the food humans were eating up to the beginning of the century. So you can see, there is nothing odd or cranky or indeed new about organic foods at all.

As organic fruits and vegetables are grown with few synthetic chemical sprays, they end up being much lower in *Chemical Calories* than their intensively grown counterparts. Organic animals are reared with minimum drug treatment and are given food that is itself organically produced to a high degree, so they too have fewer *Chemical Calories* in their meat, milk or eggs.

But hang on, you might say: if few chemicals are deliberately added, why should organic foods possess any *Chemical Calories* at all? Well, unfortunately, due to the extensive presence of pollutants in our environment, no organic foods will now ever be totally *Chemical-Calorie*-free – despite possessing a much lower level of contamination than conventionally grown equivalents. Some organic certification bodies may permit a minimum level of synthetic chemicals in certain circumstances. Also, natural fertilizers and pesticides do contain chemicals, albeit naturally occurring ones.

So, sadly, we have to accept that organic foods are now probably the closest we will ever get to food that is truly *Chemical-Calorie*-free.

Now that you know what organic foods are, how can you tell by looking at an item of food whether it is organic or not? Well, to help you identify them, all organic produce available in the shops should have a symbol on it to show that it has been certified by one of the official organically registering organizations. This is your guarantee that the farm where the food is produced is regularly inspected and meets the standards legally required. In addition, any grower selling produce locally should also be able to show you their organic certification.

The leading organic certification body in the UK is the Soil Association, but there are other organizations too, which possess their own legally binding symbols used on food packaging.

WHY IS ORGANIC FOOD DIFFERENT?

Probably the most important features distinguishing organic foods from conventionally grown foods are:

- Improved flavour and food texture.
- Increased nutritional content.
- Lower levels of toxic heavy metals, organochlorines and pesticides.

It wasn't until I tasted my first organically grown apple that I knew something was seriously wrong with our food industry. It was so different from all the other apples I had eaten over the previous twenty years. They had left a strange aftertaste in my mouth, but the organic apple tasted simply great, taking me back to my childhood when we picked our own apples from the trees in my parents' garden. From then on I was hooked.

Curiously, it took a long time before I decided to try that first apple. I used to fool myself that somehow I could eat chemically treated foods without coming to any harm. And there were hardly any organic products in the supermarkets. The few bits of organic fruit and vegetables that were on sale looked so much less glossy and appetizing than the perfect produce on the other shelves, and they cost so much more!

Since then my understanding has totally changed. Instead of marvelling over the superficial unblemished beauty of conventional foods, I think about how many chemicals have been used to get them to look large and perfect. I am even happy when I find the occasional bug on organic fruit and vegetables, as this is some evidence that my food has not been sprayed with nasties. If that bug can survive, then nothing on the food is likely to harm me.

BETTER FLAVOUR AND SUPERIOR TEXTURE

You don't have to be a vegetarian or on a weight-reduction programme to enjoy organic produce. Foodies have already discovered that the taste and the quality are far superior. Fruit and vegetables taste sweeter, porridge oats taste creamier, chocolate is sensational and meat and chicken have real depth of flavour. Even pasta, rice and bread taste slightly sweeter and more flavoursome.

This is not just a marketing ploy: there are two very good reasons why organic food really does taste better. First, organic produce tends to be higher in natural sugars (approximately 21 per cent more than in conventionally grown foods).[1] This is thought to be because the chemicals and nitrates in fertilizers interfere with the plant's own metabolism, particularly by reducing its level of natural sugars. Without interference from excessive amounts of artificial fertilizers, organic foods with their higher levels of natural sugars really do taste sweeter.

Second, pesticides appear to alter the sensations the brain gets from the taste-buds, distorting flavours when we eat, and also damaging our sense of smell. Common pesticides (such as carbamates) significantly reduce taste and smell, and can leave a metallic or bitter flavour in the mouth.[2]

From personal experience I can vouch for this effect. Since I now eat mostly organic foods, I seem to have become far more sensitive to the presence of chemicals in my food. And on certain occasions when I have eaten particular non-organic foods at other people's houses, I have felt a sort of burning, tingling sensation in my mouth, lasting for hours, which I never previously encountered before going organic. In the light of their known taste-altering effects, I have put these experiences down to the additional presence of chemicals in the food.

The texture of organic meat also appears to be much superior. This is probably because the animals are reared slowly, are fed more natural foods, are not treated with growth hormone and have more exercise. This appears to be most evident in pork and poultry produce, possibly due to the artificially forced growth rates in non-organic meat production.

Even my husband, who normally eats what he is given without question, recently refused to eat some chicken in a restaurant because it lacked both taste and texture. Over the years his palate has become used to high-quality organic food, so that he could not stomach the lack of texture and flavour in that piece of processed chicken.

I've found this difference to be most noticeable with organic bacon, which I think tastes out of this world. But listen, don't just take our word for it, try it out for yourself!

PACKED WITH SLIMMING NUTRIENTS

It's official. According to a scientific study by nutritionist David Thomas, based on published data from *The Composition of Foods*, a comprehensive study of the content of all major foods dating back to 1940, conventionally grown fruits and vegetables have been found to have fewer nutrients than they had fifty years ago.[3] It seems that modern farming methods, using large amounts of agrochemicals and artificial fertilizers, have effectively depleted the soil of essential minerals.

This means that the quantities of essential minerals in our foods have been reduced alarmingly. Levels of magnesium, iodine, potassium, zinc, calcium and iron have plummeted, and as we desperately need these to power our natural *Slimming System*, this can directly influence our weight.

By comparison, a recent review of forty-one studies comparing organic and conventionally grown foods concluded that, overall, organic farming methods really do appear to produce foods that contain higher levels of minerals and vitamins.[4] This is thought to be because the soil is treated with naturally balanced fertilizers which contain a more balanced spread of minerals. And in addition, crops tend to be more robust because their metabolism is less damaged by pesticides, so they can also produce more vitamins. In particular, vitamin C, which is a carbohydrate and so particularly at risk from damage in conventionally grown plants, is commonly found in higher quantities in organic foods.

But the differences don't stop there – the proteins found in organic fruits and vegetables are also of higher quality.[5] So by eating organically your body can luxuriate in larger amounts of high-quality 'slimming' nutrients that are vital in keeping your weight low and stable.

FEWER *CHEMICAL CALORIES*

Our planet is so polluted now that is not possible to reduce our intake of *Chemical Calories* to zero. All our crops are exposed to and contaminated by chemicals in the atmosphere, and in particular by PCBs from air and rainwater. Organically grown foods are just as likely as non-organic foods to be contaminated in this way.

However, organically grown fruit and vegetables are far less polluted with *Chemical Calories* added during growth and storage. In addition, natural farming methods mean that organically grown crops tend to be less polluted with heavy metals and artificial fertilizers drawn from the soil.[6] Contaminated soil grows contaminated crops. So by buying organic fruit and vegetables, you will be reducing your *Chemical Calorie* exposure to the lowest levels possible.

Buying organically reared animals and organic dairy products will also make a huge contribution to reducing the *Chemical Calories* in your diet. Some organic producers use feed that needs to be up to, and preferably above, 80 per cent derived from organically produced sources.[7] Since additives in what an animal eats will build up in its body over time, a less contaminated food source will result in fewer *Chemical Calories* in the resultant meats and dairy products.

In addition, organically reared animals are not treated with growth-promoters, so when eating a piece of organic steak or chicken you know that it doesn't have unwanted residues of those same chemicals that could fatten you up too.[8]

Sadly, all animals raised for food can be particularly affected by environmental pollution. Certain environments are now so contaminated that the livestock kept there will have far higher levels of *Chemical Calories* than livestock in other areas, even if it is raised organically.

For example, our seas are now so polluted that all carnivorous fish (even if they are organically reared) are likely to be heavily contaminated by the water they live in and by the smaller fish they eat. However, organically raised fish will still have an advantage because at least they will not be contaminated with the chemical cocktail often used for conventionally farmed fish.

WHY DOESN'T EVERYONE EAT ORGANIC FOOD?

So if it is so good, why doesn't everybody eat organic food? Well, as with everything in life, there are pros and cons. Price and availability have been major barriers for many people in the past, though this is changing all the time. To help you get more of a feel for the issues, some of the most commonly quoted reasons for and against buying organic foods are listed below.

ADVANTAGES OF ORGANIC FOOD

- Generally much lower levels of *Chemical Calories* (to aid weight control).
- Higher levels of essential nutrients (to boost the *Slimming System*, your health and possibly even your time on this planet).
- Environmentally friendly farming adds far less to environmental pollution than conventional farming does.
- Organic farming appears to be more humane for animals.
- Organic food has superior taste.
- A lower toxic chemical intake will enhance rather than injure your general health.

DISADVANTAGES OF ORGANIC FOOD

- Generally 20–30 per cent more expensive than conventionally produced food.
- Restricted availability in shops and supermarkets.
- A smaller choice of foods (particularly convenience foods).
- Reduced shelf life.
- Sometimes less visually appealing.
- Few organic restaurants for eating out.
- Increased preparation time, since meals are mostly made from fresh ingredients.

WHERE TO FIND ORGANIC FOODS

So now you have heard all about organic foods and are keen to start using them in order to help you lose weight, but where can you find them? Fortunately, as demand grows, organic foods are becoming more and more mainstream. As a result, the major supermarkets are increasing their organic ranges all the time and it is now possible to find an organic version of a large number of the items on your shopping list in your regular superstore.

In addition, many specialist shops, farm shops and home delivery schemes will offer you a wide choice of high-quality items. Some suppliers advertise in food magazines and there are also organic guidebooks to tell you about local shops and restaurants that offer organic foods. So you can see that it is becoming easier to find more choice across the whole range of foods.

Practically everything I have suggested on my diet is now available organically, most of it from major supermarkets. It may take a bit of time to change your shopping habits, but it will undoubtedly be worth every moment's thought and effort that you put into it.

Of course, the best way to get fresh organic fruit and vegetables is by growing your own, because you can eat it at its best. But if you lack the time and space, an organic box delivery from a local grower will give you the same seasonal variation of fresh produce.

EATING ORGANICALLY IS THE IDEAL WAY TO LOSE WEIGHT

With lower *Chemical Calories* and higher levels of slimming nutrients, eating organic food is the ideal way to eat to lose weight. A few years ago my husband started complaining that his trousers no longer fitted him. After only eight months of eating largely organically grown foods, he had lost approximately 10 per cent of his body weight without even trying. He now fits into all the clothes he wore when he was a good ten years younger! Not surprisingly he has become a total convert to organic foods.

While in the ideal world we would probably all eat organically, unfortunately not everyone is able to do this, for a whole host of different reasons. If this is the case, the next chapter is designed for you, as it will provide invaluable advice which will help you to prepare and cook foods so that your potential exposure to *Chemical Calories* can be slashed.

Even if you already eat 100 per cent organically, the following chapter will still prove to be essential reading because it also covers the ways in which even the purest foods can become contaminated with *Chemical Calories* on the long journey from shop to plate. So read on to discover yet more indispensable secrets about how to achieve a diet low in *Chemical Calories*.

9. Eating Low in *Chemical Calories*

How to Choose, Store and Prepare Your Food to Minimize *Chemical Calories*

So you have just gone out and bought your first supplies of organic food. Well, congratulations! You are at the starting point of your transformation into a new slimmer you. But in order to maximize your weight loss, you need to know that there is actually a bit more to it than just eating organically. However careful you are about the food you buy, there are plenty of ways in which *Chemical Calories* can still sneak into your foods before you eat them, transforming even the purest of organic foods into a seething mass of synthetic chemicals.

This chapter will tell you not only how to avoid these extra unwanted *Chemical Calories* that enter our food after being produced, but also how to reduce the *Chemical Calorie* loading of both conventionally grown and organically raised foods.

Believe me, there is a great deal you can do to reduce that exposure to an absolute minimum. By adopting the following suggestions, not only will you lose weight more readily, but you will be able to stay slim for the rest of your life.

HOW TO SELECT FOOD LOW IN *CHEMICAL CALORIES*

After reading the previous chapters, and armed with your *Chemical Calorie* charts (see Chapter 18), you will now be able when you go shopping to make informed choices about which foods are high in *Chemical Calories* and which are not. And if it is just too expensive to buy organic versions of everything on your shopping list, you will be able to choose which products are likely to be the most contaminated and limit your organic shopping to that group.

To be honest, this is probably the most sensible way to go. As long as you abide by the advice in this chapter, and indeed in the rest of the book, you will still be able to achieve the body you want even if you have very little or indeed no access to organic foods at all. You just need to put a bit more effort into ensuring that your foods are as low in *Chemical Calories* as you can reasonably make them.

To start you off, I would like to provide some general rules to help you select foods with the lowest possible levels of *Chemical Calories*:

- When it comes to animal produce, buy organic or less intensively farmed produce whenever you can.
- Keep animal fats low – choose low-fat milk and leaner meats even if the food is organic. (Low-fat is especially important if the produce is not organic.) Make sure that the low-fat food and indeed any processed food that you buy is not also high in additives.
- Soft fruits and more delicate vegetables are likely to be more polluted than robust fruits and vegetables that store well.
- Choose products in natural packaging materials (cardboard, paper, glass) or remove plastic packaging as soon as you can.

WHY IT IS BETTER TO KEEP YOUR INTAKE OF ANIMAL FATS LOW

Limiting your animal fats is generally a sensible policy. This is because most environmental pollutants accumulate in animals, and tend to be stored in their fatty tissues. So by cutting down on all types of animal fats you will be automatically reducing the transfer of *Chemical Calories* to your body.

In this way, simply buying semi-skimmed milk rather than full-fat milk, or eating naturally low-fat cottage cheese rather than full-fat hard cheese, will reduce the potential amount of *Chemical Calories* from environmental pollutants likely to be present in your foods. As you can imagine, this applies to both organic and conventional foods.

While it is relatively easy to choose meat with less visible fat, or low-fat dairy products, it becomes much more difficult to determine how much and which types of fat have been used in processed foods. For example, fish oils, which tend to be particularly heavily contaminated with *Chemical Calories*, may be used in all sorts of products.[1]

You could easily be forgiven for thinking that fish oils would be too smelly to use in anything other than processed fish, but you would in fact be wrong. Fish oils are common in baked goods, margarine, ice-cream, animal foods and even some cosmetics. Next time you pick up a ready-made meal, make sure you look at the label before you buy it. On the whole, if given the choice, select products made with vegetable oils, as they are potentially less risky than animal fats.

One more point: whether you buy organic produce or not, it's important to realize that most pesticides tend to be absorbed into your body far more readily if they are mixed with fats.[2] Because of this, you can limit to some extent the amount of pesticides you absorb from a food by lowering the overall fat content of the meal.

For example, if you buy a mixed non-organically grown salad, make sure that you serve it with low-fat or no-fat dressing. If you really love tinned salmon or tuna, but want to keep down the *Chemical Calories*, buy it stored in brine rather than vegetable oil, and never, never stored in its own oils.

WHY THE PACKAGING REALLY MATTERS

Cutting down *Chemical Calories* doesn't stop with the kind of food that you buy, it also extends to how it is packaged. Unfortunately the materials now commonly used in packaging can add loads of extra chemicals to our food.

Once upon a time foods were sold in traditional natural materials such as glass, paper and cardboard. But now most foods are sold in plastic, because it is cheap to produce, weighs very little, is tough-wearing, waterproof, 'hygienic' and won't break like glass.[3] The problem is that, unlike the natural materials, plastics readily leach chemicals into foods, which can add significantly to the total *Chemical Calorie* loading.[4] On top of this, the act of printing can be the source of yet more *Chemical Calories* because modern inks now contain a large number of synthetic chemicals which can readily pass through the wrappings and into the food.[5]

At present, there is no obligation for producers to list any of the materials used in the packaging, whether the food is organic or not. So to help you pick the lowest *Chemical Calories* option, we need to understand which types of packaging cause a problem and in which situations.

WHERE *CHEMICAL CALORIES* CAN BE FOUND IN PLASTICS

Before we can understand how plastics add *Chemical Calories* to our foods, we need to know what a plastic actually is.

Plastics are made up of two main components. First, the plastic itself, which is a long chain of monomers, identical chemicals that join up to make a strong continuous link.[6] Second, a large number of toxic additives which give plastics their characteristic flexibility and strength.[7]

The plastic monomers include the 'styrene' of polystyrene[8] and the chemical bisphenol.[9] Both these substances have significant numbers of *Chemical Calories*. They are both used widely in food-packaging, as well as in catering. Think about it: which one of us has never had a hot drink out of a polystyrene cup?

Although we are less aware of them, plastics made up of bisphenols are also widely used in food-packaging, for example in the plastic inner lining of metal food cans, as sealants on cartons and in numerous other products.

Now for the additives themselves. Among the many additives used in plastics, possibly the most important are the group of chemicals known as the phthalates. These substances appear to be high in *Chemical Calories* and are present in virtually all plastics, giving these materials their characteristic flexibility. They are also commonly used in printing inks.[10]

Another common group of additives are fire-retardants, such as PBBs (polybrominated biphenyls), which can increase the *Chemical Calorie* loading even further. In fact, plastics can contain a whole number of other additives which are high in *Chemical Calories* such as organophosphates and heavy metals such as lead.[11] In addition, the level of additives can also vary greatly. For example, the plastic known as PVC contains a much larger amount of additives than, say, polyethylene.[12]

While it is possible to get 'safer' plastics which are lower in additives, and indeed chemical-free ink (which some organic producers already use for labelling), for practical purposes it is currently virtually impossible to tell what type of plastic or ink your food is packaged in just by looking at it. So unless you know any different, you should treat all plastic wrappings with the same degree of caution. As a rough guide, however, the more flexible the plastic, the higher the content of plasticizers.

SITUATIONS WHICH AFFECT THE EXTENT OF 'PLASTIC-RELATED' FOOD CONTAMINATION

If all the chemicals found in plastics just stayed in the packaging, there would not be such a problem. The reality is that many of these chemicals can readily leach out and enter the enclosed foods. The extent of this contamination will depend largely on the following factors:

- Heat – or anything that increases temperature (such as microwaving or storage in a hot environment) – can significantly increase the leaching of plastics and additives into food.[13]
- Length of storage time – longer storage times will increase the migration of plastics and additives into food.[14]
- Proximity of food to the plastic – food in direct contact with plastic (such as milk in plastic bottles) will increase the level of contamination.[15]
- Percentage fat content of the food – the greater the proportion of fats, the greater the extent of food contamination (due to the extreme fat solubility of most of these chemicals).[16]

This means that if a food is high in fats, is stored for a long time, is in intimate contact with the plastic, and is then subjected to high temperatures, the chances of the food being contaminated are going to be relatively high. In order to keep the contamination to an absolute minimum, you will need to consider changing some of your food storage and preparation habits.

In particular you should avoid storing food in clingfilm made of PVC, a particularly toxic plastic,[17] and if possible also avoid using the 'safer' 'low migration' PVC clingfilm as, despite its name, it too has been found to contaminate foods to above safety levels.[18] Microwaving food covered with clingfilm makes the problem even worse, and for the same reasons you should avoid cooking ready-made meals in their plastic containers.

Fortunately non-fatty produce appears to be far less affected by plastic packaging. So fruit and vegetables stored in plastics (for example apples stored in cardboard trays with thin sheets of bubble wrap between them, or produce bagged in plastic) will have relatively low levels of contamination.[19]

Storing food in aluminium foil doesn't appear to add too many *Chemical Calories*, but it can taint food that is particularly salty[20] or acidic (such as cooked fruit).[21] However, foil can be safely used for fatty foods, grain products and vegetables.

WATCH OUT FOR HIDDEN 'PACKAGING' SOURCES OF *CHEMICAL CALORIES*

One more important thing to remember is that the use of plastics and other additives may not always be particularly obvious. Packaging that appears to be made of natural materials can still contain plastic parts. Here are some examples:

- Substances used to seal up bags of foods, such as sugar, contain plastic additives that can migrate into food. (When bags of sugar were stored at 40 degrees, 80 per cent of the phthalates migrated into the sugar.)[22]
- Printing inks on paper wrappers can contain phthalates that migrate into food. (Many snacks, biscuits and confectionery items have also been found to be contaminated by the printing ink.)[23]

- Drinks in glass bottles or waxed cardboard pots of yoghurt may have caps or seals containing plasticizers that seep into the contents.
- Cardboard cartons can be lined with plastic inside.
- Tinned foods can be lined with a plastic coating.[24]

So you have just bought food in the supermarket, and some of it is wrapped in plastic: what do you do next? Whether or not you remove the wrapping, the cooler the place you store your food, the better. So putting plastic-wrapped foods in the freezer will greatly reduce the potential degree of contamination. And if the fat content of the food is very high, it might be advisable to transfer the foods from plastic into a *Chemical-Calorie*-free container before you put them in the fridge.

I use a set of glass dishes with lids, which lets me see the contents without opening them, and I transfer fatty liquids such as milk into a glass or ceramic jug. I also remove any layers of clingfilm before I put the food away. While you cannot undo what has already been done, it is perfectly possible to limit further contamination – it just takes a bit of extra thought and effort on your part.

HOW TO REDUCE *CHEMICAL CALORIES* IN FOOD PREPARATION

As previously mentioned, you don't have to go organic to eat low in *Chemical Calories* (although it helps) – with the right know-how, you can dramatically reduce the number of *Chemical Calories* by the way you prepare and cook food. And while these techniques are particularly useful for conventional foods, they will also ensure that you get the most benefit from your organic produce too.

WASHING AND CLEANING: The most obvious way to rid your fruit and vegetables of pesticide or plastic residues is to wash them off. There has actually been quite a significant amount of scientific investigation into the effectiveness of removing chemicals by washing produce in plain water and by washing it in water and detergents. On the whole, the results appear to depend largely on the kind of chemicals present.[25] Some pesticides are designed to stay on the surface, but others are specifically intended to infiltrate into the very heart of the food. As you can imagine, washing will only deal with chemicals found on the surface. But it has variable success even within that group, as some chemicals are water-soluble and will wash off with plain water, while others are fat-soluble and can only be removed by using detergents.

It has to be said that few people would relish using washing-up liquid on their fruit and vegetables! Quite apart from the taste, certain detergents even have their own *Chemical Calorie* content. However, it is now possible to buy naturally derived products that claim to specifically remove many surface toxins from fruit and vegetables.

Despite proving more effective in some cases than others, washing your fruit and vegetables is a good first line of defence. However, for foods that absorb a certain amount of chemicals, such as strawberries, grapes, oranges, peaches, spinach and tomatoes, washing is a good start, but we need to realize that a significant amount of chemicals may still persist.

PEELING: Compared to washing, peeling fruit and vegetables can be a really dramatic way of lowering the *Chemical Calorie* content of food. Take, for example, an orange. If the peel is included (as orange zest, for example) it is one of the most polluted of all foods, but the simple act of peeling it will reduce the *Chemical Calorie* count very considerably. This is because most of the chemicals in an orange are in its thick skin.[26]

The same applies to apples: unpeeled they can be very highly contaminated, yet once the skin is removed the contamination is radically reduced.[27] Although a peeled apple cannot compare in flavour and goodness with organic apples, which you should feel free to eat peel and all, it is far safer and contains significantly fewer *Chemical Calories* than an unpeeled conventionally grown one.

The same holds for vegetables such as tomatoes and, in particular, potatoes. So if you are eating non-organic fruit and vegetables, you can still make a really big difference by getting the peeler out!

PREPARING MEATS AND FISH: I've already talked about the ways that *Chemical Calories* can accumulate in animal fat, so you can see that by cutting off all visible fat as you prepare meat, poultry or fish, the *Chemical Calorie* content could potentially be greatly reduced.[28] In the case of fish, it is particularly beneficial to remove the skin before cooking if there tends to be a lot of fat just underneath it – which should help make all you fish fans out there a bit happier.

REDUCING *CHEMICAL CALORIES* THROUGH COOKING

Since heat can break down certain chemicals and can also lower levels of others, food is usually lower in *Chemical Calories* after it has been cooked. Generally speaking, the higher the temperature and the longer the food is cooked, the more effective cooking will be in reducing the overall *Chemical Calorie* level.[29]

For example, if you are making marmalade with non-organic oranges (which you should only do with Seville oranges and never dessert oranges or non-organic citrus fruit), cooking it for a long time in an open pan on top of the stove is much more effective than the quicker lower-temperature method using a microwave oven.[30]

At the other extreme, some foods, such as vegetables, are cooked for only a short time – even so, many of the chemicals will still be washed off into the water. While this makes the vegetables safer to eat, it can make the vegetable water more contaminated. So if the potential level of *Chemical Calories* present in the vegetables is high, it may be best not to use the leftover water for making gravies or sauces.[31]

Some chemicals are more heat-stable, and are not destroyed by cooking – indeed, in some cases cooking can actually make less toxic chemicals more toxic (which appears to be the case with one of the pesticides commonly found on tomatoes).[32]

The more persistent chemicals, such as the organochlorines, can be virtually unaffected by cooking – not too surprising in view of their heat-resistant properties.[33] Indeed, some of the plastic additives and veterinary drug residues found in meats (such as products to treat the animal for worms) may not be destroyed either.[34]

In these cases, the main benefit of cooking is to remove some of the fat from meats and fish, as most of the above persistent chemicals tend to remain in these fats. Grilling and throwing away the fat is one option. Roasting is another, provided that the fat is not used in gravy. Another way is to cook meat or fish in vegetable oil, and then throw all the oil and fat parts away.

I do think it is sad that things have come to this, since natural animal fats can really improve the flavour of many dishes, but if you don't know how badly the fats are contaminated, it is probably your best option. If on the other hand you are pretty sure that the meats are relatively 'clean', all this becomes less essential.

Apart from the extra preparation involved, there is another down-side to all this peeling and cooking. Even though these techniques can be very effective in lowering the total levels of *Chemical Calories*, they will also tend to lower the nutritional value of the food, as vitamins are particularly heat-sensitive. If you choose to use these methods, you must ensure that you are still getting enough nutrients by using supplements as recommended in Chapter 15.

HOW TO AVOID ADDING *CHEMICAL CALORIES* DURING COOKING AND SERVING

Although cooking can actively lower the *Chemical Calorie* content of food, it can itself be a potential source of *Chemical Calories*. This can happen if hot foods or liquids are in close proximity to heated plastics, as the plastics and their additives will be transferred into your food in double-quick time. Think of the times you drink hot coffee from a polystyrene cup,[35] after adding milk from a plastic carton, then stirring it with a plastic spoon. You might even eat hot food from a plastic bowl or plate (fast food is an obvious example).

By heating your ready-made meal in a plastic container, by microwaving food in plastic bowls, by using plastic cooking implements or even plastic non-stick pan coatings, you will unwittingly be eating not just the food, but potentially an extra dose of *Chemical Calories* from the plastic.

To avoid any unwanted additions to your food, it is worth making an effort to use glass, ceramic or even paper plates and metallic knives, forks and spoons, as this will lower your overall dose of *Chemical Calories*. And if they are not available in restaurants, why don't you make a special request? You never know, the next time you visit them they might be able to offer you the lower-*Chemical-Calorie* option.

You can now see that it really is possible to keep your exposure to *Chemical Calories* in your diet to an absolute minimum, even if you have limited access to organic foods. However, there is one more significant area which I have not yet touched upon.

Apart from food, there is one other major source of *Chemical Calories* in our diet – and that is our water supplies. To find out more about how much of a problem this poses and how it can be tackled, let's proceed to the next chapter.

10. Pure Water, the Slimmer's Friend

To maximize the full slimming benefit of lowering our intake of *Chemical Calories* from food, we need to cut back on all the other ways in which our bodies are exposed to potentially harmful toxins.

After food, water is one of the main sources of *Chemical Calories*. And as we are exposed to water in so many different aspects of our lives, we can't afford to let it bypass our scrutiny. If we do, it will be to the detriment of our figures, and of course of our general well-being.

This chapter will explain how our water has come to be so polluted and will outline what we can do to lower the levels of *Chemical Calories* in our own domestic water supply. Then it will explain how we can accelerate weight-loss simply by drinking lots of *Chemical-Calorie*-free water. Sounds good? Now find out why!

HOW CLEAN IS YOUR WATER SUPPLY?

Since the creation and wide-scale use of synthetic chemicals, some-what shockingly, over 350 synthetic chemicals have been detected in tap water. Not surprisingly, many of these substances have also revealed themselves to be very high in *Chemical Calories*.[1]

The alarming contamination of our water supplies has largely occurred over the last 100 years, following years of industrial, agricultural and environmental pollution. As a direct result, every day, as we eat, drink, wash, cook, clean and go about our daily lives, we will now be exposed to and absorb whichever chemicals happen to be in our water supplies at the time.

The level of contamination varies a lot, depending on where you live, but a certain number of chemicals can be found universally and they include the following groups:

- Pesticides
- Heavy metals
- Solvents
- Environmental pollutants (e.g. industrial pollutants)
- Environmental pollutants
- Plastics

In order even to start to tackle the problem, we need to understand how these toxins get into our water in the first place. This will give us a better idea of how to improve the quality of our existing water supplies as well as reduce future contamination at its source.

1. SEEPAGE FROM THE SURFACE: Whenever we use chemicals on the land, for any reason, it will usually lead to pollution of our underground water sources as well as of our rivers and oceans. Chemicals used to clear weeds, improve crops or poison pests seep into the earth, where they then pollute the ground water. In addition, wind and rain sweep the chemicals off the surface of the land into the rivers and the sea.

The most obvious example is the contamination caused by pesticides sprayed on to the fields by farmers in the process of growing crops. Not surprisingly, year after year these pesticides end up in our drinking water. It's particularly shocking that this poisoning of our water supply is caused by legitimate use according to all the proper recommendations, and is not just due to accidents, spillage or carelessness.

Pesticide levels are now so high that the Chief Scientist of Anglian Water (operating in a well-known UK agricultural area) was quoted in a national newspaper as saying that 'about half our water supplies exceed the EC limits for pesticides'.[2]

2. INDUSTRIAL WASTE: This is another huge source of toxic chemical contamination. Waste from factories is commonly poured into rivers, or it can enter the water supply from the atmosphere or leak out from ill-managed toxic waste dumps. Once chemicals enter the water supply, they can cause persistent damage for a

surprisingly long time. A prime example of a persistent pollutant is the dry-cleaning substance and industrial solvent trichloroethylene, which is also very high in *Chemical Calories*.

Another persistent pollutant, especially in the US, is a chemical called MTBE (Methyl, Tertiary-Butyl Ether). It was added to fuel in the late 70s in an attempt to make gasoline burn cleaner, but it had no real effect on curbing air pollution. Still, no one expected it to cause real harm.

Several years ago, however, the sleepy village of Napoleon, Michigan, was the scene of a major unwanted discovery. In the course of drilling a new well for the church, it was found that the ground water was so contaminated that it was actually unsafe to drink. It appeared that the underground storage tanks of three gas stations had been leaking and the gasoline had seeped into the local aquifer, contaminating most of the wells in the vicinity.[3]

After the alert was sounded, many other regions were also found to face the same problem. Quite apart from the pollution issues, MTBE appears to be very high in *Chemical Calories*.[4]

3. INTENTIONAL ADDING OF CHEMICALS: Not all the contamination in our water is accidental, since certain chemicals, such as chlorine and aluminium, are deliberately added to the supply. Aluminium is added in water-processing plants to 'clear' the water. Although it is not particularly high in *Chemical Calories*, it does damage some aspects of our *Slimming System* and it has also been linked to Alzheimer's disease.[5] Chlorine is another chemical that is deliberately added to water as a disinfectant. Although it is not particularly high in *Chemical Calories*, chlorine binds to other chemicals forming trihalomethanes, which are thought to be cancer-forming substances. It also destroys proteins in the hair and skin, as well as making water taste, in my opinion, disgusting.

4. ENVIRONMENTAL POLLUTION: As mentioned previously, certain chemicals such as PCBs and other organochlorines can evaporate into the air, particularly in warm countries. They may then be carried around the world's atmosphere and fall back on to

the ground in cooler countries, particularly via the rain. In this way, even the most remote water sources have become polluted.

5. CONTAMINATION FROM WATER PIPES AND STORAGE CONTAINERS: Sometimes the storage and distribution system itself can add significant amounts of *Chemical Calories* to our water. Lead pipes (although these are being replaced) can add significantly to the *Chemical Calorie* loading of water. Lead pipes are also linked to damage to children's IQs.[6]

Sadly, the replacement plastic pipes used are also full of *Chemical Calories*, which leach out into the water. This is particularly problematic if the pipes are made of PVC, one of the worst offenders. If drinking water is then bottled in plastic, as it commonly is, the levels of *Chemical Calories* will increase again.

This was clearly shown in vol. 4 of *Chemical Sensitivity* by Professor W. Rea, a highly respected authority on environmental medicine.[7] He tested a very large number of samples from water bottled in plastic and found them all to be contaminated to some extent by the plastic containers.

6. NATURAL CONTAMINATION: Water sources may be contaminated by heavy metals occurring naturally in the soil, particularly if the water is acidic.

The result of all this collective contamination is that it has been reported that millions of families drink water containing toxic chemicals in excess of international limits.[8] Our children's intelligence has been reported damaged by the levels of lead in millions of homes,[9] and our elderly are being exposed to the dangers of aluminium deliberately added to our water. Finally, to top it all, many of the chemicals we are exposed to in water could also be making us fat!

So exactly how do we absorb *Chemical Calories* from water, and how can we reduce our exposure to them?

HOW DO WE ABSORB *CHEMICAL CALORIES* FROM WATER?

Most people will think that the main way we absorb *Chemical Calories* from water is by drinking it. I certainly did before researching this book, but it wasn't long before I discovered that this is not in fact the whole story.

There are two very important but less recognized routes by which *Chemical Calories* in water can enter our bodies – via our skin and our lungs. In fact, about half of all the chlorine we absorb from water is thought to be through the lungs and skin,[10] and this contamination occurs every time we take a shower or bath in contaminated water.

As chlorine is not the only chemical present in our bath water, the chances are that many others are absorbed in this way too. This illustrates the importance of pure water for bathing as well as drinking in order to keep our total exposure to *Chemical Calories* as low as possible.

The next obvious question is: how do we achieve this?

REDUCING THE LEVEL OF *CHEMICAL CALORIES* IN WATER

Fortunately, we can do quite a lot to lower the *Chemical Calorie* content of water. Let's start by outlining a couple of these protective measures:

- Before using the water, let cold taps run for a few minutes to flush out any lead that has leached into the water from the pipes.
- Use only the cold tap for drinking water and cooking, as there is a greater probability that the hot water contains lead, asbestos and other pollutants from the hot water tank, if you have one.
- If you drink bottled water, buy it in glass rather than plastic bottles. If there is no alternative to plastic, make sure the bottles are stored in a cool place.
- Use water filters to filter both your drinking water and your household supply.

Many people now invest in a home water-treatment system to ensure that all the water they use is as pure as possible. Many different methods are currently used to clean up water, but I will concentrate on the more commonly used ones.

JUG FILTER: Possibly the most commonly used type of water filter is the jug filter. These are relatively cheap to buy and easy to use, and are generally designed to remove harmful chlorine and make the water taste better. However, they are pretty ineffective in lowering the levels of other *Chemical Calories*.

You should follow the instructions on the jug filter carefully to make sure that it does not contaminate the water. For example, if you do not change the filter according to the guidelines, it can dump many of the chemicals it has filtered out back into the water. Since jug filters remove the chlorine from drinking water, bacteria will grow rapidly in the filtered water, and the plastic jug itself may add to contamination.

If you have a jug filter, make sure you keep it in the fridge – lower temperatures will reduce the amount of bacterial growth and the contamination by plastics.

FILTRATION SYSTEMS: There is a bewildering range of water filters designed to provide filtered water on tap. Some of them are installed under the sink and work through a separate drinking-water tap placed next to the existing taps. Other systems treat all the domestic water coming into the house from the main supply, filtering the water for washing and cooking as well as that for drinking.

These systems use a whole range of different methods, such as simple filtration, resins, deionization, distillation and reverse osmosis. Some are better at removing one type of chemical than others, and your choice may to some extent depend on the main pollutants in your water. Generally speaking, though, the following methods are the best at removing overall levels of *Chemical Calories* from your water.

Distillation: This is possibly the most effective way of removing *Chemical Calories*, but it is very slow and energy-consuming because the water has to be heated up and then cooled. It will take up to six hours to produce 4 litres of water. This type of system is more suited to producing drinking water, but larger models can be obtained for offices or bigger buildings.

Filtration: This is a cheaper and more practical method of removing pollutants. The water goes through a filter, which removes particles too large to pass through. Although most manufacturers claim that the filter removes 98 per cent of bacteria, chlorine, metals and pesticides, the amount of chemicals removed really depends on the size and the type of filter used. As many of the pesticide particles can be very small, they may not be caught in the filter.

Also, the active part of the filter tends to last for around six months to a year before it needs to be changed. If this does not happen on time, the filter will lose its usefulness.

The advantages of this system are that it is relatively quick and efficient and you can filter large amounts of water straight off the mains supply in 'real time', making it well suited for a total household supply. I have one of these systems installed on the mains supply into my house to keep my entire household water low in *Chemical Calories*. Since getting it fitted, I have really noticed the difference, not only in the absence of a chlorine smell but also in the general improvement in my sons' skins.

Reverse osmosis: This method works like a filter: water is passed through a very fine membrane by applying pressure on one side of the membrane so that the water comes through the other side. Manufacturers claim that this method is very effective in removing between 80 per cent and 98 per cent of total dissolved solids, with different minerals having different reduction rates. The filtered water is stored in a tank, which could be made of plastic, but it is possible to buy units made of less polluting materials.

Since the water needs to be stored and is not filtered as fast as it comes in from the mains supply, this type of filter may be more suited to drinking water only.

★

One last word on the subject of water filters: the more effective the filter, the more *Chemical Calories* it will remove. However, in removing the baddies it will also remove some of the beneficial minerals from drinking water. As water is an important source of certain minerals in our diet, you should make sure that you also take the mineral supplements recommended in Chapters 15 and 24.

HOW PURE WATER HELPS YOU TO LOSE WEIGHT

Once you have got your *Chemical-Calorie*-free water, you should drink lots of it. When my older sister Julia was in holiday in Italy and asked for mineral water, it was assumed that she was doing it to keep her slim figure. Well, this assumption was absolutely right, since water can positively help to enhance weight loss in several different ways including:

- Flushing toxins out in sweat and urine.
- Enhancing energy levels by staying hydrated.
- Burning higher numbers of conventional calories.
- Reducing water retention.

By drinking lots of water, you will be enhancing your body's natural ability to rid itself of *Chemical Calories* in your sweat and urine. And the more you drink, the more you will flush out your system. About eight glasses of pure water a day is ideal to expel toxins.

You might not realize it but our bodies are largely made up of water – 75 per cent if you are an adult. In order to work properly, all these tissues need to be fully hydrated, as even a tiny 2 per cent loss in the water surrounding the cells will mean a 20 per cent fall in your energy levels.[11] This will reduce the amount of energy you can expend and therefore reduce your ability to lose weight.

Before I go any further, when I say the body needs water, I don't mean tea, coffee, fizzy drinks or alcohol. Herb tea is fine, as is fruit juice, but all the other drinks mentioned act as diuretics, forcing water out of the body. Thus for every alcoholic drink you consume, you will lose the same volume of water. It is best to cut out these drinks, but if you can't resist them, do make sure that you drink an extra glass of water for each of these 'diuretic drinks' you take in.

CHEMICAL CALORIES, WATER AND WEIGHT

By making the effort to reduce your daily intake of *Chemical Calories* from water, you will be helping yourself to lose weight by allowing your *Slimming System* to function more smoothly. A pure water supply will also help you lose weight in another way.

As well as reducing the rate at which the body burns off energy, many pollutants can cause swelling and oedema by actively reducing levels of the body's natural diuretic hormone, vasopressin (ADH, anti-diuretic hormone). The less chemical damage the body has, the higher the level of vasopressin and the less excess fluid your body will carry.

Finally, I found an interesting fact in an academic paper that made a lot of sense to me. It showed that the simple act of drinking water actually speeds up the metabolic rate. This is probably caused by the body's need to heat itself up after drinking a relatively cool liquid. So by drinking cool pure water, you can actually increase the amount of calories you burn off, as well as helping your *Slimming System* to get rid of more weight.[12]

So now we have talked about how to reduce our exposure to *Chemical Calories* from food and water. The next two chapters will deal with the other ways we are exposed to *Chemical Calories* – in our homes and in the environment. The bottom line is that once you have tackled all the main sources of *Chemical Calories* in your life, you will be well on the way to achieving the body of your dreams, and keeping it.

However, as our major source of persistent fattening chemicals comes from our food, you may choose to bypass the next two chapters temporarily and go straight to Chapter 13: Repair and Revitalize Your Natural *Slimming System* – returning to them after you have finished reading all about the diet. Whatever you decide to do, put a water filter on your shopping list, pour yourself a glass of water, and read on!

11. *Chemical Calories* Lurk All around You

Identifying *Chemical Calories* in Your Home and Environment

By now you will have well and truly realized that you are playing by a whole new set of dieting rules – but to succeed you will have to pace yourself. It will take time to take all this new information in and then make the changes necessary to create a lifestyle low in *Chemical Calories*, and by taking one step at a time, everything will suddenly become less daunting and more do-able.

I have already made a number of suggestions about the way in which you can lower the level of *Chemical Calories* in both your water and your food, so try not to be fazed by all the additional information in these next two chapters. You really don't have to do everything at once to achieve weight loss, and you certainly don't have do everything I recommend in this and the next chapter to successfully lose weight.

As the greatest number of persistent *Chemical Calories* will originate from your diet, lowering your intake of *Chemical Calories* in your food and drink should be your No. 1 priority. A substantial amount of weight loss can be achieved by dietary and supplement changes alone.

Once you have got the hang of this, you can spend more time in reducing your exposure to *Chemical Calories* in the environment. My philosophy is to give you all the information you need – the number of changes you make and when you choose to make them will be up to you.

One thing you may discover is that as your daily intake of *Chemical Calories* gets lower, your body's ability to reduce its lifelong burden of stored *Chemical Calories* will markedly increase. This is because your detoxification system suddenly becomes freed up from dealing with the daily onslaught of *Chemical Calories* it is regularly exposed to and can, perhaps for the first time, start to remove these built-up stores – making a world of difference to your ability to lose weight.

Time and time again, once people experience the incredible slimming benefits for themselves, they actively look for more and more ways to cut out *Chemical Calories* from their lives. This is why I have given you so much information at once: not so that you can change everything right now but so that you can progress to different areas when the time is right for you.

Now for more about this chapter. The fact is that we are increasingly being exposed to more and more *Chemical Calories* in our lives. We absorb them in large quantities from the cosmetics and cleaners used in our homes, from the sprays we use in our gardens, from contaminated air, public transport, the workplace and even at the dentist!

While we have to accept that we will never now be completely free from them, there are a huge number of measures we can take to limit our exposure. Think of it this way: the more *Chemical Calories* we avoid, the closer we will get to achieving our goals of permanent weight loss and better health.

This chapter will help you achieve just that by flagging up the highest non-food sources of *Chemical Calories*. The next chapter will tell you how to slash your exposure to the vast majority of these identified problem areas. So don't fret, there are lots of things which can be done to remedy the situation.

HOW NON-FOOD *CHEMICAL CALORIES* ENTER OUR BODIES

As you would imagine, you will absorb more *Chemical Calories* by eating plastic residues in contaminated foods than by, say, walking past a plastic toy. Nevertheless, the levels of airborne *Chemical Calories* produced by plastics and other synthetic substances are significant and real. We are exposed to them all the time.

Some synthetic substances are volatile and evaporate into the air.

Others 'out-gas' which means that they emit gases which contain *Chemical Calories*. Out-gassing is usually more common in newer objects, which is why carpets and other new furnishings are more pungent in the first few weeks and months, after which this becomes less noticeable.

The warmer the environment, the more synthetic substances will out-gas even if they are years old. When you smell the characteristic smell of new carpets or a new car, the chemicals will not just have activated the smelling sensors in your nose, they will also have entered your lungs and from there moved directly into your blood-stream as *Chemical Calories*. And there they will remain until they are processed by your liver.

Chemical Calories can also readily enter your body through your skin, triggered by the simple act of walking barefoot on treated carpets, by wearing synthetic clothes, or by using chemically loaded cosmetics.

Although we are exposed to a generally lower amount of chemi-cals via our skin and lungs, these can in fact be just as toxic to our *Slimming System* as those we eat in food (if not more so). Because although they will be detoxified to a certain extend in the skin, in bypassing the gut they have effectively avoided all the powerful acids and enzymes that we use in our gut to break down and neutralize chemicals in food.

E. J. Routledge and his colleagues at Brunel University in Eng-land found this to be the case for the chemical preservatives known as parabens.[1] Parabens are widely used in a whole range of foods, cosmetics and toiletries, but they appear to be more toxic if they enter our bodies through the skin rather than in food. It seems that the gut can break down parabens to an extent that decreases their overall toxicity.

So in this case, the non-food routes of contamination could in some cases be even more dangerous than encountering certain chemicals in food.

HOW TOXIC IS YOUR HOME?

The chances are that if you did not build your house yourself or know the people who lived in it previously, it will be very hard to assess how contaminated it is with *Chemical Calories*. Unless the previous owners were known for their environmentally friendly ways, then it is likely that the products used in the house will have been the 'conventional' ones, which may have been heavily treated with chemicals.

To some extent, the age of the house will also determine what types of chemicals were used. Thirty or forty years ago, carpets and wood were treated with very persistent chemicals such as the organo-chlorines. As a result, unless you have the paperwork detailing what has been used in your house, you may need some expert help.

If you really want to find out the extent to which your house is contaminated with chemicals, it can be done by calling in an environmental house doctor (see Useful Contacts, page 353). This is exactly what I did to discover how contaminated my house was and to see whether there were any particular problem areas. A sample of household air was collected over twenty-four hours, in addition to a bottle of tap water. These were then sent off for analysis.

Fortunately my house appeared to be relatively uncontaminated, which was a great relief, particularly because of my young family. As a matter of fact, the largest amount of chemicals detected were plant-based citrus ones from the low-toxicity cleaning products that I use!

The main drawback of this type of investigation is the cost, as the more things you test the more expensive it becomes. I did it because I live in a very old house and I have only been here for a few years. I wanted to know about any problem areas so that I could deal with them. While the tests were useful, they are definitely not essential. And even if you do consult an environmental house doctor, you still need to find out where the contaminating chemicals are, so that you can take positive action.

The rest of this chapter is targeted at identifying the areas of our lives (including the home and the workplace) where we are now exposed to potentially high levels of *Chemical Calories*.

Owing to the sheer diversity of chemicals found in different products, it is virtually impossible to be specific about the chemicals in your own home or workplace. However, there are some chemicals that turn up again and again in similar situations. At the very least, the following information should alert you to most of the potential *Chemical Calorie* hot spots that now exist.

WHAT LURKS IN THE AVERAGE ROOM?

The main sources of *Chemical Calories* in any room stem from the use of the following groups of substances. Unfortunately they are now used in far more places than most of us could imagine. The four worst offenders are:

- Pesticides
- Plastics
- Flame-retardants
- Solvents

As you can imagine, building materials or furnishings that incorporate these offenders will be potentially loaded with *Chemical Calories*. Because of this the average room can have many potential hot spots.

A prime example is interior wood that has been treated with preservatives. Think about it: if you have wood treated to prevent woodworm or dry rot, the treatment will be guaranteed for a certain number of years. What this really translates down to is that the pesticides inside the wood will be present and active in sufficiently high doses for all those years and will also contaminate the surrounding air and dust.

Dry rot, along with other infestations, can strike fear into the heart of the homeowner, but fortunately there are now natural alternatives available both for providing preventive treatment and for dealing with existing fungal or insect damage problems.

Staying on the subject of woodwork in modern houses, fibre-board or chipboard tends to be more commonly used nowadays than solid wood. Unfortunately these can cause a problem from their mixture of adhesives and solvents, which out-gas fumes into the air.

Generally anything treated with flame-retardants (chemicals which slow down the rate of burning) can also be high in *Chemical Calories* – particularly if the extremely persistent chemicals known as polybrominated biphenyls (PBBs) have been used.

Another major source of *Chemical Calories* is plastics, particularly since they are not just used in obvious places such as PVC window frames but are also used in cement, glues and adhesives. As a result, all these products will potentially out-gas *Chemical Calories* into the air.

One further hot spot is the electric wiring of older houses, where the organochlorines known as PCBs may have been used as insulation. Unfortunately PCBs can contaminate the air quite significantly, and in some cases old electric wiring in a house can account for up to one third of the inhabitants' daily PCB exposure.[2]

FLOORING: You may be surprised to discover that a natural prod-uct such as wool carpet can often contain more *Chemical Calories* than some synthetic carpets. This is because the manufacturers may have used pesticides to mothproof the wool. The carpet backing of wool and synthetic carpets alike, and even the underlay, all contain *Chemical Calories* from the plastics and other solvents used in their manufacture.

If the carpets have been in place for a long time, the overall amount of toxic fumes will be significantly reduced. However, many old carpets made in the mid-eighties were manufactured using longer-acting and persistent organochlorine pesticides such as lindane, which are loaded with *Chemical Calories*.

Other 'fattening' forms of flooring include vinyl flooring. Again this releases the greatest amount of fumes into the air during the first few months after being laid. Wood and laminated flooring can also introduce *Chemical Calories* if glue or plastic underlay are used, and so can the synthetic-based wood sealants used to give your wooden floor that beautiful shiny polished look.

WALL-COVERINGS: Wall-coverings also contribute their share of *Chemical Calories* to the air inside your house. As a general rule, any product that contains vinyl or plastic is particularly likely to be high in *Chemical Calories*.

Paint is one of the worst offenders, as it can contain a whole variety of different chemicals, such as solvents, synthetic colours and plastics. Although lead was commonly added to older paints, this practice is much less widespread now.

Wallpaper, especially if it is intended for kitchens or bathrooms, can often contain plastics which will off-gas. In addition, the paste used to apply wallpaper to the walls can contain fungicides.

And while ceramic tiles are fine, the adhesives and grouting used when applying them to the walls can be home to a whole cornucopia of chemicals – as I discovered when looking at a pot of the stuff just recently.

SOFT FURNISHINGS AND FABRICS: Soft furnishings and curtain fabrics can add a great deal to the attractiveness of a room – unfortunately they can also add significantly to the toxic chemical cocktail. This is because the law requires that the fabrics used on furniture should pass certain standards of fire-resistance.

This can entail a whole number of flame-retardant chemicals being added, to slow down the speed at which a product will burn,[3] and unfortunately many of these chemicals can be particularly high in *Chemical Calories*. The level of *Chemical Calories* will be even higher if the furniture is also padded with flame-retardant foam.

Now I am not telling you that you should choose fabrics without flame-retardants, I am just giving you the facts so that you can make an informed decision weighing up all the potential risks according to your individual situation. The problem with buying furniture in particular is that you can't tell the level of contamination just by looking at the product, and the labels rarely help. Sometimes the information is in the form of coded messages that seem positive and are commonly used as selling points.

Look out for information revealing that the products have been heavily treated. If, for example, it is guaranteed mothproof or fireproof, you will know that a whole lot of potentially toxic and fattening chemicals have been added; however, it will then be up to you to choose whether you would rather have the qualities that these chemicals bestow, or fewer *Chemical Calories*.

WHAT LURKS IN THE BATHROOM?

The typical bathroom can be a relative minefield of *Chemical Calories*. You may not realize it, but behind the hype many beauty products are far from natural. In fact, many are stuffed with synthetic chemicals. Consequently the simple act of taking a bath with your favourite scented bath products can increase your *Chemical Calorie* loading. Afterwards, as you generously cover your skin with your favourite moisturizing cream, you could be adding to it even more!

We are constantly told how one product will give us shiny healthy hair and that another will stop our skin from ageing. Whether these claims are true or not, one thing is increasingly clear. More and more personal care products contain significant levels of *Chemical Calories*. Plastics lurk in hair sprays, nail polish, perfumes, hair mousse and a whole range of cosmetics. Surfactants (cleaning compounds commonly derived from petroleum) are found in detergents, bubble bath and shampoos.

The trend is for products to be sold in plastic containers rather than glass, so the plastics are likely to contaminate the product even further. And the longer these products hang around in their plastic containers, the more likely they are to contain leached plastics.

Synthetic preservatives are yet another source of *Chemical Calories*. Most toiletries and cosmetics contain some sort of preservative that will add to the *Chemical Calorie* content. Scientists know that our bodies can absorb much of what we put on our skin. For example, Dr Philippa Darbre of Reading University, England, has found that the lipid-soluble chemicals organochlorines PCBs readily penetrate skin, then enter the body's circulation. This makes products containing lipid-soluble toxic chemicals a potentially significant source of *Chemical Calories*, if we apply them directly to our bodies.[4]

The other main source of *Chemical Calories* in your bathroom is likely to be your medicine cabinet. I am not talking about prescription drugs here and I am certainly not encouraging anyone who is ill to stop taking their medication. The products that I want to warn you about are the 'medicated' shampoos specifically designed for head infestations such as nits, and head and crab lice (not dandruff).

These may contain powerful insecticides such as organophosphates which are extremely toxic as well as high in *Chemical Calories*. As they are intended to be put directly on to the skin, a proportion of the chemicals can be absorbed straight into our bodies. What's worse, those preparations are frequently used on children because they are the ones with the highest risk of infestation.

Your doctor, pharmacist or alternative health-care specialist may be able to recommend alternatives such as fine-tooth combing and natural remedies, which are just as effective as these potentially highly toxic medicated formulae, if not more so.

WHAT LURKS IN THE KITCHEN?

I think you will agree with me that I have already exposed the hiding places for most of the *Chemical Calories* in the kitchen. But what I haven't dealt with is the cleaning cupboard, which you will shortly discover is a real *Chemical Calorie* hot spot! By taking a look at the labels, you will discover that many household products are quite frankly downright scary in the number of toxic chemicals they contain.

Needless to say, quite a few products are particularly high in *Chemical Calories*, from the concoction of preservatives, perfumes, solvents, plastics, detergents, surfactants and emulsifiers that they possess. While I don't suggest you put down all your cleaning tools, I would advise that you use more natural alternatives, about which there are a number of suggestions in the next chapter.

Many kitchens also contain common household pesticides. You may not think you use pesticides, but in reality very few houses are without them. You probably have them in the form of fly-killers, ant poisons, mosquito sprays, rodent controls, insect-repellent, and all the many forms of pet products such as flea powder, flea sprays and shampoos for fleas, lice and mange.

All these products are high in *Chemical Calories*, but the good news is that as with cleaning products, there are plenty of alternatives. After all, these problems have been around for a very long time, long before synthetic chemicals were ever created.

WHAT LURKS IN THE BEDROOM?

The bedroom is a particularly important room, as most of us spend over one third of our lives there. Consequently if any room needs to be free of *Chemical Calories* this should be the one. Let's start with the bed.

Because of the current fire regulations, most mattresses are now covered with flame-retardants, which we now know can act as a major source of contamination. But the mattress is not alone here: the coverings and pillows can also be treated with flame-retardants, adding further to the overall *Chemical Calorie* loading of the bed. And if the structure of the bed is made of plastic and the mattress filling is foam, you will inhale even more *Chemical Calories* while you sleep.

As mentioned above, if you have a relatively high fire-risk factor, for example if you smoke or have an open fire in your bedroom, it will be best to keep the flame-retardant items but minimize the *Chemical Calorie* effect by using the methods described in the next chapter.

Apart from the bed, your wardrobe tends to be the other major source of *Chemical Calories*. Some will originate from clothes that contain plastics, such as synthetic leather or waterproof clothing.

Other clothes will have *Chemical Calories* added in the manufacturing process – look out for labels that say 'fire-resistant', 'easy care' or 'easy iron'.

You can even be responsible for adding *Chemical Calories* yourself if you dry-clean your clothes (because of the solvents used in cleaning), or if you use certain chemically treated mothballs to prevent insect damage.

THE CHILDREN'S PLAYROOM

Go into any toy shop and you will be greeted by a strong smell of plastics wafting through the air. Take a good look around you and you will soon see why. The vast majority of new toys are made from highly toxic PVC and a whole range of other plastics, replacing more traditional materials such as wood.

Although some countries have withdrawn plastic toys designed to be chewed during teething, there appear to be no restrictions on PVC being used in other children's products. Remember that if your children have plastic toys, these will to a certain extent out-gas into the air, exposing the whole household to fattening and toxic chemicals.

I am not suggesting for one moment that you throw all their toys out – first this is not necessary and second it might just trigger an internal revolution (I know it would in our household anyway!) – but just that you should make sure they are stored properly and that the rooms they are stored in are well ventilated.

Other children's products high in *Chemical Calories* include glues used in all kinds of art and model-making, paints, felt tips, plastic play mats, protective plastic sheeting, bath books, laminated board books and soft toys.

THE GARDEN SHED AND GARAGE

The garden shed, or anywhere that you store DIY and gardening materials, can be a huge source of *Chemical Calories*. Old pots of paint and varnish are highly volatile and can contain a large number of synthetic chemicals such as plastics, surfactants, lead, styrenes and solvents. Most DIY areas can also contain toxic glues and adhesives for use all over the house as well as wood preservatives for garden fences and furniture. On a warm day you can really smell these toxic substances because they will evaporate into the air more quickly.

Garages are not particularly healthy places, on the whole, as they tend to contain lots of *Chemical-Calorie*-rich sources such as oil, petrol, solvents and detergents, which tend to evaporate. On top of this, oil, petrol and diesel are also adulterated with a whole range of additives including lead, organophosphates, plastics, detergents and a whole lot more highly toxic and fattening chemicals.

The problems get worse if your garage is connected to the house and the overall ventilation is poor, as the chances are that the fumes will waft straight into your home. And if you park your car in an integral garage, then by starting up the engine in this confined space you are likely to send yet more fumes into your living space.

Moving onwards and outwards to the garden – far from being a natural and relaxing environment, the modern garden is becoming a toxic battlefield! *Chemical Calories* abound in the ordinary garden shed – pesticides to kill insects and weedkillers to remove unwanted plants from your paths, flower-beds or lawn.

These chemicals are bad enough in the garden, but did you know that lawn herbicides, for example, can be tracked indoors on your shoes, as well as by your children and pets, and can contaminate carpets for a long time? What's more, dogs that roll around on herbicide-treated lawns tend to be more prone to getting a certain type of cancer (non-Hodgkins lymphoma).[5]

These facts are starting to be more widely appreciated, and many gardening books and programmes now recommend organic methods to control weeds and pests. Any changes you make in this direction will make your garden and home a safer place too.

WHAT LURKS IN THE WORKPLACE?

As you can imagine, different occupations will vary greatly in their exposure to *Chemical Calories*. Certain factory workers, painters and decorators, hairdressers and mechanics tend to have a relatively high exposure. In most cases the majority of this contamination is via their lungs and skin. But they are not the only ones at risk, for even office workers can be regularly exposed to chemicals in stationery or newly fitted carpets, or in the cleaning solutions used on the office furniture.

On top of this, some buildings are regularly sprayed with insecticides to prevent infestations and this could increase your exposure to *Chemical Calories* quite dramatically. To find out more about your particular working environment, you need to make inquiries about which chemicals are used, and how often. Be warned though, the results may shock you.

CHEMICAL CALORIES AT THE DENTIST

Advances in dentistry and dental awareness mean that we tend to keep our teeth for much longer than our ancestors did. In order to achieve this, dentists now use a whole range of substances to patch up or replace broken teeth. The problem is that any substance on our teeth is likely to be ground up and swallowed with the rest of our food.

Recently I had to embark upon a long course of treatment originating from breaking one of my teeth on a piece of organic homemade popcorn – yes, ironic, isn't it! This experience really opened my eyes to the substances dentists now use routinely. For instance, I discovered that most of the materials used by dentists as temporary fillings or sealants contain a mixture of chemicals and plastics. The materials used to get dental impressions are also plastic, white fillings contain plastic, and amalgam mercury fillings contain heavy metals.

Even if you choose the safer option of repairing teeth with

porcelain, the repair is usually inserted with plastics, unless you request otherwise. Even false teeth are made with plastics! All these materials will leach *Chemical Calories* into your mouth. The amount of chemicals seems small, but because repair materials are constantly wearing away in your mouth and being ingested, the level of contamination from many of these interventions can actually be measured in your blood.

In the *Canadian Dental Association Journal* Dr M. Levy suggests that more research should be carried out into the potential health effects from certain dental materials, such as dental amalgam. And he also suggests that in the meantime more of an effort should be put into preserving healthy teeth and that the restorative dental materials in current practice should be used judiciously.[6]

While I definitely don't want to stop you going to the dentist, it is worthwhile finding out from your dentist the options open to you and then choosing the safest treatment (I opted for the porcelain repair).

CHEMICAL CALORIES ARE EVERYWHERE

Finally, *Chemical Calories* bombard us from all directions as we walk, shop and take part in local activities. If you live in the middle of a city or close to a motorway, particularly if it has stationary or slow-moving traffic for much of the day, the chances are that the air outside and inside your house will be polluted with *Chemical Calories* from exhaust fumes.

Green and welcoming city parks may in fact be heavily sprayed with herbicides, since this is a cheap method of keeping down weeds. Additional pollution belches out from factories, chemical plants and power stations. All these factors do their bit to rack up the total levels of *Chemical Calories* in the environment.

But cities are not the only danger zones – agricultural areas where food is grown intensively can also be very polluted with pesticide sprays. If you consider that as little as 1 per cent of the spray can go on the crop where it is needed and that the rest either stays in the air or falls to the ground,[7] you will realize that the countryside can have its problems too!

So now you know where the problems are. The next chapter will help you deal with them by telling you about the easy ways in which you can significantly lower the *Chemical Calorie* content of your home. It won't take too long before you realize that it is possible to make a significant difference without too much expense or upheaval. So don't be too depressed, as there really is light ahead!

12. Beating the *Chemical Calorie*
Lowering Your Overall Exposure

The beauty of reducing the amount of *Chemical Calories* in your home is that by lowering your overall exposure to them you will be making real advances in preventing further damage to your *Slimming System*. Over time, this is what will help you achieve and maintain your ideal weight, so it's worth making a real effort to discover how it can be done.

Since I started to cut down on *Chemical Calories* in my food and home, I no longer have any fear of the scales. My *Slimming System* is now strong enough to maintain my weight on its own. In fact, despite not actively dieting, and still having some of my favourite foods daily, I am still continuing to lose weight – slowly, I admit, but the trend is still downwards. I am delighted, as I now have a figure which I am very happy with and which requires very little effort to maintain.

Now it's your turn to discover my secret!

WHERE TO BEGIN – AIR YOUR AIR

As I previously mentioned, the first thing you need to do is pace yourself. It is simply not possible to create a *Chemical-Calorie*-free environment overnight, and in any case it is not necessary to endure the time, cost and inconvenience of ripping everything out and starting all over again. There are lots of simple ways to significantly reduce the *Chemical Calories* around your home which will require very little effort.

For example, as a large number of *Chemical Calories* in your home will be airborne, the quickest way to get rid of them is simply to open the windows. Try to make sure that you open windows at the front and back of the house, as this will increase the flow of air. This is particularly valuable in new houses, as many of them are now hermetically sealed. Ventilating the house for just half an hour can really make all the difference.

Even if you live in a city, indoor air still tends to be far more polluted than city air, so it is still a good idea to allow some ventilation. Of course, if you live next to a very busy road it would be wise to close the windows during peak-hour traffic. If the outside air is exceptionally polluted, you could always consider investing in an air filter, which filters out pollutants, many of which will contain *Chemical Calories* from exhaust fumes.

Another way of reducing *Chemical Calories* is by filling your home with plants. It has been found that spider plants, Boston ferns, elephant-ear philodendron, English ivy and aloe vera appear to be particularly efficient 'air filters', and are very good at removing solvents from the atmosphere.[1]

GET RID OF HOUSEHOLD PESTICIDES

One of the really positive things you can do to lower the *Chemical Calorie* content of your home is to get rid of all your pesticides. By that I mean your fly sprays, insect-repellents, flea powders, flea shampoos, headlice shampoos, weedkillers, ant and slug killers and all other types of home and garden pesticides. But don't put them down the sink where they will poison the water supply – dispose of them responsibly. Many local authorities provide safe disposal for these toxic chemicals at council dumps and waste-recycling centres, so if you clear out these chemicals from your kitchen or garden shed, there is a place where they can and should be disposed of safely.

Next you will need to find alternative treatments. For example, if your dog has fleas, then rather than spraying the whole house with toxic chemicals you could use a herbal shampoo or spray and buy a herbal flea-collar, which contains natural repellents such as pennyroyal or eucalyptus oils. There are even herbal flea powders to use on carpets and furnishings. They usually contain pyrethrum (a plant extract) or borax.

Throughout the rest of the house, you can use citrus oils to repel flies. Try spraying the room with a solution of essential citrus oils and water. Cockroaches can be eliminated by mixing equal parts of baking soda and powdered sugar. Spread this mixture where they congregate and repeat every one to two weeks until they are gone.

To eradicate ants you can use mint – they despise it. Mix one cup of water with two teaspoons of essential oil of peppermint and spray the mixture wherever the ants come in – on windowsills, countertops and along skirting boards.

There are so many natural remedies, and I don't have the space to cover them all here. I suggest you consult a local health shop or herbalist, or look on the Internet. You will find that because of health worries from modern-day pesticides, many of the long-forgotten traditional ways of pest-control are being rediscovered and are coming back into favour.

ALTERNATIVE CLEANING SOLUTIONS

The vast majority of domestic cleaning products contain a cornucopia of toxic and fattening chemicals, so the best thing is to try to find alternatives. To be honest, cleaning a home doesn't need complex ingredients: white vinegar, baking soda, or borax diluted with water in liquid or paste form all make cheap and safe cleaning products. Vinegar and water is excellent for cleaning windows. Lemon juice will work wonders washing dishes or cleaning your loo (just look how many artificial products still use lemon juice).

If this approach doesn't appeal to you, you'll find plenty of alternative cleaning solutions in your local health shop or supermarket. If there are particular products you really can't find a replacement for, it's a good idea to seal them up in an airtight container such as an old biscuit tin. This will significantly reduce the amount of vapour they release into the air, which will otherwise end up in your lungs.

LOW-*CHEMICAL-CALORIE* COSMETICS
AND TOILETRIES

One of the most direct ways to absorb *Chemical Calories* is to put them straight on to your skin in creams and cosmetics, so a good rule of thumb is to try to use natural or organic products without artificial scents, colour or preservatives. Now be warned: you have got to keep your wits about you here, as the way that products are marketed can be very misleading. Some natural-sounding products can in fact be heaving with chemicals.

To see whether a product really is what it claims to be, take a look at the label. If the product suggests that it is organic, it must by law list all the ingredients as organic and contain the relevant organic certification mark. If it doesn't, it will not be organic in the 'chemical-free' sense of the word, although it may be organic in the sense that it is made up of animal- or plant-based products – which, as you can imagine, is a completely different thing.

As more and more people are becoming aware of the importance of truly natural beauty products, the range on the market is exploding. While it may take you time to seek out new favourites, the rewards will most definitely be worth it.

If on the other hand you really can't bear to get rid of certain favourite cosmetics, why don't you just cut right back on the amounts you use? Another strategy would be to ask whether the company has any plans to lower the amount of additives. Believe you me, if enough valued customers were to start demanding changes, this would probably happen very quickly!

Remember that just because a product is expensive it doesn't mean that it has more natural products and is lower in *Chemical Calories*, as often the reverse can be true.

Transfer moisturizers and other cosmetics into glass containers if they are packaged in plastic. If you don't want to do this, keep them refrigerated, as this lowers their *Chemical Calorie* loading. A lot of plastic contamination arises in the first place because people are reluctant to throw away pots of cream that they bought years ago. I used to be dreadful about doing this myself and kept some things for years. This can actually be a problem, as the longer you keep a product in plastic, the more contaminated it will be – especially if it is perched on the windowsill in full glare of the sunlight and in a warm humid atmosphere.

Recently I got a bit of a shock when I ran out of my favourite shampoo and went back to an older bottle of 'natural' shampoo. As I poured it out, I got a strong smell of plastic. As you can imagine, it ended up straight in the bin along with a whole lot of other products. If you can smell a strong whiff of plastic from anything that you intend using or even eating, throw it away.

KEEPING *CHEMICAL CALORIES* OUT OF CLOTHES AND FABRICS

In order to keep the *Chemical Calorie* content as low as possible in clothes and fabrics, you have three priorities. The first thing to do is to try to buy clothes and fabrics made of natural fibres (provided there are no residual pesticides on the latter). The second thing, if you consider yourself or the recipient of the clothing to be at low risk from fire, is to check whether it has been treated with flame-retardant chemicals. And the third is to check whether the fabric has been chemically treated to be 'easy care'.

Synthetic fabrics are in essence plastics, so they will off-gas *Chemical Calories*. Did you know that children as well as adults will have more abnormal heart rhythms and blood-pressure changes if they wear synthetic clothes, compared to those who wear cotton?[2]

For most people, switching to natural fibres is not really a problem, since the selection is pretty extensive, but you still need to be careful about chemical finishes. The ideal solution is to buy organic fabrics.

This is a pretty specialized market, but it is possible to buy natural organic untreated fabrics, clothes and other goods from a range that includes hemp, cotton, wool, silk and linen. The market for organic fabrics is growing rapidly because of environmental concerns about the vast amounts of pesticides used in growing cotton. It's sad but true that pesticides for cotton growers have been estimated at a stunning third of the entire worldwide production of pesticides.[3] If you buy organic fabrics you have a guarantee that no added pesticide residues or chemicals will be found on them and you also know that they haven't contributed to the contamination of the land. Indeed, many people who wear them are convinced that organic fabrics are not only softer but also stronger.

The main disadvantages are their limited colours and designs and generally higher price. However, things are changing on the colour front and more organic companies are looking into the use of vegetable dyes or low-impact dyeing methods. Low-impact dyeing uses synthetic dyes but minimizes the use of synthetic chemicals in processing the fibres. As with everything, pester power is the key to making these products more widely available. The more people who ask for chemical-free clothes, the more likely companies are to introduce new lines.

Even if you can't get organic clothes, you should ask whether the clothes are treated with flame-retardants, as many companies are starting to cut down on the routine treatment of clothes with these chemicals, particularly for the baby and toddler age groups.

While on the subject of clothes and fabrics – if you dry-clean clothes, curtains and other items they will be covered in a solvent that contains lots of *Chemical Calories*. Either hang your clothes out to air in a well-ventilated place for a few days after dry-cleaning, or, best of all, try to find a dry-cleaner who uses steam instead of solvents.

One last point: it's generally best to keep the amount of conditioner and detergent you use in washing clothes to a minimum, so experiment with cutting the amount you use down to as low a level as you possibly can. You could also use one of the growing number of environmentally friendly detergents that are available.

LOW-*CHEMICAL-CALORIE* FURNITURE

Most furniture now has to be treated with flame-retardants to pass current fire regulations, so the chances are that the fabric your sofa is covered with and the foam it is filled with are both loaded with *Chemical Calories*. Even furniture made from natural wood may now be treated with flame-retardants or preservatives.

If you want to avoid these chemicals, based on personal fire risk versus toxic chemical preference, buying older second-hand furniture is often cheaper and it usually tends to be of much better quality. The stuffings are all natural fibres such as horsehair or cotton, and the upholstery fabrics are not treated with chemicals – unless of course the furniture has recently been re-covered.

If you prefer newer pieces, stick with furniture made from natural substances such as wood, glass and metal. The best types of stuffing and upholstery are untreated fibres such as cotton, wool, jute and silk. Avoid especially buying furniture made of chipboard or plastic, as these will off-gas. And when you look for soft furnishings, avoid stuffing such as foam, styrene, foam chips or foam rubber.

Probably the most important piece of furniture of all is your bed. It is vitally important to ensure that this is low in *Chemical Calories*, since you spend so much time there. Because of this, the first items of 'organic' furniture I ever bought were organic mattresses for my boys, as well as for my husband and me. I think it was well worth the extra money, but if you can't change your mattress, you can significantly lower your exposure to *Chemical Calories* by putting several layers of blanket between the mattress and yourself.

So far as bedlinen, duvets and pillows are concerned, it is also far better to use natural untreated fibres such as wool, cotton, linen or silk.

You have to accept that schools, nurseries and other public places are bound by safety regulations and therefore by law need to have products treated with flame-retardants. In this case, or if there is a smoker in the family or there is a fire risk, my advice will be not to stop using flame-retardant products.

However, what you can do is be more selective in the products you buy. Choose those products which are naturally flame-resistant, which means that they don't burn at all, such as glass or metal. In addition, pick those which have not used PBBs or PBDEs, because out of all the many chemicals used, these are among the most long-lived and toxic. This will take an extra effort, as it is fairly unlikely that the chemicals used will be listed on the product as such, although they should be present on the product data sheet. Alternatively the company's representative should be able to help you out.

BASIC ROOM FITTINGS WHICH ARE LOW IN *CHEMICAL CALORIES*

So many of the things that we have in our homes contain *Chemical Calories*, making it really quite a battle to avoid them. Let's start at the bottom, and work up through a typical room.

Floors are vital in keeping down the overall level of contamination. You should avoid buying vinyl products, synthetic carpets or even woollen carpets if they are treated with pesticides. The best types of flooring are made from natural untreated woods, cork, linoleum (natural variety with no added plastics), terracotta tiles, slate, limestone or sandstone. All these surfaces are hard-wearing and will not off-gas. Just be careful not to spoil your natural wood with a plastic coating of varnish. Natural oil waxes are available and do not contain *Chemical Calories*.

Although most of these surfaces are pretty hard, they can be made softer by using untreated rugs made from natural fibres. You can even buy organic carpet and underlay which is virtually free of *Chemical Calories*. I found that the demand was so great for organic carpet that there was a very long waiting list – put it this way, I had to wait over seven months to receive the one I ordered!

If you can't get organic carpet, or don't want to wait that long, you can buy a wool carpet, so long as you make sure it has not been treated with the flame-retardants PBBs, PBDEs or with pesticides. Look under the carpet before you buy it to make sure it has been backed with natural fabrics rather than plastics.

Finally, when buying carpet underlay try to get the most natural substance available. You may even find it less expensive than the more commonly used plastic- or rubber-based underlays, which fill the air with *Chemical Calories* as soon as they are fitted!

Next we come to the walls. If you want to use wallpaper, make sure it does not contain plastics or vinyl and look for paste that does not contain fungicide, which is now available. If you choose to paint the walls, there are quite a few organic paints on the market. The range of natural colours is very good and you have the added peace of mind that they will not off-gas over time. If you can't get organic paints for your purpose, choose paints that are low in solvents.

One last point: make sure that you keep any paints and white spirit in sealed containers, preferably in a building not directly connected to your home, otherwise they will fill the whole house with *Chemical Calories*.

LOW-*CHEMICAL-CALORIE* CONSTRUCTION

This section is only applicable if you are going to rebuild part of your house or build an extension. Having building work done is always stressful, but it is really worth making an extra effort to source natural building materials that are low in *Chemical Calories*. Many current building materials are heavily treated with chemicals, and once they are incorporated into the fabric of the house they are very hard to deal with.

When I rebuilt my kitchen recently I made sure that the builder was happy to use more traditional and less treated substances. Fortunately he had done this kind of thing before and was very happy to help. He supplied me with a data sheet (a list of all the chemicals or materials contained in a product) for all the products he was intending to use. I then went through all these items checking whether they were acceptable. If not, we looked for alternative products from a shop that specialized in organic or environmentally friendly building materials.

I must say I was initially surprised at the number of everyday products that were contaminated with chemicals. Consequently, we ended up using quite a few of the specialist products. But at the end of the day I now have a kitchen that I am very happy to spend much of my time in, since it is as low in *Chemical Calories* as I could possibly make it.

Although it is impossible to offer advice on specific projects, there are a few general rules that apply across the board:

- Try to use building methods that avoid using adhesives.
- If you have to use glue, then silicon rubber glue, latex, hide glue and water washable wood glue are less toxic than epoxy adhesives.
- The best sealants are made of pure silicone or linseed oil putty.
- When using wood, use solid untreated hard wood, rather than chemically treated soft wood such as pine. Definitely avoid using plywood, MDF (medium density fibreboard) or chipboard.
- Use wooden window-frames rather than PVC fittings.
- Avoid products that are made of plastics and treated with fire-retardants if possible.

THE LOW-CHEMICAL-CALORIE GARDEN

Once you have chucked out all your herbicides, weedkillers, insect sprays and other noxious substances (responsibly of course), you will have significantly lowered your exposure to *Chemical Calories*. The next process will take a little longer, as you need to discover new techniques to discourage weeds and pests naturally.

Since agriculture played such a vital role long before chemicals were invented, there is already a mountain of information on traditional practices. Much of it has been ignored for years, but a growing number of farmers are reviving older methods to farm their land and raise their animals organically.

If you take your gardening seriously, there are now lots of books available on organic horticultural techniques. For instance, to keep down pests in your vegetable garden, you can achieve a lot with a technique known as companion planting. Some pests identify crops by scent, and a neighbouring crop with a powerful scent (such as onions) will confuse them. Even if you don't grow vegetables and want to preserve your roses, planting chives round your roses will not only protect them from disease, but somewhat surprisingly enhance their perfume too.

Another technique is to encourage your allies, the predators that feed on aphids and other pests. A pesticide cannot recognize the difference between good and bad bugs and just kills the lot. But by leaving piles of wood, stones or leaves undisturbed over winter, where many ladybirds and other predators hibernate, you can tip the balance in favour of the predators and use them to reduce the number of aphids in your garden. Did you know that one ladybird eats many thousands of aphids in a lifetime?

Birds are also excellent predators, though they tend to eat your soft fruit too! I have just created a flower garden near my vegetable patch and filled one area with flowers to encourage pollinators and another area with flowers that produce seed-heads for birds. I am also exceedingly fortunate to have an organic vegetable garden that provides us with mountains of food throughout the year. To help us achieve this we make our own compost from our kitchen household waste.

I have to say, few pleasures in life can compare with eating freshly picked fruit and vegetables which are brimming with flavour and bursting with oodles of slimming nutrients.

THE LOW-*CHEMICAL-CALORIE* WORKPLACE

Since most people spend so much of their lives at work, we need to see to it that our exposure to *Chemical Calories* at work is as low as possible.

As with your home, you need to have good ventilation, particularly if you work with chemicals. If you work in a traditional office, it is a good idea to keep inks, carbon paper, liquid paper and rubber cement in sealed containers. Bringing a plant into your office may help reduce the level of air pollution. And if the chemicals used to clean the office are overpowering, find out whether these can be changed or used more sparingly (a good argument, as this will save your employer money). It may also be a good idea to find out more about pesticides used in the buildings.

I do accept that in certain professions (such as hairdressing and painting and decorating) it may be particularly difficult to reduce the level of *Chemical Calories*. However, if there were no difference in cost, what would stop your company using products that contain fewer chemicals? It could even be a positive selling point: who would actually want to have chemicals that could possibly make them fat sprayed on to their hair?

As pesticides and chemicals endanger not only your weight, but also your health, it is actually in the best interests of employers to provide a healthy environment. So you may have more say in the matter than you might initially think.

AVOIDING *CHEMICAL CALORIES* IN YOUR ENVIRONMENT

You can do quite a lot to lower the level of *Chemical Calories* in your home, but there is relatively little you can do about air pollution outside. If you are planning to move house, the best areas to live are those away from large factories, big cities, major roadways and areas of intensive horticulture.

If you have no plans to move, there are some things you can do to reduce your exposure. If your house is surrounded by fields that are sprayed regularly, make sure that the farmer tells you when he intends to spray so that you can stay in and keep your windows closed. If you have children, going to parks may be a regular event for you. Try to find out if your local park uses lots of pesticides to control weeds. If they do, you should stay clear of the areas where they spray, and stay away altogether while the spraying is going on. The same holds true if you live in an agricultural area. Never walk through a field just after or during spraying.

Even when you are driving in your car you can be exposed to large amounts of *Chemical Calories* from the other cars on the road. Much of the exhaust fumes from the car in front will go straight into your car if you are driving too close behind it. Try to stay more than four car lengths behind the car in front of you, as this gives the exhaust some time to disperse before you drive through it. Not to mention giving you more time to react in case of an accident ahead! You could also invest in a filter on your air inlet and recycle air around your car if you have to stop in a traffic jam.

THE NEXT STEP FORWARD

Now you know how to lower your exposure to *Chemical Calories* in many different areas of your life, and by gradually introducing these changes you will be well on your way to achieving that goal of permanent weight loss. However, it will still take your body time to rid itself of all the *Chemical Calories* that it has built up over the years.

Most people will prefer to see quicker results, and the good news is that there are many other ways in which this process can be not only speeded up but also greatly enhanced. These revolve around using supplements, foods, diet and exercise.

Part Three of the book will tell you how the proper use of the above methods can not only significantly enhance the functioning of your natural *Slimming System* but can also accelerate the rate at which *Chemical Calories* are removed from your body. Unlike most diet books, which are simply based around methods involving starving yourself of calories, the whole emphasis here is based on feeding and protecting your natural *Slimming System*. The next chapter is brimming with all the information you need to revitalize your natural *Slimming System*, simply by feeding it the foods and supplements it needs.

PART THREE

Detoxify and Lose Weight

13. Repair and Revitalize Your Natural *Slimming System*

By now you know a great deal about avoiding exposure to *Chemical Calories*. While this aspect is important to the success of the programme, it is only part of the overall strategy to lose weight. Now we need to turn to the next major task, which is to optimize your own natural *Slimming System*.

If your *Slimming System* were in perfect working order, it would take on all the work of dieting for you, adjusting your appetite and metabolism so that your body would lose weight without any conscious effort. In other words, by rebuilding your natural *Slimming System* you will be working with your body and not continually battling against it to lose weight and keep it off – effectively releasing yourself from a lifetime of dieting and deprivation.

So what does it take to rebuild the *Slimming System*? Fortunately, most of the work can be done by a combination of the right foods and supplements. The chances are that you got into this predicament because your body, overloaded with *Chemical Calories*, badly lacks many of the essential slimming nutrients that it needs because of the increased demands made on it.

To help pull your *Slimming System* out of intensive care and back to full health, I will go through all the foods and nutrients which it needs in order to have new life breathed into it. Then watch those excess pounds just melt away!

HOW CERTAIN FATS CAN MAKE YOU SLIM

Fats have unfortunately got themselves a very bad name and are often seen as the enemy of dieters. But in fact the right kinds of fats are absolutely essential in achieving weight loss, as without them our *Slimming System* would fail to work properly.

You may not realize it, but not all fats are the same. Your diet will actually contain two different kinds of fats: most of them will be saturated (bad) fats, typically animal fats, but only a few will be the essential (good) fats, typically fish oils or fats from nuts and seeds. Saturated fats are not essential in our diet, since we can make them ourselves. In fact, most people's diets contain far too many saturated fats. But worlds apart are the essential fats.

These polyunsaturated fats are quite literally essential to our diet. This is because our bodies cannot manufacture their own supply, and therefore are totally reliant on us eating them in food. They are also vital to the smooth working of the *Slimming System*. To put it bluntly, without them we would simply not be able to lose weight efficiently.

Although the very idea that fats can make us lose weight is counter-intuitive, they achieve this in the following ways:

- Massively increasing the rate at which we burn up our body fat stores.[1]
- Increasing the levels of energy we can produce from food (the more energy we create, the fewer calories we store as fats).[2]
- Stabilizing blood sugar levels and so reducing sugar cravings (also preventing the development of diabetes).
- Boosting the levels of slimming hormones, in particular the hormones that suppress our appetite for fats (catecholamines).
- Raising our body's sensitivity to slimming hormones, so speeding up the rate at which calories are burned up.
- Improving our ability to retain slimming vitamins and minerals in our bodies.[3]
- Suppressing free radical production and so preventing damage to our *Slimming Systems* (particularly in the more crucial high-fat-containing parts).[4]

If you are not getting enough essential fats, your ability to lose weight will greatly pick up if you start taking them. Despite most people's diets containing a huge chunk of fat (typically 40 per cent of the total calories), little of this is essential fats. The hard reality is that, unless you are making a special effort to include these fats in your diet, the chances are that you will be deficient in them – disastrous news for your ability to lose weight!

THE IMPORTANCE OF THESE ESSENTIAL OMEGA-3 AND OMEGA-6 FATS

So why are these essential fats so important? Well, it all stems from many thousands of years ago, when humanity was in its infancy. At that time we were a shore-dwelling people and tended to eat large quantities of fish as well as scavenging for nuts and seeds. As all these foods contained large amounts of omega-3 and omega-6 oils, which are the essential fats that possess these slimming actions, so our bodies adapted to use these fats extensively – and we still need them just as much today.[5]

However, over the years our diet has changed dramatically – our intake of nuts and fish has decreased and our food has become more processed. As a direct consequence, the total quantity of essential fats in our diet has fallen right away.

Modern-day living also conspires in other ways to lower the level of fatty acids in our diet. Heat not only rapidly destroys the slimming benefits of essential fats but transforms them into harmful substances known as trans-fats, which prevent you absorbing any of the remaining essential fatty acids (olive oil and butter, however, are safe for use in cooking as they contain fats which don't tend to form trans-fats).

So by eating fried foods such as chips, you could actually be reducing the absorption of the essential fatty acids that you do manage to eat in your diet. Other types of food-processing also produce these trans-fats, such as the process of turning vegetable oils into margarine (hydrogenation).

Making a bad situation worse, few processed foods and ready-made meals contain any beneficial essential fats. This is because they tend to go off more quickly, reducing the shelf life of foods that contain them. So you can see that because of our changing lifestyles and habits, most of our bodies will now be crying out to be fed more essential fats.

HOW TO RESTORE THE SITUATION

Omega-3 fats are the ones that you are most likely to be deficient in, particularly since they are easily damaged in their natural form. They also appear to play a more important role in lowering our weight. Many people already take omega-3 supplements in the form of fish oils, but since some of them have been found to be heavily polluted with *Chemical Calories* I would not advise using them.[6] Saying this, some manufacturers acknowledge that there is a problem and are actively removing some of the contaminants from fish oils and so making them safer, but you should not assume they are all doing it and to a similar extent.

Organic flax (otherwise known as linseed oil), on the other hand, is a rich and unpolluted alternative source. Its importance has been recognized for years, as it is one of the earliest crops known to be cultivated and its name in Latin translates to 'the much needed'. You can buy it in liquid form to take off a spoon, or in capsules, since you may not find the taste particularly pleasant (for the recommended dose see Chapters 15 and 19). I have to admit, the first time I took it I gagged. But after uncovering so much powerful and positive information about its benefits, I have got more used to it and now can take it quite readily.

Remember to keep essential oils in the fridge, as they are so easily oxidized. One more thing, don't take them last thing at night, as they may increase your energy levels so much that they could stop you from going to sleep!

Another sensible way of boosting your intake of omega-3 fats is by taking them in your diet, as they are found in seeds such as flax and pumpkin and in certain nuts, such as walnuts. To a lesser extent they can also be found in wild meats such as venison and in some other meats, particularly if they are organic. This is because the higher the animal's diet is in omega-3 fats, the higher the level found in the meat.

Just a word of caution here: I have also seen some eggs advertised as high in omega-3 fats. But before you rush out and buy them, make sure that the hens have not been fed with fish oils, otherwise you may get a large dose of *Chemical Calories* too.

Omega-6 fats are found more widely, and on the whole we tend to have larger amounts of these fats in our diet because more foods contain them. For example, most vegetable oils contain far higher levels of omega-6 oils compared to omega-3 oils, and they are also found in flax oil, seeds, nuts and meats.

Consequently, there is not such a great need to supplement omega-6 fats, but to ensure you are getting enough on this programme I advise that you do take evening primrose oil. The message is: eat more essential oils and less saturated fat and you are more likely to lose weight.

THE ROLE OF CARBOHYDRATES IN THE
SLIMMING SYSTEM

Recently a whole new generation of diet books has virtually demonized carbohydrates, blaming them for weight gain and a host of other problems. Certainly excessive carbohydrates will cause weight gain, but moderate levels of carbohydrates are essential for the smooth running of the *Slimming System*. They are the body's basic fuel for energy, and without them a whole range of body functions begins to shut down. So let's find out a bit more about what carbohydrates are and where they can be found.

Carbohydrates can be divided into three main groups, ranging from simple sugars to the complex carbohydrates:

1. Sugars, commonly found in fruit and a whole range of
   other foods, are very easy nutrients for the body to
   convert into energy.

2. Starches (or polysaccharides) are long chains of sugars, which the body needs to break down before it can convert into energy.

3. Fibre (soluble and insoluble) is made up of sugars but they are bound together in such a way that the body cannot digest them, so they have no nutritional value, but aid the body's waste-disposal systems.

Carbohydrates play an absolutely vital role in powering the *Slimming System*, because they:

- Ensure your muscles are packed with readily accessible sugar stores, so you have plenty of energy to power exercise.
- Increase energy levels and so encourage exercise.
- Greatly raise your metabolic rate, as they strongly stimulate the sympathetic nervous system, promoting the release of the slimming hormones catecholamines, epinephrine and norepinepherine. This results in converting up to 20 per cent of the original energy value (calories) of all the carbohydrates you eat into heat that is then easily lost.
- Suppress the appetite for more carbohydrates, preventing potential bingeing.

Although the system was designed to work smoothly, the presence of *Chemical Calories* has changed all this by damaging the ways in which the body metabolizes carbohydrates.

I have experienced this myself. For years before I took supplements or ate organic foods, my own ability to control my sugar levels was appalling. If I didn't eat something every two or three hours, my blood sugar would take a dive. I would get into a real state. My concentration would go first, then I would get very sweaty. And if I didn't eat something straight away, I would get even worse. My husband quickly came to recognize the signs – he could spot a crisis-in-the-making way before I could and made sure I had something to eat immediately.

Now, since I have lowered my exposure to chemicals and started taking supplements, I really don't have this problem at all, as my body now seems to be able to regulate my blood sugar on its own.

I was therefore not too surprised when on examining the relevant research I discovered that chemicals appear to damage carbohydrate metabolism in a number of different ways.

- The appetite for carbohydrates increases, caused by a number of factors such as damage to a whole range of hormones that control the appetite for sugar.[7]
- Chemicals interfere with the process of converting glucose into usable energy. In other words, the body is less able to use up carbohydrates.[8]
- Dieting exacerbates this damage. People, particularly women, tend to eat need more sugary foods rather than starchy foods after dieting.[9]

The damage caused by *Chemical Calories* could explain why over-weight people appear to have a reduced ability to break down carbohydrates. When overweight people, who generally as a group tend to have high levels of chemicals in their bodies, go on a fast they use approximately half as much carbohydrate as lean people use.[10] Even when they are given readily usable glucose, overweight people still tend to draw on fats for energy rather than carbohydrates.

This diminished ability to metabolize carbohydrates fully also explains why there has been a rash of very low carbohydrate diets on the market. But while the idea seems like a good one on the surface, there are many problems associated with the exclusion of virtually all carbohydrates from the diet.

THE PROS AND CONS OF LOW-CARBOHYDRATE DIETS

By cutting right back on carbohydrates, you will certainly reduce the amount of excess carbohydrates which can be converted to weight. You will also lower the levels of insulin, and this increases mobilization of the body fat stores. Superficially this seems like a very plausible idea and will probably achieve good temporary weight losses.

However, the presence of fattening chemicals is another signifi-cant cause of weight gain, and cutting carbohydrates out of the diet will definitely not treat this. In truth, there are many disadvantages to a very low carbohydrate diet and they include the following:

- Increased absorption of pesticides, as pesticides are far more readily absorbed from high-fat foods rather than high-carbohydrate foods.[11]
- Reduced ability to metabolize toxic chemicals, as this process needs carbohydrates.[12]
- Reduced stimulation of the sympathetic nervous system, resulting in reduced fat burning.
- Huge carbohydrate cravings, caused by low blood sugar which will trigger the release of hormones.
- Shrinkage of lean muscle, as your body needs to break down muscle to produce readily usable sugars.
- Reduced levels of slimming micronutrients usually found in carbo-hydrate-rich foods such as fruit and vegetables.
- Increased release of fat-soluble toxins, as more fats are mobilized.
- High risk of arteriosclerosis, as high levels of mobilized fats and choles-terol in the blood in combination with prolonged low insulin levels is known to increase the likelihood of heart disease and strokes.

So while too many carbohydrates may make us fatter, too few will have the same effect in the long term and more serious damage is also possible. The ideal is to eat carbohydrates in moderation and to choose complex carbohydrates, as they release their sugars over several hours rather than in one massive rush. And the simple sugars that you do eat should be mainly in the form of fruit.

You have to realize that until your chemical loading is tackled, you will still crave sweet foods. Though, as the levels of *Chemical Calories* drop, your ability to handle carbohydrates, like mine, will greatly improve. And as well as significantly reducing your sugar cravings it will also mean that you start burning up carbohydrates more efficiently.

THE PROTEINS THAT KEEP YOU SLIM

Virtually all aspects of the *Slimming System* are controlled in some way by substances or structures containing protein. So an upset in protein metabolism or a shortage in any particular protein can result in damage to any one of the numerous mechanisms vital in controlling our body weight. So what types of proteins are we talking about?

Starting from the basics: a protein is a large complex molecule, which is made up of units known as amino acids. There are approximately twenty-nine different amino acids in the body, of which eight are 'essential', meaning that the body cannot manufacture them and must get them from food and supplements.

Despite their name, many of the 'non-essential' amino acids are absolutely vital for the smooth functioning of the body, but we can usually manufacture them ourselves if we do not get enough from other sources. So how do they control our weight?

In brief, proteins are used in the *Slimming System* to:

- Form the structure of the most important slimming hormones.
- Speed up the metabolism (protein-rich foods can lift the metabolic rate to 30 per cent above normal for 3–12 hours).
- Allow energy production to take place.
- Build muscles so we can burn off body fat during exercise.

HOW CHEMICALS DAMAGE PROTEINS

The problem with toxic chemicals is that they appear to damage virtually every aspect of the way our body handles, absorbs and creates proteins as well as increasing the rate at which they are lost from the body.[13] They even directly damage the proteins themselves.

So although we may think we are eating enough proteins, chemical damage means that our bodies can fail to extract and use the proteins they need to allow our *Slimming System* to work properly. This chemical damage is caused in the following ways:

- Lowering levels of amino acids that we specifically need to create our slimming hormones (catecholamines and thyroid hormones).[14]
- Damaging the way our body responds to slimming hormones.
- Upsetting our body's natural rhythm. Billions of carefully timed sequences are put out of sync, making the whole metabolic system less effective. This will also severely reduce the body's ability to burn off excess fat.[15]
- Hindering the creation of all types of body proteins, including those essential in energy production and calorie burning such as body muscle.[16]

WHAT YOU CAN DO ABOUT IT

We all need to eat a moderate and balanced amount of protein in our diet to keep the *Slimming System* in peak working order. So where can we find the proteins we need? Most people assume that we get most of our proteins from meat, dairy products and eggs. While these are very rich sources, they are not the only ones – a whole range of fruit, vegetables, nuts, beans and pulses also contain proteins. OK, although these sources can be less rich, in combination they are still well able to supply the protein needs of the *Slimming System*.

However, the presence of toxic chemicals makes it more difficult for the body to get and create all the proteins it needs from food alone, so it is a good idea to supplement key slimming proteins in the diet. I believe that it is really only necessary to supplement four slimming proteins.

The first is methionine, because it is the amino acid most damaged by chemicals. It plays one of the most essential roles in promoting energy metabolism, so it is particularly important to ensure you get enough. The next is glutathione, the main role of which is chemical detoxification and which is therefore always in great demand.

Thirdly, tyrosine – this forms the base structure for the most important slimming hormones of all, the catecholamines and the thyroid hormones. Many of us tend to be short of this vitally important protein because we are unable to create enough of it ourselves due to chemical damage. It is better to take tyrosine supplements in the morning, as it will help boost your energy levels.

And finally, we need more serotonin. This powerfully suppresses the appetite. So if the body's levels run low, this will result in food cravings and binge eating. As serotonin is also readily damaged by the presence of chemicals, it is definitely worthwhile supplementing. Ideally you should take serotonin, in the form of its precursor L-5 hydroxytryptophan, before you go to sleep, as it can make you drowsy.

The good news is, as your loading of *Chemical Calories* falls, your ability to use and create new proteins will increase and your need for these supplements will be reduced. For most people, whose bodies are loaded with *Chemical Calories* right now, protein supplements will be of great benefit in helping to get their *Slimming Systems* back into shape. A healthy *Slimming System* will soon be followed by a shapely body!

VITAMINS AND MINERALS

By now you will already have heard quite a lot about our need for vitamins and minerals. You will also have realized that they play a crucial role in our *Slimming Systems* and that our need for them is greatly increased by chemicals. But before I go on let's start with some basic information. What exactly are vitamins and minerals and where can they be found?

Vitamins and minerals are naturally occurring substances which are essential for normal growth and nutrition. They cannot be synthesized by the body, so we must get them from our diet or from supplements. Because we need only very small amounts, they are commonly described as micronutrients. Although they are usually described together, their structures differ greatly.

Vitamins are complex substances which are made by plants, tend to be fragile and are easily destroyed by heat. Minerals are substances found in the earth's crust. They are absorbed into plants, which use them for their own growth. Although these micronutrients have no calorific value as such, they are vital ingredients in a healthy diet because they are used as catalysts for most of the processes needed for life.

They enhance growth and energy production, quicken our metabolism, allow detoxification to take place, activate our immune system, facilitate reproduction, promote longevity – and among other things they also help to keep us slim.

HOW VITAMINS ARE ESSENTIAL IN POWERING THE *SLIMMING SYSTEM*

Vitamins and minerals play a pivotal role in weight control. Because of their role as catalysts in speeding up the millions of reactions taking place daily in our bodies, they allow us to convert foodstuffs and body fat into energy. So, to a large extent, they actually determine our ability to burn up calories.

For example, Vitamin A is absolutely essential in order for fat to be burned up and converted into heat. But it is also essential in processing chemicals. So if the body is exposed to larger levels of chemicals there will be less vitamin A left to burn up fat, and this situation will encourage weight gain. As the presence of some chemicals can actually halve the body's store of vitamins, this effect simply cannot be ignored.

But it is not just vitamin A that is important – many other vitamins and minerals play an equally vital role in powering our *Slimming System* and ridding our body of *Chemical Calories*.[17] This is why in this book I have on many occasions described these micronutrients as slimming, as that is often just what they do.

WHY WE NEED MORE AND MORE VITAMINS

Astonishingly, the majority of the population are deficient in at least one vitamin or mineral according to current government recommended guidelines,[18] despite nutritional supplements commonly being taken. This is largely due to changes in diet and the presence of chemicals, resulting in the need for certain vitamins and minerals escalating. So if the supplement tablets don't give us all the micronutrients we need, we will still be deficient in the ones they give us short rations of.

This shortfall of vitamins has massively reduced our ability to keep excess weight off. It has also increased the vulnerability of our *Slimming System* to chemical damage. Bad news for us girls, as women appear to be particularly vulnerable because we tend to eat less food. This reduces even further the opportunity to extract all the micronutrients we now need. Perhaps it also helps to explain why women are gaining twice as much weight as men every year.

OPTIMIZING YOUR NUTRIENT LEVELS

The micronutrients that play a crucial role in powering the *Slimming System* include vitamins A, B1 (thiamine), B2 (riboflavin), B6 (pyridoxine); C, E, Co-enzyme Q10, magnesium and zinc among others. (The charts showing recommended levels for the diet and in the long term can be found in Chapters 15 and 24.)

Even if you cannot get all the micronutrients you need just from your food, it is still a good idea to eat foods that are high in slimming micronutrients, such as uncooked vegetables, salads and fruits. The highest levels of slimming nutrients appear to be found in organic produce and the fresher the produce the better, since levels of vitamins will fall during storage, and plummet during cooking. So a fresh salad of organic fruit and vegetables will take some beating for providing plenty of slimming nutrients.

As well as their micronutrient content, unprocessed raw foods also appear to contain a whole range of other nutrients, known as phytonutrients, which also seem to have some role in enhancing our *Slimming System*.

In addition to eating a certain amount of fresh raw organic produce every day, it is now essential to supplement your diet with tablets containing a good level of vitamins and minerals. This will ensure that, whatever your food intake, you are getting all the micronutrients you need to power your *Slimming System*.

Because a whole range of micronutrients are essential in the smooth running of your *Slimming System*, it is best to take a multi-vitamin and mineral supplement. You can top this up with larger individual doses of certain micronutrients if necessary. However, if you take one or two large doses of individual vitamins or minerals without a good general multivitamin, they will be far less effective and possibly unbalance your *Slimming System*.

So we now need supplements, not just at levels aimed at preventing deficiencies (the Recommended Daily Amounts) but at levels that will optimize the *Slimming System*. By ensuring that your rate of vitamin and mineral supplementation is sufficient, you will be helping your body to slim. Fortunately, as much of the harm done by low levels of micronutrients can be reversed, it is never too late to start!

So now we know what to feed our *Slimming System* to optimize its efficiency. Next we need to deal with the *Chemical Calories* already stored in our bodies that continually damage our *Slimming System*, particularly when we actively cut down on food.

Please understand this: no longer do you have to be stuck with a body full of *Chemical Calories* for life, as it is now possible to remove them from your body safely. Once this is achieved, your *Slimming System* will be boosted to a new level of efficiency, converting your dream of permanent weight loss into reality.

14. Shed Your Body Stores of *Chemical Calories*

Now we know how to cut out *Chemical Calories* from our food, homes, water and environment. Nevertheless, before we can benefit fully from these actions we need to get rid of the massive amounts of *Chemical Calories* which are already present within our bodies and which have been building up throughout our lives.

Fortunately for us, there are safe ways in which we can remove the most persistent and fattening *Chemical Calories*. This chapter will tell you how to shed this build-up safely. Not only will this revitalize your *Slimming System*, but the health- and energy-giving benefits could also be very substantial, allowing you to get the utmost enjoyment out of your new slimmer and fitter body.

HOW DID THE BUILD-UP GET THERE?

Over the last 300,000 years or so, our bodies have evolved to deal with a huge variety of toxins in our food and environment. For centuries our immune systems have protected us by neutralizing and then excreting thousands of poisons in the course of our everyday lives.

The process worked well until very recently, but now our immune systems are facing a new challenge and they are struggling. Today, the food we eat at every meal is laced with all the industrial chemicals, pesticides, fungicides, antibiotics, growth hormones and other drugs used at every stage of food production. Many of these chemicals are extremely toxic, highly persistent and long-lasting.

Our bodies cannot break them down, process them, excrete them or get rid of them by any of its current resources. So it takes the only other option – which is to store them in its tissues. Consequently these unprocessed toxins remain with us, stored in our fat, liver, blood and even our bones, and they are continually building up.

The use of extremely toxic synthetic chemicals in the food chain has resulted in every man, woman and child being permanently contaminated, as some of the more persistent (and highly fattening) chemicals can remain for decades.

We even store and build up some of the less dangerous *Chemical Calories*, which the body could process if it had enough resources.[1] But to process them, the body's waste-disposal mechanisms would need far higher amounts of vitamins and nutrients than it receives even in the most 'balanced' of diets.

For example, to get enough vitamin E to deal fully with these toxins, we would have to eat impossibly large amounts of fat-rich foods.

THE REAL BADDIES

Knowing your enemy is the first step in defeating it, so it is time to talk about the most fattening *Chemical Calories* of all, the persistent, fat-soluble organochlorines. The simple fact is that we have no efficient natural way of breaking them down and removing them from our bodies. They are very stable, highly soluble in fat, and tend to 'take up residence' in the body's fat stores.

Because toxic chemicals are stored in body fat the myth has grown up that they are relatively safe. But body fat is not just inert, or there for life. Over the course of each two to three weeks the entire body fat stores are broken down, circulate in the bloodstream and then are re-created. As it is virtually impossible to separate these chemicals from fat, wherever these fats go, so will the organo-chlorines.

CONVENTIONAL DIETING CAN MAKE YOU FATTER

I think most of us who have ever been on a diet will know from experience that while we might achieve a temporary weight loss, after a few months not only will we have regained all the weight we lost but the chances are that we will weigh more than we did before we even started. What's worse, most of this extra weight tends to be fat. Why does this happen?

It all stems from the fact that when a person goes on a conventional diet they eat less food. Our bodies then urgently need to produce energy from somewhere and, as one of the most readily available sources of energy is body fat, this is used as an energy source. If the energy demands are too great, however, our body fats will be broken up far too rapidly, resulting in large amounts of stored toxins, which have accumulated over the years, being released into our bloodstream. These then circulate and cause increased damage throughout the body.[2]

Crucially, because many of the most essential parts of our *Slimming System*, such as our hormone-producing glands and our brains, have such a good blood supply as well as a high fat content, they are exceedingly vulnerable to damage from these highly fat-soluble chemicals.

Common ways in which we experience this poisoning in the short term are nausea, fatigue, headaches and general unwellness.[3] This may explain why people can feel unwell or get headaches for the first few days of a diet.

The weight problems come from the damage done to the *Slimming System* which follows this exposure. The greater the damage done, the higher your weight set-point is likely to become, which means that your weight will stabilize at a higher level. This tendency to damage the *Slimming System* is one of the main reasons why conventional diets tend to cause weight gain in the long term.

WHY FASTING CAN ALSO BE DANGEROUS

It is not just dieting which can be dangerous – the more extreme forms of food-restriction, such as fasting, can be too. Over the centuries, different cultures and religions have developed their own techniques to help the body detoxify itself, and until fairly recently they were very successful. Most of these techniques depend on fasting, drinking only water or spending a few days drinking fruit and vegetable juices. Some methods incorporate particular herbs or foods.

In a world without chemical loading, fasting was a spiritual experience as well as a bodily purge. Now that our bodies store such harmful chemicals, however, these techniques can be extremely dangerous. I find this very sad, particularly since fasting has been practised for many years and can have great religious importance.

The risk from fasting can be more than that from dieting alone, as the level of food-restriction is more extreme: when people fast they usually totally deprive their bodies of food rather than just cutting back. The resultant level of toxins mobilized can be up to 300 per cent above the normal blood levels, far greater than that brought about by dieting alone, and this may potentially cause greater damage to our *Slimming System*. (If you need to fast for religious reasons, there are ways in which it can be made safer and these will be discussed later, in Chapter 20.)

THE HARMFUL NATURE OF DIETING – MY PAINFUL STORY

A few months after my second son was born, I was absolutely desperate to lose weight and get into my old clothes again. The very sight of my maternity clothes was almost too much to bear.

As I was extremely busy with two young and very demanding boys, I fell back on a diet that I had used before, based on a very low carbohydrate intake. However, I quickly discovered that it was totally unsuitable for me, as it proved far too restrictive and I had huge cravings for carbohydrates coupled with an almost continual headache. When the headache finally wore off I experienced general muscular aches and fatigue for months. I gave up on the diet but in the meantime I felt so ill that I sometimes had to stay in bed when I most wanted to get out and enjoy my family.

This is definitely not what you need at one of the most enjoyable but stressful periods in your life. I know now that I experienced, at first hand, many of the toxic effects that stored chemicals have on our bodies when they are mobilized. Although I have never felt better than I do now, I certainly never want to experience that illness again, as I felt I lost a chunk of my life in the process.

HOW THESE PERSISTENT *CHEMICAL CALORIES* CAN BE REMOVED FROM OUR BODIES

However, there is a bright side. Personally experiencing the effects of *Chemical Calories* first of all reinforced the fact to me that they were a real problem, then spurred me on to understand exactly how and why the problem occurs. And once you understand how it happens, it suddenly becomes possible to find a workable solution.

There are actually many different ways in which we can shed these *Chemical Calories* from our bodies. Curiously, many of the early studies were performed not with humans but with cows and other farm animals which had been contaminated with organochlorines from their feed. Farmers had to remove the chemicals from the animals or be faced with the expensive consequence that they could not be used for human consumption.

Tests showed that animals given extra rations of specific vitamins and minerals were much more able to get rid of these chemicals from their bodies. In some cases the rate of excretion of certain organochlorines more than doubled.[4] While this technique was obviously safe and very useful, it was still relatively slow. An additional method needed to be found.

It soon became apparent that one of the best techniques was to take advantage of the natural recycling of fats in the gut. As fat is broken down it is released into the blood, taking with it its collection of organochlorines. Some of the fats are then secreted from the blood into the gut in the gastric juices and travel through the gut until they are absorbed back into the blood again in the small intestines. These reabsorbed fats are then put back into the body stores. This forms a 'fat cycle' from the fat stores, round the gut, and back to the fat stores. Fortunately it also creates a window of opportunity, while these chemicals are in the gut, for removing them,[5] as we too recycle fats in our gut.

This window of opportunity can be grasped by using substances, given by mouth, which bind in the gut not just to the recycling fats but also to the pesticides and other fat-loving synthetic chemicals.

Once they are firmly bound to these 'carriers' the pesticides will not be reabsorbed further down the gut. Instead, they are carried out of the body with the rest of the waste products.[6]

This method of feeding 'binding' substances to highly contaminated animals, to make them 'safe' to eat, has actually been highly effective in ridding animals of persistent *Chemical Calories*. The main substance used in previous research studies was charcoal. Indeed, one study showed that charcoal was so effective in reducing the level of the very fattening chemical DDT (an organochlorine) that it also resulted in the animal losing fat.[7] In the eyes of the farmer, any weight-loss effect was not likely to be appreciated, and this was commented upon in the study as being a potential problem!

Looking at it from the dieter's point of view it is fantastic news, as it indicates that by ridding your body of persistent *Chemical Calories* it is possible to lose fat as well.

The conclusions from these findings are clear. The extensive contamination of our bodies with *Chemical Calories* means that the whole way we diet now needs to change. Any attempt to lose fat must now include a detox programme. If we don't deal with the very high levels of toxins released, ordinary methods of dieting which use food-restriction alone will not only damage the *Slimming System* and make us fatter but could also potentially ruin good health in the process (see Chapter 22), something we could all do without.

Anyone who is really serious about losing weight needs to adapt the way they diet to our more polluted environment. Only by doing this will we ever be successful in losing weight permanently. So how do we do it? To be able to answer this we need to know a bit more about the ways in which our bodies detoxify.

THE TRIALS OF DETOXING

The ability to detoxify will vary greatly from one individual to another. The extent to which *Chemical Calories* build up in a person's fat and other body parts depends not only on how much they have been exposed but on how efficient their bodies are in chucking these chemicals out.

Genetic make-up is one very important factor. Some people will be better at detoxifying than others because they are born with more powerful enzyme systems that are better able to break down chemicals. This could result in some families, less able to detoxify, being far more vulnerable than others to chemical-related problems such as excess weight and to chemical-related illnesses such as cancers and allergies.

As well as differences in inherited resistance, what you eat will also largely determine how good your natural detoxification system is. If you have a highly processed diet deficient in many essential nutrients, then the chances are that your detox system will be struggling.

In our caveman days we probably used to consume many times more vitamins and minerals in our foods than we do now because of the large amounts of raw foods that were eaten. Despite the wider ranges of foods available today, the amount of raw nutrient-rich food in our diets has dramatically fallen, so we are functioning on levels of vitamins and minerals far lower than they have ever been. As the amount of food we eat falls and our diets become more and more deficient in essential nutrients, we end up having substantially fewer resources available for detoxification – resulting in the accelerated build-up of toxins over time.

BY UNDERSTANDING THE PROBLEM, WE CAN TURN THIS SITUATION AROUND

Luckily, unlike our genetic make-up, which we cannot change, we can actually do something really positive about this situation. The simple act of taking certain nutrient supplements can allow our detoxification systems to work to their best ability and therefore boost the rate at which these toxins are excreted from our bodies.

Another problem arises from the fact that much of our diet is so highly processed. As well as being low in slimming nutrients, these processed foods will also reduce our natural ability to detoxify because when they break down they will increase our body's acidity levels.

As an acidic environment significantly slows down the rate at which our detoxification enzymes can work, an increased level of processed foods will make detoxification just that bit more difficult.

Other acid-producing foods include meat and dairy products. On the other hand, alkaline-producing foods such as fruit and vegetables or certain supplements will optimize our ability to detoxify.[8]

As well as genetic make-up, our age also plays an important part in how vulnerable we are to chemical damage and our ability to detoxify. Those who are very young or very old are the most vulnerable. Young immune systems are not fully developed and so are less able to kick chemicals out. Consequently they are damaged by far lower levels of chemicals than those needed to cause damage in adults.[9]

At the other end of the age scale, the ability to detoxify will fall significantly with age due to an overall reduction in efficiency of all the detoxification systems.[10] The good news is that you can boost the efficiency of your detoxification system at any age and, as a result, lose weight. So how do we set about it?

HOW TO SHED *CHEMICAL CALORIES* SAFELY

The most important way to start is to minimize any further build-up of *Chemical Calories* in your body. This can be achieved by eating organic foods or those low in *Chemical Calories*, and by cutting down your exposure to *Chemical Calories* in your household and environment (see Chapters 7–12). By not continually adding to your load, you will be giving your body a chance to deal with its 'chemical' backlog.

Next you will need to help your body to use its natural detoxification system to the full by giving it all the nutrients it needs to perform optimally (see below).

Then you need to start actively ridding your body of the most persistent *Chemical Calories* with which they are contaminated by providing your body with extra help in the form of 'binding' substances which you can then excrete naturally.

ALL ABOUT BINDING SUBSTANCES

Although charcoal is one of the more important of these binders, another widely available substance is soluble fibre. This is not the type of fibre that tends to be known as roughage, but a kind of fibre that can form a gel-like consistency when mixed with water.

Soluble fibre includes substances such as psyllium husks, the fibre commonly found in beans and oats, and other naturally occurring plant fibre such as pectin, found in many fruits. There is also one other major type of binder – clay-based substances such as bentonite. All these binding substances can be readily bought as supplements from good health food shops, and I will be explaining later how you should use them.

Together, charcoal, soluble fibre and some of these clays are invaluable tools in removing the most persistent *Chemical Calories* from your body. They have a powerful ability to bind themselves to dangerous toxins which you can then excrete safely.[11]

I will just mention here that not only can these substances bind the most persistent *Chemical Calories*, they can also bind some of the essential slimming nutrients that we need.[12] So while taking any of these detoxers you will need to ensure that you are getting a generous amount of vitamins and minerals in the form of supplements. Ideally, take the vitamins and minerals at least half an hour or preferably an hour after the detoxing binders. This should ensure that you are getting enough nutrients to optimize your *Slimming System*.

Once you have slowed down your intake of *Chemical Calories* and boosted your ability to get rid of existing ones using nutritional supplements, you are well on your way in tackling any excess weight. With this new way of using natural substances to absorb mobilized *Chemical Calories* in the body, it now becomes much safer to diet.

In fact, if performed with a mild degree of food-restriction and by stepping up your exercise regime, the rate at which you will shed *Chemical Calories* from your body will be accelerated. As long as you follow the advice carefully, by combining a mild food-restriction diet with 'binding' substances in the form of supplements and foods you will create an extremely effective way of eliminating *Chemical Calories* from your body.

The presence of these binding substances will also keep the level of blood-borne *Chemical Calories* low, reducing any potential damage to our *Slimming System*. As a result, the toxins and your excess weight should gradually disappear together, leaving you lighter, healthier and re-energized. By adopting this system, we can adapt the way we lose weight to the problems of the twentieth century.

WHAT WE NEED TO DO TO SHED *CHEMICAL CALORIES*

So, to sum up, the five-step process for shedding even the most persistent *Chemical Calories* is as follows:

1. Keep your chemical load down. The less exposure your body has to *Chemical Calories* the better it will be able to deal with processing the *Chemical Calories* it already has.
2. Feed your detoxification system with nutrients. The right nutrients will help you shed *Chemical Calories* faster and protect your natural *Slimming System* from toxic damage.
3. Take 'binding' substances to draw the most persistent *Chemical Calories* out of the gut, as these very fattening chemicals are not easily removed by any other means.
4. Use mild 'food-restriction' to mobilize toxins stored in body fat.
5. Exercise to mobilize fat stores and enhance your detoxification processes.

SUPPLEMENTS ARE ESSENTIAL FOR ENHANCING DETOXIFICATION

Many supplements will be needed in larger quantities to maximize the rate at which we can break down these *Chemical Calories*. One of the most important organs where this breakdown occurs is the liver, so to achieve maximum rates of detoxification, we need to ensure our liver is getting enough nutrients.

Our liver needs a whole range of vitamins, minerals, amino acids, essential fatty acids and sufficient supplies of carbohydrate to effectively power, permit or speed up the thousands of different reactions that are taking place around the clock. The more stress placed on the liver by higher levels of *Chemical Calories*, the more nutrients the liver will need to do its job.

But it is not just the liver which needs feeding: the very presence of *Chemical Calories* in our bodies will create another need for nutrients because of the increased production of free radicals. For example, many *Chemical Calories* trigger the release of free radicals into our tissues. So what are free radicals?

FREE RADICALS

A free radical is a particle with an attitude.[13] It knocks around the tissue in which it finds itself and tries to destroy all the structures present.

The body can soak up these tissue-wreckers but it needs to use up some of its precious supply of antioxidants (such as vitamin C and E) to limit the damage. This results in smaller levels of antioxidants available from our food being left to power our *Slimming System*.

The drain that *Chemical Calories* make on many of our essential nutrients doesn't stop there, as these substances can in themselves reduce our ability to absorb nutrients from our food by damaging the complex mechanisms involved. What's worse, they can even increase the rate at which many of these slimming nutrients are excreted from our bodies.[14] In other words, stored *Chemical Calories* leave us with even fewer nutrients for detoxification and repair. So the more damage we have done in the past, the more nutrients we now need to put it right.

But before you rush out to buy your supplements, you need to know one thing so that you are prepared if it happens: some people who start to take vitamin and mineral supplements may temporarily feel mildly worse for the first few weeks before they feel better. This may come as a surprise, but can easily be explained. For the first time in years the body will actually have sufficient resources to start dealing with the massive build-up of stored chemicals.

This unexpected side-effect is quite real and I experienced it myself. When I mentioned it to a knowledgeable professor friend of mine, he said that it was because I was detoxing. I must admit that at the time I was highly sceptical, but since then I have seen the same thing happen in many people when they start taking nutrients. The temporary ill-effects are most probably caused by the increased mobilization of chemicals which are in the process of being broken down.

Don't be disheartened if this affects you. On the contrary, you should realize that it is happening because the supplements are having the desired effect. Keep on going and this phase will soon wear off – you will soon be rewarded with a higher level of health, which is of course accompanied by permanent weight loss.

FEED YOUR DETOX SYSTEM

Many multivitamins that you can buy from your local shops, i.e. those that follow the current RDA (recommended daily average), are thought to be insufficient for optimizing your ability to detoxify. This is because the recommended levels are the minimum amount you need to prevent vitamin deficiencies.

It is getting clearer that our need for certain vitamins has increased because they are the ones that are excreted more rapidly from our bodies by chemicals or are used up in larger quantities when we process toxins. More recent studies have shown that we now have an increased need for vitamins A, C and E at levels way above those stated in the RDA.[15]

So to boost your ability to kick out *Chemical Calories* and prevent any damage to your *Slimming System* in the process, the supplements that you take need to have higher levels of these particular vitamins that tend to get used up more quickly.

If these particular nutrients were really 'slimming' vitamins, you might expect those people who are deficient in them to be overweight. Well, several studies have shown this to be absolutely true. In fact the more overweight a person is, the lower the level of these vitamins will be in their bodies.[16] This is probably related to the fact that overweight people will tend to use these nutrients up faster and/or simply don't get enough in their food. These lower levels will then impair the running of their *Slimming Systems*, which will result in weight gain.

So by taking the right supplements, which are readily available, you can easily ensure you are getting enough nutrients. For the doses that I recommend, see Chapters 15 and 24.

THE NUTRIENTS WE NOW NEED TO ENHANCE REMOVAL OF *CHEMICAL CALORIES*

If someone is concerned for their health, the typical supplement that they will consider taking tends to be one made out of vitamins and minerals. The problem is that our need for other nutrients, besides vitamins and minerals, has also increased, due to the presence of *Chemical Calories* and our increasingly processed diets.

As many of these other nutrients play a vital role in boosting the functioning of our detoxification and of our *Slimming System*, it is essential to ensure that we get sufficient levels of these other nutrients too. I will now give more detail about what these other substances are and how they can enhance our ability to detoxify.

AMINO ACIDS: As seen earlier, the problem with chemical pollutants is that they damage the way our bodies break down, absorb, use and manufacture amino acids. This is why people who are damaged by chemicals are frequently deficient in amino acids, despite seemingly adequate levels in their diet.[17]

Certain amino acids are absolutely crucial to our ability to detoxify ourselves of chemical pollutants, particularly the harder to shift organochlorines.[18] They include methionine, cysteine, taurine and glutathione. These can be found in many of the foods listed on the *Slimming System* detoxification diet, but to ensure that you are receiving optimal levels you could always supplement some of them (see Chapters 15 and 24).

LIPID SUPPLEMENTATION: As previously discussed, although eating fats takes some getting used to for people who want to lose weight, the right fats are absolutely essential for successful slimming since they allow your slimming hormones to work fully.

The fats you eat also have a significant effect on the toxicity of chemicals by altering your ability to break them down. Diets that are deficient in certain essential fatty acids, such as omega-3 and omega-6, make people less able to detoxify chemicals.[19] Flax oil, for example, will greatly improve your ability to break down *Chemical Calories* and will make them less toxic. Consequently these fats play a crucial role in powering our detoxification systems. On the other hand, saturated fats, such as animal fats, appear to have no such protective actions.

Our need for these essential fatty acids becomes even greater when we are dieting. High levels of newly mobilized *Chemical Calories* will readily destroy essential fats, possibly because of the increased levels of free radicals created. This destructive effect could be reflected in the fact that dieting has been associated with a fall in the body's level of omega-3 fatty acids.[20]

To prevent any drop in essential fatty acids, we need to increase our intake of them during times of food-restriction. This will prevent any drop in our levels of essential fatty acids just at the time we need them the most. The recommended doses for these highly effective and vital 'slimming' fats can be found in Chapters 15 and 24.

PH BALANCE: Although most people know about the need for certain nutrients in our diet, very few know that pH is also crucial. The pH balance of your body is the relative level of acidity/ alkalinity and is vitally important in allowing the detoxification enzymes to work properly.

Unfortunately most people's food intake is too high in acid-producing foods (meat, cheese, etc.), and too low in alkaline-forming foods (fruits, and particularly vegetables). This means that in most people, the enzyme systems do not function properly. As a result, their ability to detoxify *Chemical Calories* is seriously reduced.

This is why an alkalinization supplement is useful for people who are actively dieting – as this will promote more effective and rapid removal and processing of *Chemical Calories*.

If you already eat a diet high in vegetables and fruit, or indeed the diet in this programme, you may not need this supplement. If you want to check, you can test your own urine to see whether it is alkaline or acidic by using a piece of litmus paper, which is provided with most alkalinization supplements. If you are already hypertensive (have high blood pressure) or have a renal (kidney) or cardiac (heart) impairment, then you should not take this supplement but should drink vegetable juice instead.

BINDING AGENTS: This is a general name for substances used to draw out toxic *Chemical Calories* from the body. They play an exceptionally important part in my programme because they are among the few substances which can lower the level of virtually all the different types of *Chemical Calories* found in the body.

Soluble fibre is the most popular kind of binding agent. You can buy it in supplement form as psyllium husks, fruit pectins and gums, widely available in health food shops. It has been estimated that we eat far too little dietary fibre in our daily diet. The average UK citizen eats just over 12 grams per day, whereas the Department of Health's Committee on Medical Aspects of Food Policy recommends that the total level of dietary fibre in an adult's diet should average 18 grams per day and go up to 24 grams per day. In fact they implied that additional benefit could be gained by eating up to 32 grams a day.[21] So you can see that we could all do with eating significantly more fibre then we currently do!

Charcoal is another well-tested substance that binds to persistent *Chemical Calories* in the gut. As well as reducing the level of certain persistent *Chemical Calories* over time, these substances are also able to reduce the amount of chemicals absorbed from a meal high in persistent *Chemical Calories*.

Another useful substance is clay. Certain clays such as bentonite are able to bind to a whole range of toxic pollutants.[22] Although markedly less palatable, they can be made more attractive by mixing them with fruit juice. Charcoal and bentonite supplements are available from good health food shops.

When and how to take these binding agents: A good time to take these substances is immediately after waking up and before breakfast, as your night's fast will have mobilized your fats and increased your blood levels of *Chemical Calories*. They can also be taken with meals throughout the day, especially when following the *Slimming System* detox diet, as mild food-restriction will increase the mobilization of *Chemical Calories*.

Although there have been worries about the mineral-depleting effects of dietary fibre, the above-mentioned Committee from the UK Department of Health has found that these mainly apply to insoluble fibre, such as wheat bran, rather than the soluble types I am recommending. Populations who consume large amounts of dietary fibre in their diet do not on balance show a significant reduction in minerals. In fact the only people who tend to be affected are those whose diets are likely to be low in minerals, such as the elderly. The levels the Committee recommends, as shown above, should not cause any adverse effects on adults.

As a precautionary measure, however, it is best to take vitamin and mineral pills separately from binding agents, particularly if you are taking charcoal and clays. Also you should drink plenty of fluid with soluble fibres, in particular with psyllium husks, as they tend to absorb lots of water.

I like to mix up the fibre powder with water before I drink it. Despite having the consistency of wallpaper paste, there is no real taste to it. The added bonus is that I am confident that it will start to act in removing my *Chemical Calories* almost immediately.

HERBAL REMEDIES: There is a large range of other natural substances which can be used for their ability to improve detoxification and which can also be used during the detoxification diet. Perhaps the best known is milk thistle, which is a powerful antioxidant and a great tonic for the liver. Others include burdock, red clover, fenugreek, echinacea, yellow dock, dandelion root, ginkgo biloba and ginger root.

Strictly speaking, none of these substances are essential nutrients for our body but they do seem to improve our ability to detoxify and so could be beneficial.

WATER: It is vitally important to drink water in sufficient quantities to help wash away some of the *Chemical Calories* from the system, particularly if you are mobilizing *Chemical Calories* from your fat by dieting or exercising. I would suggest that an intake of at least 2–3 litres per day is vital, and if you are food-restricting then you should increase this to at least 3 litres every day.

Don't forget, if your body becomes mildly dehydrated by just a few per cent, the level of energy you can produce will drop by 20 per cent.

CARBOHYDRATES: Although you might not expect it, carbo-hydrates appear to be absolutely essential for our ability to detoxify. This is because many of the individual reactions taking place need a certain amount of readily available sugar.

Consequently, very low-carbohydrate diets can actually hinder our body's ability to detoxify, as they effectively starve the detox-ification enzymes of their food so that they cannot work fully. As a result, food-restriction diets should always include a certain amount of carbohydrate and very low-carbohydrate diets should be avoided.

USE FOOD-RESTRICTION, EXERCISE AND OTHER METHODS TO ENHANCE DETOXIFICATION

If you cut out *Chemical Calories* from your life as well as going on all the supplements I have previously mentioned, you will be well on your way to significantly lowering your inner *Chemical Calorie* levels and as such enhancing your long-term weight loss. This is fine for people who have not much weight to lose, or who don't mind it taking a longer time to bring about weight loss. But for those of you who want to speed up this process there are now several ways in which this can be done safely. All involve approaches which combine taking the above-mentioned supplements, in addition to using ways of mobilizing body fats, and they include the following.

FOOD-RESTRICTION: Severe food-restriction, and fasting in par-ticular, can be very toxic, as it greatly increases the levels of *Chemical Calories* released into the blood circulation without providing an exit route for them.

However, if you follow a mild food-restriction diet with increased levels of vitamins, supplements and binding agents, it can be a great way of detoxifying and speeding up the safe removal of highly toxic and fattening chemicals.

EXERCISE: Exercise, if performed for a long period of time, can create the same effect. This is because extensive periods of exercise will increase the amount of fat burnt up, which will therefore increase the amount of *Chemical Calories* released.

Exercise also has the added bonus of increasing the oxygen supply to the body, which will greatly help the detoxification process.[23]

The best general advice here is to take it steadily, and if you are on a food-restriction diet, don't overdo the amount of exercise in the first few weeks. This is because the levels of *Chemical Calories* are likely to be at their highest during the first few days of a food-restriction diet. So it is best not to increase these high levels still further by undergoing excessive periods of exercise. This doesn't mean you should totally stop all forms of exercise – far from it – just that you should initially refrain from undertaking excessively vigorous spells of exercise for hours on end. (See Chapter 21 for more detailed advice.)

One more comment: to get the maximum detoxification value out of the exercise you do, you need to be taking the supplements recommended in Chapters 15 and 24. This will also ensure that your *Slimming System* is protected from the increased levels of free radicals released by exercise.

HEAT TREATMENT: Taking a sauna or a steam bath has the effect of mobilizing *Chemical Calories*. As with exercise, you can use this method to boost detoxification, particularly if you take the supplements recommended for this programme.[24] Remember to keep drinking lots of water though.

I would also recommend body scrubbing or dry skin brushing, as this will accelerate one of the few natural ways in which the body can rid as itself of persistent *Chemical Calories* – the shedding of dead skin cells. Many people also recommend colonic irrigation, but there is a risk of removing good bowel bacteria so it wouldn't be my first choice for detoxing.

Now that we have dealt with the extremely important subject of how to shift your body's stores of persistent *Chemical Calories* safely, it is time to progress rapidly to the diet itself.

By now you will understand that synthetic chemicals have changed the ways our bodies work. As a result, all the previous diets which have ignored their effects are not only obsolete, but potentially downright dangerous. Anyone who seriously wants to shape up will need to bring the way they diet into the twenty-first century. Fortunately we now have the know-how to achieve this dietary revolution. Read on to discover the exciting new secrets of how to lose weight, not just for a few weeks but for the rest of your life!

15. Guide to the Detox Diet

We can now see that the whole concept of weight-loss diet has been radically changed. In the new scheme of things, the food-restrictive element of the diet, once the be-all and end-all of dieting, is not the only method we have of achieving weight loss.

Food-restriction is still a very important tool, however, as it can be used to remove very large amounts of existing *Chemical Calories* from the body – which will result in significant weight loss, because the *Slimming System* will be less suppressed and better able to burn up excess fat.

Now I will explain more about how food-restriction can help us to lose weight, as well as discussing who should now use the food-restrictive element of the diet. Then I will go through all the other things we now used to do to haul the way we diet slap bang into the twenty-first century.

WHAT DOES IT MEAN TO 'GO ON A DIET'?

Previously, 'going on a diet' meant that the person was intending to cut down their intake of calories from food. They hoped that their body fat stores would be used up to replace the calories that they needed, but didn't consume as food. Go into your local bookshop and you will find that almost any diet book will be based on this principle.

In fact the only difference between the abundance of different diets will be in the combination of foods used to achieve this goal – low fat, high protein, low carbohydrate, high fibre, raw foods, low sugar, cabbage soup, wheat-free, dairy-free, strict calorie-counting and so on. You could say that virtually every combination of foods under the sun has been used to claim dieting success.

While it is true that many of these diets will indeed help you lose weight, this will only be for as long as you can stick to the diet: in the long term, all these methods will probably fail. When you get tired of the diet, you tend to regain the weight you lost, because cutting down the amount of food you eat only treats the symptom of excess weight, not the actual cause.

As so many of you have already found out, for this type of dieting to be effective in the long term you would need to be on a diet for the rest of your life. And if you do this, your own natural *Slimming System* will tend to become less and less effective with each dieting attempt. As a result, the number of calories you need just to stay the same weight will become lower and lower, so unless you keep getting stricter about what you eat, you will begin to gain weight again. Not at all something to look forward to.

IT DOESN'T HAVE TO BE LIKE THAT

My philosophy about food-restriction in dieting is totally different. I believe food-restriction still has a major role to play in helping us to lose weight, but its function has totally changed from that of being used just to produce a shortfall of calories. In my programme, food-restriction is now used for its powerful ability to remove the massive build-up of *Chemical Calories* from the body.

The presence of *Chemical Calories* has changed the way we diet for ever. Now when we cut down on food we release high levels of *Chemical Calories* into the bloodstream and they are carried all round the body. If we fail to control the release and neutralize the toxic effects of these *Chemical Calories*, they can cause extensive damage to our *Slimming System*.

On the other hand, by gradually mobilizing these chemicals into the bloodstream, we have a fabulous opportunity to get rid of them for good. This can only be achieved by eating the right foods and taking the right supplements. As we lose our fattening stores of chemicals, the body's own natural *Slimming System* will be rejuvenated, and the body will regain its natural ability to control its own weight!

So by restricting your food, you will be able to shift more

Chemical Calories from your body stores than you would without the extra effort. And losing those unwanted *Chemical Calories* will work to lower your body-weight set-point even further.

FOOD-RESTRICTION AND THE DETOX DIET

Because of this *Chemical-Calorie* shifting ability, the Detox Diet is based around a 28-day programme of a mildly food-restrictive 'diet'. If there is a large amount of weight to lose, this 28-day programme can then be repeated several times until you get close to your ideal weight. In between each 28-day block, you should spend two weeks following the advice in Chapter 24, which essentially follows the same principles as the Detox Diet but is without the food-restrictive element.

You must bear in mind throughout that it has probably taken many years for you to get to the weight you are, so don't have unrealistic expectations of massive overnight weight losses. The more overweight you are, the longer you should expect to be on the programme. But on the plus side, if you lose weight in a controlled way, the chances are that you are more likely to keep it off over the longer term – which after all should be your main goal. So remember to pace yourself.

By adopting these new methods you can, for the first time, use food-restriction to actually treat the main cause of excessive weight gain – toxic chemical build-up.

CUTTING DOWN SAFELY

Just as the reason for restricting what you eat has changed, so too has the best way to carry it through. If you are going to limit what you eat, you need to make sure that your diet is safe and effective.

The first thing you need to do is to lower your exposure to *Chemical Calories* in your food, and preferably in your environment as well. This will reduce the body's daily burden of new *Chemical Calories*, allowing it to concentrate on eliminating the old *Chemical Calories* released into your bloodstream from your body as you cut down on what you eat.

The second thing you need to do is eat foods and take supplements to enhance your *Slimming System*. This is vital, in order to protect your *Slimming System* from damage when food-restriction releases *Chemical Calories* from the body stores.

The third thing is to eat the foods and take the supplements that will remove *Chemical Calories* from your body. During this time, regular exercise will boost your ability to detoxify and will enhance the performance of your *Slimming System*.

So while it may have been knocked off its high pedestal, conventional dieting, in combination with these new methods, can still play a crucial role in weight loss.

WHO SHOULD USE FOOD-RESTRICTION TO LOSE WEIGHT?

Adults who are genuinely overweight should use food-restriction as part of their weight-loss plan. By including a mild food-restrictive element they can get down to their target weight in a much shorter time. Then, when they are close to their target weight, they can drop the food-restrictive element of the diet and lose the last few remaining kilos just by following the advice on how to maintain your weight-loss given in Chapter 24. However, not everyone needs to cut down on their food intake to lose weight.

If you are just a few pounds heavier than you want to be, you can probably lose them, again just by following the advice in Chapter 24, which involves taking supplements and adopting a regular exercise routine. These measures will strengthen your *Slimming System* and lower your weight set-point. The main drawback here will be the time it takes to lose those few kilos.

If you are happy with your weight, but just want to improve your shape and muscle tone, again this gentler method is for you.

On the other hand, some people, for example young children, pregnant women or those who are breastfeeding, should not go on a food-restriction diet even if they want to lose weight. In pregnancy the baby is especially vulnerable to damage from chemicals, so any sort of food-restriction would not be a good idea.[1] On the other hand, eating foods that are low in *Chemical Calories* and naturally high in slimming nutrients and soluble fibre can only be good for you and your baby.

The same is true of women who are breastfeeding. It is a time when most mothers are desperate to lose weight, as I know only too well from experience. However, if they restrict their food and release massive amounts of *Chemical Calories* from their fat stores, it is very likely that the chemicals will concentrate in the fat-rich breast milk and be passed to the baby.[2]

The good news is that even people who cannot restrict their food can follow the other principles of the programme, and I will talk more about these issues in Chapter 20.

STARTING THE *SLIMMING SYSTEM* DETOXIFICATION DIET

At this point I have already covered most of the principles behind the Detox Diet. In the rest of this chapter I will lead you through the stages of putting the whole programme together. The first stage is to buy the supplements, and start taking them in the recommended quantities (see below).

You should start taking the supplements at least two weeks before starting the diet. This is vitally important for several reasons:

- It allows you to source all the supplements and get into a routine of taking them at the right times of day. As there are quite a few supplements to take, this will give you one less thing to contend with when you start the diet.
- Your body will have a chance to get rid of some *Chemical Calories* that are easily removed, reducing the burden of detoxification when you start to diet.
- The body's natural *Slimming System* will be strengthened by the supplements and be more able to protect itself from potential damage when the diet starts.

If you already take supplements, but not all those suggested, it is still better to give your body a week to prepare itself properly. Don't forget, in this time you will also be learning the lifelong habits you need to stay slim, as well as improving your ability to lose weight, so it really is worth getting into the routine.

STEP I: SUPPLEMENTS FOR DIETERS

Below is a list of vitamins, minerals and other supplements which you can take to enhance your weight loss while restricting your food intake. You may end up taking combinations of supplements, as few will contain the exact levels you need. In this case, the best option is to take a high-potency multivitamin and mineral formula, flax seed oil and soluble fibre, and then add the extra supplements to bring the quantities as close as you can to the figures below.

The levels of recommended supplements are based on a very extensive amount of published research, but in particular on the research of Dr E. J. Cheraskin, who over a fifteen-year period established the Optimal Nutrient Allowances for vitamins in over 10,000 Americans.[3] It is also based on Dr W. Rea's work in treating over 20,000 chemically sensitive patients at the Environmental Health Center, based in Dallas, in the USA.[4] And finally it takes into account some of the values recommended by the UK Department of Health.[5]

I'm afraid you are going to rattle with the number of supplements you now need to take, but if you are really serious about wanting to lose weight, this is the way to go. You must also accept the fact that it may be very difficult to find all the supplements recommended, let alone the exact recommended doses, but don't worry, just do the best you can for now. If you can only get the essentials, i.e. a good multivitamin and mineral tablet, the flax seed oil and the soluble fibre, this alone should make a significant difference. Then you can build on that as and when you have an opportunity.

Essential supplements	Total daily amount
Vitamin A (retinol or betacarotene)	5,000–10,000ius*
Vitamin B1 (thiamine)	10–50mg
Vitamin B2 (riboflavin)	10–50mg
Vitamin B3 (niacin)	25–50mg
Vitamin B5	25–50mg
Vitamin B6	25–100mg
Vitamin B12	10–50mcg
Vitamin C	500–3,000mg
Vitamin E	200–400ius
Folic acid	200–400mcg
Choline	25–100mg
Zinc	15–30mg
Magnesium	200–400mg
Iron	15–20mg
Co-enzyme Q10	10–50mg

*If pregnant or trying to conceive, do not exceed 10,000ius of retinol a day.

Essential fats	Total daily amount
Omega-3 essential fats	
Linseed oil	5–15g (approx.1–3 teaspoons)
and	
Omega-6 essential fats	
Evening primrose oil (or equivalent)	500–1,000mg

Amino acids (protein)	Total daily amount
Tyrosine	200–500mg
L-5 hydroxytryptophan (5HTP, a natural precursor of serotonin)	25–50mg
Methionine	200–500mg
Glutathione	200–500mg

It may be very difficult to source the above amino acids (particularly 5HTP and methionine). Again, don't worry: just take the ones you can get hold of for now.

Detoxers	Total daily amount
Soluble fibre*	
Grapefruit pectin	up to 3g before meals (3 times a day)
or	
Apple pectin	up to 3g before meals (3 times a day)
or	
Psyllium seed husks	up to 3g before meals (3 times a day)

*All soluble fibre supplements must be taken with water as instructed.

Charcoal (optional, but particularly useful when actively restricting food intake)

Activated charcoal	up to 500mg taken before each of 3 meals

Clay (again optional, but useful when restricting food intake)*

Green clay	1 to 2 teaspoons daily in a glass of water
or	
Bentonite	1 teaspoon daily in a glass of water

*I must admit, I find clay very difficult to take with water alone and so tend to mix it up with fruit juice to make it more palatable.

NB: iu = international units; mcg = micrograms; mg = milligrams; 1,000mcg = 1mg

AN IMPORTANT NOTE ON TIMING SUPPLEMENT DOSES: If you prefer, you can take all the supplements, essential fats and amino acids in the morning. But if you can manage it, split the dose by taking some the morning and some in the evening. A split dose is particularly useful for vitamin C, which lasts for only about 8 hours in the body. If you take the total daily amount in two doses you will give your *Slimming System* better protection from free radicals.

One thing to remember: whenever you take the supplements, it is important not to take them at the same time as the detoxers. This is because if you take the supplements and detoxers too close together then there is a chance that the detoxers may 'soak up' some of these essential nutrients.

Ideally you should take the detoxers with some water as soon as you wake up in the morning, then by the time you have got dressed and had breakfast you can take the supplements, leaving at least 30 minutes between the two, and longer if possible.

If you want to split the vitamin doses through the day, then taking the detoxers before meals and the supplements after meals will allow sufficient time between them. I can imagine that if you have never taken a supplement before this whole thing may seem rather daunting. To help you put all the supplement advice into action, Chapter 17 will show some suggested meal plans and provide guidance on how to fit these supplements into your daily routine. And to make it easier for you to obtain the most suitable supplements for this programme, visit our website at www.chemical-calories.com.

Don't forget, the more effort you make here, the more effective the results will be.

STEP 2: CUT DOWN *CHEMICAL CALORIES*

While you are sorting out which supplements to take, it would be a good time to find out where to buy organic foods and other household products low in *Chemical Calories*. Organic products come in the usual different brands, shapes and sizes and it may take a little while for you to find everything that you'll need for the diet. Changing your cosmetics and household products will probably take weeks or months rather than days, but as and when you need to replace items, try to look out for the low-*Chemical-Calorie* version.

Water is another item that you'll need to consider in the few weeks before you start the diet. For example, you could research the best water filtration unit to fit on to your taps. Again it may take time to find out what is currently available, but it will really be worth it in the long run. Don't forget, the effort you put in now will contribute to keeping you slim throughout the rest of your life.

STEP 3: EXERCISE

At this point you should also be considering how you can fit a certain amount of exercise into this programme. Ideally, you should start exercising before you begin to restrict what you eat. Don't worry, I am not talking about a major intensive exercise programme here, just enough to enhance detoxification and boost the *Slimming System*. I will be discussing the exercise element more fully in Chapter 21.

STEP 4: RECORD-KEEPING

One of the best ways to keep yourself motivated during a diet is to keep a close record of the progress you have made. So before you start, find time to weigh and measure yourself and write your vital statistics into the charts in Chapter 19.

These measurements could make the world of difference to your morale for the rest of the diet. In addition, you will really kick yourself later if you don't, because you won't be able to see how far you've come!

Now we come to the diet itself. Here we go . . .

16. The Detox Diet

The Detox Diet has been specifically designed for those who want to lose weight more quickly than they would normally expect to do by cutting down on their *Chemical Calorie* intake alone. This is because a period of mild food-restriction can accelerate the rate at which *Chemical Calories* can be removed from the body. Its aim therefore is to provide a safe way in which the body's ability to shed its load of *Chemical Calories* is maximized. And food-wise, I have tried to make it a very easy diet to follow, whether you like cooking or prefer to keep food preparation simple.

It is a mildly food-restrictive diet and this means that, unlike many other diets, every day will not be a battle between you and your appetite. It is also designed to give your *Slimming System* the foods it needs to maximize its efficiency – in other words, you will be helping it to shift your excess body fat at the fastest rate possible.

From previous experience, I have found that the more rigid the diet, the less likely I have been to stick to it. Because of this I have kept the rules very flexible. This is a massive advantage, as we all have different preferences and different degrees of access to organic foods, and therefore need an equally flexible diet that we can follow at work, at home or eating out.

If you find menu suggestions helpful, however, Chapter 17 has a complete eating plan worked out for fourteen days, including advice on how to fit the various supplements into your daily routine. So however you want to do it, the choice is yours!

PRINCIPLES OF THE DIET

1. FEED THE BODY'S DETOXIFICATION SYSTEM: The intention is to provide your body with the resources it needs to detoxify. So the emphasis will be on eating sufficient quantities of the right foods, rather than just cutting down on food in general. It is also vital that you take the supplements recommended in Chapters 15 and 24.

2. EAT THE RIGHT FOODS: Your intake of raw foods, particularly vegetables, should be maximized. They boost your ability to detoxify for all the following reasons:

- They contain masses of valuable slimming nutrients.
- They are high in fibre and will act like an internal broom.
- They are alkaline, which aids detoxification.
- They contain enzymes which play an important role in digestion, reducing the burden on the body to produce its own enzymes for breaking down foods.

3. KEEP *CHEMICAL CALORIES* LOW: It is very important to reduce your exposure to *Chemical Calories* throughout the time you spend dieting. This will enable the body to put all its energy into removing persistent chemicals from its body stores. You should be selecting foods that are known to be low in *Chemical Calories* (see Chapter 18), or prepared in such a way that they become low in *Chemical Calories* (see Chapter 9).

Virtually all the foods referred to in the diet can be produced organically, and because organic food availability varies widely I have designed my diet to be very flexible so that you can make the most of the produce in season.

As we absorb far more *Chemical Calories* into our bodies from fats compared to carbohydrates, it is best to keep down your fat intake when eating conventionally grown foods which are potentially high in *Chemical Calories*, even if the fats or oils used are organic.

Another way of ensuring that your intake of *Chemical Calories* is kept as low as possible is to combine foods potentially high in *Chemical Calories* with a food high in soluble fibre. Beans, lentils and other pulses, oats and fruits such as apples and oranges will soak up extra *Chemical Calories* from other ingredients so that you absorb less into your body.

4. MILD FOOD-RESTRICTION: The aim of this diet is to restrict food mildly rather than dramatically. If fat stores are mobilized too quickly the body will not be able to detoxify quickly enough to keep pace.

So don't expect to lose too many pounds each week. Set your sights at a maximum of 450g per week or 1 per cent of your body weight. If you lose weight much faster than this you will probably be losing not fat, but muscle and water, which definitely won't make you slim in the long run. In addition, the less you are overweight, the slower your progress will probably be. Just take things according to your own situation.

FOODS TO EAT FREELY

Now before I launch into the nitty gritty of the diet itself, here is the good news. You can eat freely any of the following foods, provided they are organic or low in *Chemical Calories*:

- Herbs, spices, mustard, chillies, garlic, pepper, salt, soy sauce, lemon juice, vinegar, Worcestershire sauce, yeast extracts, stock cubes, fat-free vegetable soup.
- Unlimited amounts of the following vegetables, eaten raw, steamed or as fat-free vegetable soup: asparagus, aubergines, bamboo shoots, beansprouts, green beans, beetroot, broccoli, Brussels sprouts, cabbage, carrots, cauliflower, celery, Swiss chard, Chinese cabbage, courgettes, cucumbers, endive, green leafy vegetables, leeks, lettuce, mushrooms, okra, onions, green, red and yellow peppers, radishes, tomatoes, watercress, yellow squash, water chestnuts.
- Caffeine-free coffee or tea, coffee substitutes, herbal teas, filtered water.

Organic lemon or lime slices can be added freely. You can add milk, but only if it is taken from your daily allowance.

TOP TIPS TO ENSURE SUCCESS

Here are a few ideas to help you deal with temptation when the going gets tough:

- Keep some prepared raw or cooked vegetables in your refrigerator at all times, for emergency snacks.
- Eat a bowl of fresh salad every day.
- For a hot filling snack, have a mug of fat-free vegetable soup. You can make it in batches using the vegetables listed above and keep it in the fridge or freezer as an instant filler in emergencies. Take some with you in a flask when you go to work or travel. See Chapter 17 for recipe suggestions.
- Drink a large (225ml) glass of filtered or bottled water before every meal and throughout the day. As well as keeping you well hydrated, drinking plenty of water will also help to flush away unwanted chemicals released by your weight loss. To aid detoxification even more, drink mineral water and flavour it with lemon or lime juice.
- Remove all visible skin and fat from meat and fatty fish when preparing them for cooking.
- Don't eat the skin or fat on cooked meats.

HOW THE DIET IS DESIGNED

You can choose what you'd like to eat every day from three different groups – proteins, carbohydrates and fats. You have an allowance from each group and within that allowance you are free to make your own selection from the choices offered. Provided that you keep to the recommended portions, the nutritional value of the foods has already been counted for you, so you can relax on that front.

It is also a good idea to weigh out the portions at the beginning, as this will help you to estimate the right quantities involved. Don't forget, you can combine your allowances with as many items as you want from the 'Foods to eat freely' section shown above.

But whatever selections you make, you should try to keep a record of all the food you eat as you go along. This will make it much easier to remember how much of your allowance is available as the day goes on and will really help you to stick to the diet.

Towards that aim, Chapter 19 will provide a blank record which you can copy or adapt as your own food diary. Many people find this very useful. Not only does it take seconds to do, but it also helps to keep you in total control of your food intake and so greatly improves your overall chances of dieting success.

Group 1: Carbohydrates

Altogether you can have 8 portions of carbohydrate every day, 4 from the fruit section and 4 from the starch section.

FRUIT SECTION

Every day you can choose 2 portions of fresh fruit and 2 other items from the list. That's a total of 4 portions of fruit or fruit products every day. These are great for giving you instant energy if you need a quick pick-me-up.

A typical portion of fresh fruit is: an apple, an orange, ½ a grapefruit, 2 medium plums, a nectarine, a peach, a small banana or 100g of any other fruit. Choose two of these.

Make 2 more choices from the following options:

- 20g dried fruit
- 125ml fruit juice
- A portion of fresh fruit, raw, stewed or baked without sugar (approx. 100g)

STARCH SECTION

You can choose 4 portions every day from the following options. You can select the same option more than once (except breakfast cereal, where women are allowed a maximum of 1 a day and men a maximum of 2). Spread these throughout the day to ensure your energy levels remain high.

- 80g cooked (30g dry weight) pulses – lentils, kidney beans, peas, chickpeas, etc.
- 100g cooked baked beans in tomato sauce
- 120g potatoes, boiled, steamed or baked in their skins
- 25g flour or grain (preferably oats, but also barley, bulgar wheat, buckwheat, wheat, couscous, rye, rice, quinoa)
- 30g breakfast cereal – either low-sugar muesli or bran flakes or crisped rice or cornflakes
- 30g bread (approx. 1 slice)
- 70g boiled rice (25g dry weight)
- 70g cooked egg noodles (25g dry weight)
- 75g cooked pasta (25g dry weight)

Group 2: Proteins

You can choose 2 portions of protein every day. If you choose one of the dairy products (for example cheese or yoghurt), your other protein selection that day should be a non-dairy product (unless you are a vegetarian). Vegetarians should also try to combine pulses with a grain product to make a complete protein meal.

- 100g cooked lean meat (venison, beef, lamb, chicken, pork, ham, turkey or game)
- 160g cooked pulses (60g dry weight) – chickpeas, peas, beans and lentils
- 200g baked beans or other types of beans in a ready-made sauce
- 200g Quorn pieces
- 125g tofu (raw and firm)
- 100g tempeh

- 55g hard cheese
- 200g cottage cheese
- 250g natural yoghurt (low-fat) or 200g fruit yoghurt (low-fat)
- 2 eggs (NB not more than 4 eggs allowed per week)

Group 3: Fats

It's particularly important to measure out these portions of fats and keep within the quantities given. For example, measure out your daily allowance of milk every morning and remember that your daily allowance of oil, butter or other fats should not be exceeded. Choose 1 portion of each of the following:

- 1 tablespoon of oil (using olive oil for all cooking purposes and any type of oil such as walnut oil, sesame oil, olive oil, etc. for salad dressings)

  or

  1 teaspoon of butter (or seed/nut spread) and 2 teaspoons of olive oil (or other oils, or seed/nut spread)

  or

  20g non-roasted nuts or non-roasted seeds, or 20g of a combination of nuts and seeds (particularly pumpkin seeds and walnuts)

  or

  1 small avocado

OPTIONAL
- Up to 200ml (8 fl oz) semi-skimmed milk or unsweetened soya milk.

INCREASED ALLOWANCES FOR MEN

In an attempt to keep things simple, I created this plan for the needs of a relatively inactive woman trying to lose weight. It is based on providing approximately 1,500 kcal a day. That's fine for many of us, but will not be sufficient for men.

To keep things equal, men should add an extra portion of protein, and 2 more portions of starchy carbohydrates. Examples of typical menus for men have been included in Chapter 17.

VEGETARIANS AND VEGANS (OPTIONAL)

If you follow a vegetarian or vegan diet, you can have 15g of nuts or seeds in addition to the basic diet plan. This will increase the range of proteins in your diet as well as providing a little more fat, which is particularly important if you do not eat eggs or dairy products. This allowance can be used by all vegetarians in addition to any other supplements you qualify for.

HOW MUCH FOOD SHOULD YOU EAT?

When you first start you will probably find that you need all the calories that are listed and you should make the most of the foods that can be eaten freely, particularly the soup.

But as the weeks go by and you are getting nearer your ideal weight, you will find it easier to eat less. Do realize, it is perfectly fine to cut back slightly on your allowances if you find you don't need so much food. Just because you have a certain allowance of a food, it doesn't mean you have to eat it all. In other words, you should eat what you need, then stop.

FOODS AND DRINKS TO AVOID

There are some foods that you should definitely avoid on the Detox Diet, because they slow down or impair your ability to detoxify. They include:

- Caffeinated drinks, because they disturb the production of slimming hormones and create carbohydrate cravings (see Chapter 20).
- Alcohol, as it slows down detoxification (particularly important to avoid in the first week of food-restriction, see Chapter 20).
- Foods high in trans-fats. Trans-fats are created when polyunsaturated

oils and fats are heated in cooking. Food fried in sunflower oil, for example, is high in trans-fats; so is most deep-fried food. Limit yourself to cooking with olive oil and butter from your allowance, as these contain very little polyunsaturated fats. Many margarines are also high in trans-fats.

- Foods very high in *Chemical Calories* (see Chapters 7 and 18).

PUTTING IT ALL TOGETHER

So now you know what you can eat every day. The next chapter will hopefully inspire you by suggesting a large number of ways in which you can create tasty and interesting daily menus from the food allowances provided. As well as providing 14 days of exciting menus which can then be repeated to make up the 28-day recommended programme, it also will provide additional daily menus for men and for vegetarians. So *bon appétit* to you all!

17. Detox Diet Menus

Who says detoxing has to be hard work! Well, as you will soon see in this menu plan, that idea will be a thing of the past – because I have compiled a large number of delicious and easy-to-prepare recipes tried and tested for your enjoyment. They will make detoxing really easy, painless and fun to do.

There are fourteen standard menus for an average woman who wants to lose weight, as well as seven additional vegetarian menus, suitable not only for vegetarians but for anyone who is looking for a bit of a change. Each day is carefully balanced to include all the elements allowed on the diet, without exceeding the limits for fats, carbohydrates or proteins. For this reason, *you can't mix and match different meals between menus*. But saying that, you can repeat whole days and add in vegetarian days.

I have also provided seven menus for men, which are adapted from the first seven standard menus, incorporating the extra portions of protein and carbohydrate (see Chapter 16). This will show you how easy it is to create daily menus for men from any of the basic menu plans. There are recipes at the end of the chapter for all the items marked with an asterisk*. But before you get ready to start, here are just a few quick suggestions and reminders:

- Leave at least half an hour between taking fibre supplements and other vitamins.
- You can have unlimited herb tea or decaffeinated tea or coffee, so long as any added milk is counted from your 200ml daily allowance.
- Try to eat brown, wholemeal or granary bread instead of white bread.

- You should feel free to add any of the ingredients on the 'Foods to eat freely' lists found in Chapter 16 – for instance, you could spread yeast extract on your toast to give it extra zing.

- You can add extra portions of soup throughout the entire day, so long as it is fat-free (see recipes). And to help you keep to the diet, for the first two weeks at least, it is vital to ensure that there is plenty of fat-free soup readily available for you to eat at all times. But don't forget, one serving of *low-fat* soup will count as one teaspoon of oil from your fat allowance.

- For all the menus, try to avoid eating foods that are potentially very high in *Chemical Calories*. Although most are designed around conventionally grown foods which are lower in *Chemical Calories*, certain salads or herbs may contain higher levels. If you can't get hold of organic versions of these ingredients, substitute items which are lower in *Chemical Calories*. In all cases, use the *Chemical Calorie* Charts in Chapter 18 for guidance.

- If for religious or other reasons you can't eat certain meats, substitute the one stated with an appropriate alternative (see Chapter 16).

- You will notice that in some of the recipes I have suggested you can use tinned produce for certain foods, which is mainly for the sake of convenience. For example, not everyone has the time to soak beans overnight and then cook them, and as beans provide an excellent source of protein and fibre it would be a pity to cut this valuable food out of the diet totally for those who lack the time to cook.

- If you don't like butter, you can either go without it totally, use a nut or seed spread, or cut it out and use an extra teaspoon of oil in preparing that day's menu.

- Finally – do get a good pair of scales to weigh things out properly, as this will help to ensure your ultimate success.

Standard Menus

Menu 1

On waking up	Fibre supplements (and/or charcoal, and/or clay)
	Large glass of water
Breakfast	Porridge made with 25g oats (with milk from allowance)
	125ml orange juice
	Multivitamins and minerals, essential fats, and amino acid supplements taken at least half an hour after fibre supplements
Mid-morning	1 portion of fruit
Pre-lunch	Fibre supplements (and/or charcoal, and/or clay)
	Large glass of water
Lunch	200g baked beans in tomato sauce
	2 slices of toast
	Mixed salad with red and green peppers and unlimited vegetables, dressed with lemon juice and herbs
Afternoon	1 portion of fruit
Pre-dinner	Fibre supplements (and/or charcoal, and/or clay)
	Large glass of water
Dinner	100g grilled steak
	120g baked potato
	Green beans
	Apple, walnut (20g) and *green salad, dressed with lemon juice
	Any additional supplements

Menu 2

On waking up	Fibre supplements (and/or charcoal, and/or clay)
	Large glass of water
Breakfast	2 slices of toast with 1 teaspoon of butter

1 portion of fruit

Multivitamins and minerals, essential fats, and amino
   acid supplements

Mid-morning   1 portion of fruit

Pre-lunch   Fibre supplements (and/or charcoal, and/or clay)
               Large glass of water

Lunch   120g baked potato
               55g grated cheese or 200g cottage cheese
               Tossed salad with unlimited vegetables from list,
                  dressed with lemon juice and herbs

Afternoon   1 portion of fruit

Pre-dinner   Fibre supplements (and/or charcoal, and/or clay)
               Large glass of water

Dinner   *Lemon chicken kebabs (includes 100g chicken,
                  2 teaspoons oil)
               Served with 70g cooked rice and unlimited vegetables
                  from list
               1 portion of fruit

               Any additional supplements

Menu 3

On waking up   Fibre supplements (and/or charcoal, and/or clay)
               Large glass of water

Breakfast   30g breakfast cereal (with milk from allowance)
               20g raisins or dried fruit
               Multivitamins and minerals, essential fats, and amino
                  acid supplements

Mid-morning   1 portion of fruit

Pre-lunch   Fibre supplements (and/or charcoal, and/or clay)
               Large glass of water

Lunch   55g Cheddar cheese grilled on 1 slice of toast (with
                  Worcestershire sauce, optional)
               Green salad*, dressed with lemon juice

Afternoon   I portion of fruit

Pre-dinner   Fibre supplements (and/or charcoal, and/or clay)
                 Large glass of water

Dinner   Vegetable soup★ (low-fat)
                 ★ Stir-fried pork and vegetables (includes 100g
                     pork, 100g chopped pineapple, 2 teaspoons of
                     olive oil)
                 Served with 140g cooked rice

                 Any additional supplements

Menu 4

On waking up   Fibre supplements (and/or charcoal, and/or clay)
                 Large glass of water

Breakfast   2 slices of toast with 1 teaspoon of butter
                 125ml orange juice
                 Multivitamins and minerals, essential fats, and amino
                     acid supplements

Mid-morning   I portion of fruit

Pre-lunch   Fibre supplements (and/or charcoal, and/or clay)
                 Large glass of water

Lunch   120g baked potato
                 55g grated cheese or 200g cottage cheese
                 Tossed salad with unlimited vegetables from list,
                     dressed with lemon juice and herbs

Afternoon   I portion of fruit

Pre-dinner   Fibre supplements (and/or charcoal, and/or clay)
                 Large glass of water

Dinner   ★Vegetable soup (low-fat)
                 Grilled chicken breast, sliced into fine strips (100g of
                     chicken with the fat trimmed off)
                 ★Fresh tomato sauce (includes 1 teaspoon of oil from
                     allowance)
                 75g cooked pasta

Green salad
1 portion of fruit

Any additional supplements

Menu 5

On waking up	Fibre supplements (and/or charcoal, and/or clay)
	Large glass of water
Breakfast	30g breakfast cereal (with milk from allowance)
	125ml orange juice
	Multivitamins and minerals, essential fats, and amino acid supplements
Mid-morning	1 portion of fruit
Pre-lunch	Fibre supplements (and/or charcoal, and/or clay)
	Large glass of water
Lunch	100g cooked ham
	1 slice of bread with 1 teaspoon of butter
	Tossed salad with unlimited vegetables from list, dressed with lemon juice and fresh herbs
Afternoon	1 portion of fruit
Pre-dinner	Fibre supplements (and/or charcoal, and/or clay)
	Large glass of water
Dinner	*Lentil and vegetable soup (made with 80g cooked lentils and 1 teaspoon of olive oil)
	120g baked potato
	55g grated cheese or 200g cottage cheese
	Green salad, dressed with 1 teaspoon of oil
	1 portion of fruit

Any additional supplements

Menu 6

On waking up Fibre supplements (and/or charcoal, and/or clay)
Large glass of water

Breakfast Porridge (made with 25g oats and milk from
allowance)
1 portion of fruit
Multivitamins and minerals, essential fats, and amino
acid supplements

Mid-morning 1 portion of fruit

Pre-lunch Fibre supplements (and/or charcoal, and/or clay)
Large glass of water

Lunch 2 eggs
1 slice of toast
1 portion of fruit

Afternoon 1 portion of fruit

Pre-dinner Fibre supplements (and/or charcoal, and/or clay)
Large glass of water

Dinner *Vegetable soup (low-fat)
Grilled chicken breast (100g of chicken with the fat
trimmed off, marinated in lemon juice or soy sauce
and spices)
Stir-fried vegetables from the unlimited list, fried in 2
teaspoons of olive oil
Served with 140g cooked egg noodles

Any additional supplements

Menu 7

On waking up Fibre supplements (and/or charcoal, and/or clay)
Large glass of water

Breakfast 250g natural yoghurt or 200g fruit yoghurt
1 portion of fruit
Multivitamins and minerals, essential fats, and amino
acid supplements

Mid-morning   1 portion of fruit

Pre-lunch   Fibre supplements (and/or charcoal, and/or clay)
               Large glass of water

Lunch   200g baked beans in tomato sauce
               1 slice of toast
               20g mixed nuts and seeds

Afternoon   1 portion of fruit

Pre-dinner   Fibre supplements (and/or charcoal, and/or clay)
               Large glass of water

Dinner   100g roast lamb with the fat trimmed off
               120g potatoes, boiled, steamed or baked in their skins
               Vegetables from the unlimited list, prepared without fat
               1 portion of fruit

               Any additional supplements

Menu 8

On waking up   Fibre supplements (and/or charcoal, and/or clay)
               Large glass of water

Breakfast   2 slices of toast with 1 teaspoon of butter
               1 portion of fruit
               Multivitamins and minerals, essential fats, and amino
                  acid supplements

Mid-morning   1 portion of fruit

Pre-lunch   Fibre supplements (and/or charcoal, and/or clay)
               Large glass of water

Lunch   100g cold roast lamb
               1 slice of bread
               Tossed salad with unlimited vegetables from list,
                  dressed with lemon juice and herbs

Afternoon   1 portion of fruit

Pre-dinner   Fibre supplements (and/or charcoal, and/or clay)
               Large glass of water

Dinner	*Vegetable soup (low-fat)
	*Chicken casserole (including 100g chicken with the fat trimmed off, and 1 teaspoon of olive oil)
	Note: Make double quantity and keep the rest for tomorrow
	Served with 120g baked or boiled potatoes
	Green beans
	1 portion of fruit
	Any additional supplements

Menu 9

On waking up	Fibre supplements (and/or charcoal, and/or clay)
	Large glass of water
Breakfast	30g breakfast cereal (with milk from allowance)
	125ml orange juice
	Multivitamins and minerals, essential fats, and amino acid supplements
Mid-morning	1 portion of fruit
Pre-lunch	Fibre supplements (and/or charcoal, and/or clay)
	Large glass of water
Lunch	Ham sandwich (made with 2 slices of bread, 100g cooked ham, 1 teaspoon of butter)
	Tossed salad with unlimited vegetables from list, dressed with 1 teaspoon of oil, lemon juice and fresh herbs
Afternoon	1 portion of fruit
Pre-dinner	Fibre supplements (and/or charcoal, and/or clay)
	Large glass of water
Dinner	*Chicken casserole (left over from the day before, includes 100g chicken and 1 teaspoon of olive oil)
	Served with 70g cooked rice and green beans
	1 portion of fruit
	Any additional supplements

Menu 10

| On waking up | Fibre supplements (and/or charcoal, and/or clay) |
| | Large glass of water |

Breakfast	Porridge (made with 25g of oats and milk from allowance)
	125ml orange juice
	Multivitamins and minerals, essential fats, and amino acid supplements

| Mid-morning | 1 portion of fruit |
| | 20g mixed seeds and nuts |

| Pre-lunch | Fibre supplements (and/or charcoal, and/or clay) |
| | Large glass of water |

Lunch	200g baked beans in tomato sauce
	2 slices of toast
	Mixed salad with lettuce, tomatoes and unlimited vegetables, dressed with lemon juice and herbs

| Afternoon | 1 portion of fruit |

| Pre-dinner | Fibre supplements (and/or charcoal, and/or clay) |
| | Large glass of water |

Dinner	100g grilled gammon steak
	100g pineapple
	120g baked or boiled potatoes
	Mixed vegetables prepared without fat
	Any additional supplements

Menu 11

| On waking up | Fibre supplements (and/or charcoal, and/or clay) |
| | Large glass of water |

Breakfast	30g breakfast cereal (with milk from allowance)
	20g raisins or dried fruit
	Multivitamins and minerals, essential fats, and amino acid supplements

| Mid-morning | 1 portion of fruit |

Pre-lunch	Fibre supplements (and/or charcoal, and/or clay)
	Large glass of water
Lunch	55g cheese or 200g cottage cheese
	1 slice of bread with 1 teaspoon of butter
	Green salad, dressed with lemon juice
Afternoon	1 portion of fruit
Pre-dinner	Fibre supplements (and/or charcoal, and/or clay)
	Large glass of water
Dinner	*Vegetable noodle soup (includes 70g cooked egg noodles and 1 teaspoon of oil)
	*Spicy stir-fried prawns and vegetables (includes 100g tiger prawns and 2 teaspoons of olive oil)
	Served with 140g cooked rice
	1 portion of fruit
	Any additional supplements

Menu 12

On waking up	Fibre supplements (and/or charcoal, and/or clay)
	Large glass of water
Breakfast	30g breakfast cereal (with milk from allowance)
	125ml orange juice
	Multivitamins and minerals, essential fats, and amino acid supplements
Mid-morning	1 portion of fruit
Pre-lunch	Fibre supplements (and/or charcoal, and/or clay)
	Large glass of water
Lunch	120g baked potato
	55g grated cheese or 200g cottage cheese
	Tossed salad with unlimited vegetables from list, dressed with lemon juice and herbs
Afternoon	1 portion of fruit
Pre-dinner	Fibre supplements (and/or charcoal, and/or clay)
	Large glass of water

Dinner   Avocado salad (made with 1 small avocado, 1 tomato,
                balsamic vinegar, salt, pepper, salad leaves,
                herbs)
                *Pasta with bacon and tomato sauce (includes 100g
                back bacon)
                150g cooked pasta
                1 portion of fruit

                Any additional supplements

Menu 13

On waking up   Fibre supplements (and/or charcoal, and/or clay)
                Large glass of water

Breakfast   Porridge made with 25g of oats (and milk from
                allowance)
                1 portion of fruit
                Multivitamins and minerals, essential fats, and amino
                acid supplements

Mid-morning   1 portion of fruit

Pre-lunch   Fibre supplements (and/or charcoal, and/or clay)
                Large glass of water

Lunch   Two-egg omelette made with 1 teaspoon of oil or
                butter
                1 slice of bread
                *Green salad

Afternoon   1 portion of fruit

Pre-dinner   Fibre supplements (and/or charcoal, and/or clay)
                Large glass of water

Dinner   *Vegetable soup (fat-free)
                Grilled chicken breast (100g of chicken with the fat
                trimmed off, marinated in lemon juice and grated
                ginger)
                Stirfried vegetables from the unlimited list with
                Chinese five spice, fried in 2 teaspoons of olive oil

Served with 140g cooked egg noodles
1 portion of fruit

Any additional supplements

Menu 14

On waking up	Fibre supplements (and/or charcoal, and/or clay) Large glass of water
Breakfast	30g breakfast cereal 1 portion of fruit Multivitamins and minerals, essential fats, and amino acid supplements
Mid-morning	1 portion of fruit
Pre-lunch	Fibre supplements (and/or charcoal, and/or clay) Large glass of water
Lunch	Grilled cheese sandwich (made with 2 slices of bread, 55g Cheddar cheese, optional Worcestershire sauce) *Green salad
Afternoon	1 portion of fruit
Pre-dinner	Fibre supplements (and/or charcoal, and/or clay) Large glass of water

Dinner	Avocado salad (made with 1 small avocado, 1 tomato,
	    balsamic vinegar, salt, pepper, green salad)
	100g grilled steak with the fat trimmed off
	120g potatoes, boiled, steamed or baked in their skins
	Vegetables from the unlimited list, prepared without
	    fat
	1 portion of fruit

Any additional supplements

Menus for Men

The following menus are intended for men who want to lose weight. They are based on the standard menus above, with 1 extra portion of protein and 2 extra portions of carbohydrate. The vegetarian menus may also be adapted in the same way, following the guidelines in Chapter 16.

Male Menu 1

On waking up	Fibre supplements (and/or charcoal, and/or clay)
	Large glass of water
Breakfast	Porridge (made with 50g of oats and milk from allowance)
	125ml orange juice
	Multivitamins and minerals, essential fats, and amino acid supplements, taken at least half an hour after fibre supplements
Mid-morning	1 portion of fruit
Pre-lunch	Fibre supplements (and/or charcoal, and/or clay)
	Large glass of water
Lunch	200g baked beans in tomato sauce
	2 slices of toast
	Mixed salad with red and green peppers and unlimited vegetables, dressed with lemon juice and herbs
Afternoon	1 portion of fruit
Pre-dinner	Fibre supplements (and/or charcoal, and/or clay)
	Large glass of water
Dinner	200g grilled steak
	240g baked potato
	Green beans
	Apple, walnut (20g) and *green salad dressed with lemon juice
	Any additional supplements

Male Menu 2

On waking up   Fibre supplements (and/or charcoal, and/or clay)
Large glass of water

Breakfast   2 slices of toast with 1 teaspoon of butter
1 portion of fruit
Multivitamins and minerals, essential fats, and amino acid supplements

Mid-morning   1 portion of fruit

Pre-lunch   Fibre supplements (and/or charcoal, and/or clay)
Large glass of water

Lunch   120g baked potato
100g baked beans in tomato sauce
55g grated cheese or 200g cottage cheese
Tossed salad with unlimited vegetables from list, dressed with lemon juice and herbs

Afternoon   1 portion of fruit

Pre-dinner   Fibre supplements (and/or charcoal, and/or clay)
Large glass of water

Dinner   *Lemon chicken kebabs (2 chicken and 2 vegetable kebabs, made with 200g chicken and 2 teaspoons of oil)
Served with 140g cooked rice
1 portion of fruit

Any additional supplements

Male Menu 3

On waking up   Fibre supplements (and/or charcoal, and/or clay)
Large glass of water

Breakfast   60g breakfast cereal (with milk from allowance)
20g raisins or dried fruit
Multivitamins and minerals, essential fats, and amino acid supplements

Morning   1 portion of fruit

Pre-lunch	Fibre supplements (and/or charcoal, and/or clay) Large glass of water
Lunch	55g Cheddar cheese grilled on 1 slice of toast (Worcestershire sauce optional) 100g baked beans in tomato sauce *Green salad, dressed with lemon juice and herbs
Afternoon	1 portion of fruit
Pre-dinner	Fibre supplements (and/or charcoal, and/or clay) Large glass of water
Dinner	*Vegetable soup (low-fat) Stir-fried pork and vegetables (includes 200g pork, 100g chopped pineapple, 2 teaspoons of olive oil) Served with 140g cooked rice Any additional supplements

Male Menu 4

On waking up	Fibre supplements (and/or charcoal, and/or clay) Large glass of water
Breakfast	2 slices of toast with 1 teaspoon of butter 125ml orange juice Multivitamins and minerals, essential fats, and amino acid supplements
Mid-morning	1 portion of fruit
Pre-lunch	Fibre supplements Large glass of water
Lunch	120g baked potato 55g grated cheese or 200g cottage cheese 100g baked beans in tomato sauce Tossed salad with unlimited vegetables from list, dressed with lemon juice and herbs
Afternoon	1 portion of fruit
Pre-dinner	Fibre supplements (and/or charcoal, and/or clay) Large glass of water

Dinner	*Vegetable soup (low-fat)
	Grilled chicken breast, sliced into fine strips (200g of chicken with the fat trimmed off)
	*Fresh tomato sauce (includes 1 teaspoon of oil from allowance)
	150g cooked pasta
	*Green salad
	1 portion of fruit
	Any additional supplements

Male Menu 5

On waking up	Fibre supplements (and/or charcoal, and/or clay)
	Large glass of water
Breakfast	60g breakfast cereal (with milk from allowance)
	125ml orange juice
	Multivitamins and minerals, essential fats, and amino acid supplements
Mid-morning	1 portion of fruit
Pre-lunch	Fibre supplements (and/or charcoal, and/or clay)
	Large glass of water
Lunch	100g cooked ham
	2 slices of bread with 1 teaspoon of butter
	Tossed salad with unlimited vegetables from list, dressed with lemon juice and fresh herbs
Afternoon	1 portion of fruit
Pre-dinner	Fibre supplements (and/or charcoal, and/or clay)
	Large glass of water
Dinner	*Vegetable soup (low-fat)
	240g baked potato
	110g grated cheese
	*Green salad, dressed with 1 teaspoon of oil
	1 portion of fruit
	Any additional supplements

Male Menu 6

On waking up	Fibre supplements (and/or charcoal, and/or clay)
	Large glass of water
Breakfast	Porridge (made with 50g of oats and milk from allowance)
	1 portion of fruit
	Multivitamins and minerals, essential fats, and amino acid supplements
Mid-morning	1 portion of fruit
Pre-lunch	Fibre supplements (and/or charcoal, and/or clay)
	Large glass of water
Lunch	2 eggs
	2 slices of toast
	1 portion of fruit
Afternoon	1 portion of fruit
Pre-dinner	Fibre supplements (and/or charcoal, and/or clay)
	Large glass of water
Dinner	*Vegetable soup (low-fat)
	Grilled chicken breast (200g chicken with the fat trimmed off, marinated in lemon juice or soy sauce and spices)
	Stir-fried vegetables from the unlimited list, fried in 2 teaspoons of olive oil
	Served with 140g cooked egg noodles
	Any additional supplements

Male Menu 7

On waking up	Fibre supplements (and/or charcoal, and/or clay)
	Large glass of water
Breakfast	250g natural yoghurt or 200g fruit yoghurt
	1 portion of fruit
	Multivitamins and minerals, essential fats, and amino acid supplements

Mid-morning	1 portion of fruit
Pre-lunch	Fibre supplements (and/or charcoal, and/or clay) Large glass of water
Lunch	200g baked beans in tomato sauce 2 slices of toast 20g mixed nuts and seeds
Afternoon	1 portion of fruit
Pre-dinner	Fibre supplements (and/or charcoal, and/or clay) Large glass of water

Dinner	200g roast lamb with the fat trimmed off
	240g potatoes, boiled, steamed or baked in their
	   skins
	Vegetables from the unlimited list, prepared without
	   fat
	1 portion of fruit
	
	Any additional supplements

Vegetarian Menus

Although they obviously contain no meat, poultry or fish, these do contain dairy products suitable for vegetarians. And as with the previous menus, these ones too may be adapted for men according to the guidelines in Chapter 16. One sample male vegetarian menu is also included to give you an idea of how to adapt the menu.

Vegetarian Menu 1

On waking up	Fibre supplements (and/or charcoal, and/or clay) Large glass of water
Breakfast	30g breakfast cereal (with milk from allowance) 20g raisins Multivitamins and minerals, essential fats, and amino

acid supplements, taken at least half an hour after
fibre supplements

Mid-morning   1 portion of fruit
15g uncooked nuts or seeds (optional)

Pre-lunch   Fibre supplements (and/or charcoal, and/or clay)
Large glass of water

Lunch   *Vegetable soup (low-fat)
1 slice of bread
55g cheese or 200g cottage cheese, or 200g baked or
mixed beans in tomato sauce, 1 tomato and/or some
cucumber

Afternoon   1 portion of fruit

Pre-dinner   Fibre supplements (and/or charcoal, and/or clay)
Large glass of water

Dinner   *Spicy stir-fried tofu and vegetables (includes 125g tofu
and 2 teaspoons of olive oil)
Served with 140g cooked rice
1 portion of fruit

Any additional supplements

Vegetarian Menu 2

On waking up   Fibre supplements (and/or charcoal, and/or clay)
Large glass of water

Breakfast   Porridge (made with 25g of oats and milk from
allowance)
1 portion of fruit
Multivitamins and minerals, essential fats, and amino
acid supplements

Mid-morning   1 portion of fruit
15g of uncooked nuts or seeds (optional)

Pre-lunch   Fibre supplements (and/or charcoal, and/or clay)
Large glass of water

Lunch	*Lentil and vegetable soup (includes 80g lentils and 1 teaspoon of oil)
	1 slice of bread and one teaspoon of butter
	250g natural yoghurt or 200g fruit yoghurt
Afternoon	1 portion of fruit
Pre-dinner	Fibre supplements (and/or charcoal, and/or clay)
	Large glass of water
Dinner	*Herb omelette (made with 2 eggs, chives and fresh herbs, and 1 teaspoon of butter)
	1 slice of bread
	Green salad, dressed with lemon juice and herbs
	1 portion of fruit
	Any additional supplements

Vegetarian Menu 3

On waking up	Fibre supplements (and/or charcoal, and/or clay)
	Large glass of water
Breakfast	2 slices of toast with 1 teaspoon of butter
	125ml orange juice
	Multivitamins and minerals, essential fats, and amino acid supplements
Mid-morning	1 portion of fruit
	15g of uncooked nuts or seeds (optional)
Pre-lunch	Fibre supplements (and/or charcoal, and/or clay)
	Large glass of water
Lunch	120g baked potato
	55g grated cheese or 200g cottage cheese
	Tossed salad with unlimited vegetables from list, dressed with lemon juice and herbs
Afternoon	1 portion of fruit
Pre-dinner	Fibre supplements (and/or charcoal, and/or clay)
	Large glass of water

| Dinner | *Chilli with rice (includes 80g cooked green lentils, 80g cooked kidney beans, 70g cooked rice and 2 teaspoons of olive oil) |
| | 1 portion of fruit |

Any additional supplements

Vegetarian Menu 4

On waking up Fibre supplements (and/or charcoal, and/or clay)
Large glass of water

Breakfast 30g breakfast cereal (with milk from allowance)
1 portion of fruit
Multivitamins and minerals, essential fats, and amino
acid supplements

Mid-morning 1 portion of fruit
15g of uncooked nuts or seeds (optional)

Pre-lunch Fibre supplements (and/or charcoal, and/or clay)
Large glass of water

Lunch 200g baked beans in tomato sauce
1 slice of toast with 1 teaspoon of butter
1 portion of fruit

Afternoon 1 portion of fruit

Pre-dinner Fibre supplements (and/or charcoal, and/or clay)
Large glass of water

Dinner *Vegetable soup (low-fat)
150g cooked pasta
*Fresh tomato sauce (includes one teaspoon of oil from
allowance)
55g grated Parmesan cheese
*Green salad

Any additional supplements

Vegetarian Menu 5

On waking up	Fibre supplements (and/or charcoal, and/or clay) Large glass of water
Breakfast	Porridge (made with 25g of oats and milk from allowance) 1 portion of fruit Multivitamins and minerals, essential fats, and amino acid supplements
Mid-morning	1 portion of fruit 15g of uncooked nuts or seeds (optional)
Pre-lunch	Fibre supplements (and/or charcoal, and/or clay) Large glass of water
Lunch	*Lentil and vegetable soup (made with 80g of cooked lentils and 1 teaspoon of oil) 1 slice of bread 40g cheese or 150g cottage cheese
Afternoon	1 portion of fruit
Pre-dinner	Fibre supplements (and/or charcoal, and/or clay) Large glass of water
Dinner	*Borlotti bean casserole (includes 160g of cooked borlotti beans, 2 teaspoons of olive oil) 15g grated cheese 1 slice of bread (Recipe makes double quantity, second portion for next day) *Green salad 1 portion of fruit Any additional supplements

Vegetarian Menu 6

On waking up	Fibre supplements (and/or charcoal, and/or clay) Large glass of water

Breakfast	2 slices of toast with 1 teaspoon of butter
	125ml orange juice
	Multivitamins and minerals, essential fats, and amino acid supplements
Mid-morning	1 portion of fruit
	15g of uncooked nuts or seeds (optional)
Pre-lunch	Fibre supplements (and/or charcoal, and/or clay)
	Large glass of water
Lunch	120g baked potato
	100g baked beans in tomato sauce
	40g grated cheese or 150g cottage cheese
	Salad with vegetables from unlimited list
Afternoon	1 portion of fruit
Pre-dinner	Fibre supplements (and/or charcoal, and/or clay)
	Large glass of water
Dinner	★Borlotti bean casserole (left over from previous day, 160g of cooked borlotti beans and 2 teaspoons of oil)
	15g grated cheese
	★Green salad
	1 portion of fruit
	Any additional supplements

Vegetarian Menu 7

On waking up	Fibre supplements (and/or charcoal, and/or clay)
	Large glass of water
Breakfast	Porridge (made with 25g of oats and milk from allowance)
	1 portion of fruit
	Multivitamins and minerals, essential fats, and amino acid supplements
Mid-morning	1 portion of fruit
	15g of uncooked nuts or seeds (optional)

| Pre-lunch | Fibre supplements (and/or charcoal, and/or clay) |
| | Large glass of water |

| Lunch | Toasted cheese sandwich (made with 2 slices of bread and 55g Cheddar cheese) |
| | Mixed salad dressed with 1 teaspoon of oil |

| Afternoon | 1 portion of fruit |

| Pre-dinner | Fibre supplements (and/or charcoal, and/or clay) |
| | Large glass of water |

Dinner	Lentil stew (based on the recipe for lentil and vegetable soup below, using 160g cooked green lentils and one or two teaspoons of oil)
	1 slice of bread
	1 portion of fruit
	Any additional supplements

Sample vegetarian menu for a man

| On waking up | Fibre supplements (and/or charcoal, and/or clay) |
| | Large glass of water |

Breakfast	60g breakfast cereal (with milk from allowance)
	20g raisins
	Multivitamins and minerals, essential fats, and amino acid supplements, taken at least half an hour after fibre supplements

| Mid-morning | 1 portion of fruit |
| | 15g of uncooked nuts or seeds (optional) |

| Pre-lunch | Fibre supplements (and/or charcoal, and/or clay) |
| | Large glass of water |

Lunch	*Vegetable soup (fat-free)
	1 slice of bread with 1 teaspoon of butter
	200g baked beans or mixed beans in tomato sauce
	250g natural yoghurt (low-fat) or 200g fruit yoghurt (low-fat)

Afternoon	1 portion of fruit
Pre-dinner	Fibre supplements (and/or charcoal, and/or clay)
	Large glass of water
Dinner	*Spicy stir-fried tofu and vegetables (includes 125g tofu and 2 teaspoons of olive oil)
	Served with 210g cooked rice
	1 portion of fruit
	Any additional supplements

Recipes

Vegetable soup

There are endless variations on this idea, so in addition to the soups below you could let your culinary skills run riot. The good news is that soups made from vegetables on the unlimited list and without any oil or butter can be eaten freely throughout the day – and a particularly good time to enjoy them is as a starter for your evening meal.

These recipes are marked FAT-FREE to show that they can be eaten freely. They will also help you to detox, as vegetable soups are largely alkaline and so will keep your body pH at an optimal level. And if you don't have time to cook, but desperately need something warm, savoury, filling and fat-free, a speedy version can be made just by dissolving a stock cube or yeast extract in boiling water. This can help fill the gap in emergencies, and is very easy to make if you are at work.

Other soups in this section are made with a small amount of oil, which means that they *cannot* be eaten freely. They are marked LOW-FAT and count as 1 teaspoon of oil against your day's fat allowance. All these soups have been designed to be made quickly, but to save even more time you could make them in large batches then either freeze or refrigerate them so that you have them quickly to hand whenever you need them.

One more thing: you will find that quite a few recipes have lots of added herbs and spices to enhance the flavour. Do feel free to modify the herbs and spices depending on their availability and of course on your own individual preferences.

Vegetable soup with Chinese leaves FAT-FREE

This recipe is not only ideal for Chinese cabbage, but can easily be adapted for any combination from the list of unlimited vegetables.

> 1 litre chicken or vegetable stock (from stock cubes, or
>   home-made stock with the fat skimmed off)
> 2 medium carrots, thinly sliced
> 2 sticks of celery, chopped
> 1 onion, finely chopped
> 3 tablespoons chopped fresh parsley (optional)
> salt and freshly ground black pepper
> 200g Chinese cabbage leaves, finely shredded
> 1 large ripe tomato, deseeded and chopped

Bring the stock to the boil in a large pan and add the carrots, celery, onion, parsley and seasoning. Bring back to the boil, then cover and simmer for about 15 minutes. Add the Chinese cabbage and tomato and simmer for a further 5 minutes.

You can make this soup more filling by adding 75g of cooked pasta or 70g of cooked rice to a single serving. This will use up 1 unit of carbohydrate from your day's allowance.

Carrot soup FAT-FREE

Carrots are naturally sweet, and make a thick substantial fat-free soup that's particularly comforting in winter. If you have a food processor, it will take only a few minutes to prepare the vegetables.

1.5 litres chicken or vegetable stock (from stock
    cubes, or home-made stock with the fat skimmed
    off)
750g carrots, roughly chopped
1 large onion, finely chopped
4 cloves of garlic, crushed and chopped
2 tablespoons fresh grated ginger (optional)
1 teaspoon ground cumin
1 teaspoon ground coriander, or 3 stalks of fresh
    coriander
pinch of cayenne pepper
salt and freshly ground black pepper
2 tablespoons lemon juice

Bring the stock to the boil in a large pan. Add the carrots, onion,
garlic, ginger and spices and simmer for about 30 minutes. Taste
the soup, and season. Leave to cool slightly, then purée using a
hand blender, liquidizer or food processor. If the mixture is too
thick, thin it with a little stock or water. Add lemon juice to taste
just before serving.

Japanese clear soup FAT-FREE

This is another very quick and easy soup. It takes only moments to
make, and is a good stand-by to satisfy urgent food cravings. It also
makes a light and refreshing change from thicker soups.

1 litre chicken or vegetable stock (from stock cubes, or
    home-made stock with the fat skimmed off)
salt and freshly ground black pepper
1 teaspoon grated ginger
2 spring onions, finely chopped
1 carrot, chopped into matchsticks
few mushrooms, very finely sliced
soy sauce to taste

Bring the stock to the boil in a large pan and add the seasoning and grated ginger. Ladle into warm bowls and sprinkle with the finely chopped vegetables. Add soy sauce to taste.

You can raise the protein content of this soup by adding tofu from your protein allowance. Dice the tofu, add it to the boiling stock, and simmer for about 3 minutes before removing the pan from the heat and continuing as above.

Alternatively you can make a more filling version by adding 25g of dried egg noodles for a single serving. Add the noodles to the boiling stock and cook for the time given in the packet directions. This uses 1 unit of carbohydrate from your day's allowance, and could, for example, be substituted for 1 of the slices of bread suggested in several of the daily menus above.

Tomato soup LOW-FAT

Despite being a little bit more trouble to make, this tomato soup is really delicious. If you are short of time, however, there are ready-made versions of organic tomato soup available to buy. If you take this route, 1 serving would still probably count as 1 unit of fat. Just check the ingredients for added carbohydrates or increased use of fats.

  1 tablespoon olive oil
  1 onion, finely chopped
  1 carrot, grated
  900g fresh tomatoes, skinned and deseeded
  500ml chicken or vegetable stock (from stock cubes, or
      home-made stock with the fat skimmed off)
  2 tablespoons fresh basil (optional)
  1 teaspoon lemon juice
  salt and freshly ground black pepper

Heat the oil in a saucepan and cook the onion and carrot until they are soft, but not brown. Add the tomatoes and stock, bring to the boil, and simmer for about 10 minutes. Allow to cool, then add the basil and blend the soup in a food processor or liquidizer. You can either reheat the soup to serve it hot, or chill it to serve it cold. Either way, add the lemon juice and seasoning just before serving.

This makes about 6 substantial servings of delicious low-fat soup. To add a different twist: on a day when you choose natural yoghurt as one of your servings of protein (see menu 7 above), you could reserve a spoonful of yoghurt from your allowance to stir into the soup.

Mushroom and shallot soup LOW-FAT

I first came across shallots when I attended a local horticultural show as a child. I remember these small golden vegetables with their dried-out stems beautifully arranged on plates. More recently I have started to grow them in my garden for their tremendous versatility. When they are young you can use them like spring onions, and when they are more mature they are perfect for soups like this.

> 1 tablespoon olive oil
> 8 shallots or very small onions, halved
> 850ml chicken or vegetable stock (from stock cubes, or
>   home-made stock with the fat skimmed off)
> 1 carrot, thinly sliced
> 1 teaspoon dried tarragon or 2 stalks of fresh tarragon
> salt and freshly ground black pepper
> 1 teaspoon lemon juice
> 85g broccoli, broken into small florets
> 115g mushrooms, cleaned and chopped
> 225g pumpkin, diced small

Heat the oil in a pan and brown the shallots, then add the stock, carrot, tarragon, seasoning and lemon juice. Bring to the boil and simmer for about 10 minutes. Add the broccoli, mushrooms and pumpkin, and simmer for 5 more minutes or until the vegetables are tender.

This makes about 4 substantial servings of low-fat soup.

Green salad

It is very important to use organically grown salad leaves and fresh herbs, or salad leaves and herbs from your own garden that have not been sprayed. Some non-organic salad leaves tend to be high in *Chemical Calories* and are not recommended on the Detox Diet. If you can't get organic lettuce for your green salad, use the following substitutes, which will be lower in *Chemical Calories*, brimming full of slimming nutrients and will make up a great salad: beansprouts, green beans (dwarf and French varieties), broccoli, cabbage, cauliflower, chicory, Chinese cabbage, courgettes, cress, rocket, watercress and spinach.

Lemon chicken kebabs

These tasty kebabs are ideal if you are having a barbecue in the summer.

> For 1 chicken kebab and 1 vegetable kebab
> 100g boneless chicken thigh meat (trimmed of fat)
> 3 shallots or very small onions
> courgette, sliced fairly thickly
> 1 green, red, or yellow pepper, cut into 2.5cm squares
> 3 cherry tomatoes
> 2 teaspoons olive oil
> 2 teaspoons lemon juice
> 1 clove of garlic, minced
> salt and freshly ground black pepper
> (You will also need 2 wooden or metal skewers)

Cut the chicken into 2.5cm cubes, thread them on to a skewer, and put them in a foil-lined grill pan. Thread the shallots, courgette slices, pepper and tomatoes on to a second skewer, and put that on the side. Mix the oil, lemon juice, garlic and seasoning and brush about half of it on to the kebabs. Grill the chicken under a high heat for about 7-8 minutes each side, and add the vegetable kebabs for the last 6 minutes of the cooking time. Baste with the remainder of the oil mixture during cooking.

Stir-fried pork with pineapple

This takes only about 20 minutes to make from start to finish, and tastes so delicious that no one would ever guess that it was good for you too!

> 2 teaspoons olive oil
> 100g lean pork, sliced into fine strips
> salt and freshly ground black pepper
> ¼ teaspoon grated ginger
> 1 small onion, chopped finely
> 1 red pepper, cut into strips
> soy sauce to taste
> 2 tomatoes, peeled, deseeded and chopped, or a few
> 　　spoonfuls of tinned chopped tomatoes
> 100g fresh or tinned pineapple cubes

If you are going to serve this dish with rice, start cooking the rice after you have chopped the vegetables, but before you begin to cook. Heat the oil in a wok, and season the pork with salt and pepper. Add the pork and ginger to the wok, and cook until the pork is brown on both sides. Add the onion, red pepper and soy sauce and cook for a few minutes, then add the tomatoes and pineapple. Check the seasoning, and add more salt, pepper or soy sauce if necessary. Serve right away.

Fresh tomato sauce

Make this sauce in double quantity (or more) and divide it into individual portions for the freezer. It's very good with pasta and grilled chicken breast or grated cheese, but remember to count these accompaniments from your day's allowance. Each portion of the sauce contains 1 teaspoon of oil.

1 teaspoon olive oil

1 onion, chopped finely

½ a small courgette, chopped finely

4 large tomatoes, skinned and deseeded and chopped,
    or 1 small tin of Italian tomatoes

salt and freshly ground black pepper

½ teaspoon dried basil or a few fresh basil leaves

Heat the oil in a non-stick pan and fry the onion until it is soft, but not brown. Add the courgette and cook, stirring, for 5 minutes. Add the tomatoes, dried basil (if using) and seasoning, cover and simmer on a low heat for 5 minutes, stirring occasionally. Serve with pasta, and garnish with fresh basil.

Lentil and vegetable soup

This hearty and filling soup contains 1 unit of carbohydrate per portion as well as oil from your allowance. The quantities given are for 4 portions. Vegetarians can easily adapt the ingredients to make a more substantial lentil stew, by doubling the amount of lentils stated in the recipe to 240g (dried weight). One portion of this stew would then be considered as either 2 portions of carbohydrate or 1 portion of protein. If extra lentils are used, you will need a little extra stock to get the stew to the consistency you like. If you use green or brown lentils for the stew, they need to be soaked before cooking.

1 tablespoon oil

1 large onion, chopped finely

1 clove of garlic, sliced or crushed

120g dried red lentils (washed)

salt and freshly ground black pepper

1.2 litres chicken or vegetable stock (from stock cubes,
    or home-made stock with the fat skimmed off)

1 carrot, chopped finely

½–1 teaspoon mixed dried herbs (optional)

3 cloves
fresh parsley and lemon wedges to garnish

Heat the oil and fry the onion and garlic gently until they are soft but not brown. Add the lentils, seasoning and stock to the pan and bring it to the boil. Add the carrot, herbs and cloves, and reduce the heat so that the soup cooks gently for about 45 minutes.

Allow the soup to cool, and remove the cloves. If you wish, blend the mixture in a food processor, adding more stock or water if it is too thick. Reheat, and garnish with fresh parsley and a lemon wedge.

Vegetable noodle soup

This soup is extremely tasty and quick to make. It is fat-free, but it contains 1 unit of carbohydrate per portion. The quantities given are for 4 portions.

1 litre chicken or vegetable stock (from stock cubes, or
   home-made stock with the fat skimmed off)
1 tablespoon grated fresh ginger
1 clove of garlic, crushed and finely sliced
½ a red chilli or 1 green chilli, deseeded and chopped
100g dried egg noodles
2 tablespoons soy sauce
2 spring onions, finely chopped
4 mushrooms, finely sliced
salt and freshly ground black pepper

Put the stock, ginger and garlic in a pan and bring it to the boil. Add the chilli, then the noodles, and simmer according to the instructions on the packet. Add the soy sauce and vegetables, Season, and serve right away.

You can also serve this soup with shredded chicken breast, counted from your protein allowance. The chicken should be grilled and added to the soup while it is still hot. (If you add cold chicken to hot soups, make sure it gets thoroughly heated up.)

Chicken casserole

To save time, make double quantity of this tasty recipe and keep the second portion in the fridge for the next day. Be sure again to reheat the chicken properly before serving.

> 1 teaspoon olive oil
> salt and freshly ground black pepper
> 100g chicken breast, with the fat trimmed off
> 1 large onion, chopped
> 200ml chicken stock (from a stock cube, or
>   home-made stock with the fat skimmed off)
> fresh parsley and thyme (optional)
> 1 red pepper, chopped

Heat the oil in a pan. Season the chicken breast and brown it thoroughly on both sides, then add the onion and stir until it softens. Add about half the stock, and bring to a simmer. Add the herbs (if using) and red pepper, cover the pan, and simmer for 20 minutes, stirring occasionally. Add more stock if the chicken seems to be drying out.

Spicy stir-fried prawns (or tofu) and vegetables

This is one of my favourite dishes because I just love the tangy, full-bodied flavour that fresh coriander lends to stir-fried foods. And if you substitute the prawns with tofu, it also makes an ideal, and very tasty, meal for veggies!

> 2 teaspoons olive oil
> 100g tiger prawns (or 125g fresh tofu, cut into 1.5cm cubes)
> salt and freshly ground black pepper
> 2 spring onions, chopped, or ½ a small onion, chopped
> 1 clove garlic, chopped
> ¼–½ teaspoon grated fresh ginger
> pinch of chilli powder

200g prepared diced or sliced vegetables, e.g. water
     chestnuts, bean sprouts, mangetout, mushrooms,
     broccoli and baby corn
2 teaspoons soy sauce
4 sprigs fresh coriander, chopped

This takes only a few minutes to cook, so if you are serving it with
rice or noodles, start cooking these before you heat the wok. Have
a hot plate ready for the prawns.

Heat the olive oil in a wok. Season the prawns (or tofu) with salt
and pepper. Add the prawns (or tofu), onion, garlic and ginger to
the wok, and cook for 2 minutes or until the prawns turn pink.
Remove the prawns to a hot plate (but if you are using tofu, leave
it in the wok). Then add the chilli powder and the vegetables to
the wok, cooking and stirring them very quickly. When ready, add
the soy sauce and coriander and serve right away.

Pasta with bacon and tomato sauce

Here's another meal that's almost instant for days when you're
tired, hungry or running late. Put the water on to boil, add the
pasta, start the bacon under the grill, and the whole meal will be
ready by the time the bacon is cooked.

25g dried pasta
100g back bacon
1 red onion, finely sliced (use an ordinary onion if you
     can't get an organic red one!)
4 large tomatoes, skinned and deseeded and chopped
fresh basil
salt and freshly ground black pepper

Put plenty of water into a large saucepan and bring to the boil. Add the
pasta, cook for the time given on the packet, and drain. Meanwhile
grill the bacon and slice it into strips. Stir the onion and tomatoes, basil,
salt and pepper into the pasta and top with the bacon slices.

Borlotti bean casserole

This is a rich and filling dish, ideal for cold days or when you're really hungry. It takes a little time to prepare if you use dried beans, but will make enough for the next day too. If you can't get hold of borlotti beans, pinto beans will work just as well. This makes enough for 2 portions.

120g dried borlotti beans, soaked overnight in
    water and drained (or 320g tinned beans,
    drained)
3 teaspoons olive oil
1 onion, finely chopped
1 clove of garlic, finely chopped
250g courgettes, diced
1 green pepper, chopped
400g tin of chopped tomatoes
1 bay leaf (optional)
salt and freshly ground black pepper

For the pesto sauce
30g grated Parmesan cheese
4 tablespoons chopped fresh basil
1 teaspoon olive oil
1 clove of garlic, finely chopped
1 teaspoon paprika
pinch of chilli powder
salt and freshly ground black pepper

Mix together all the ingredients for the pesto sauce, and set aside in the fridge. If you are using dried beans, bring a large pan of water to the boil, add the drained beans, and simmer for about 40 minutes, or until tender. Drain them and set them aside.

    Heat the oil in a casserole and fry the onion and garlic until they are soft. Add the courgettes, pepper, beans, tomatoes, bay leaf and seasoning. Cover the casserole and simmer for 25 minutes. Stir in the pesto sauce, then serve.

Chilli with rice

This tasty and satisfying dish makes enough for 2 portions. It is high in soluble fibre – great for detoxing the body. This is one of my favourite dishes – rice and kidney beans just seem to be made for each other!

    4 teaspoons olive oil
    1 onion, chopped
    1 carrot, chopped
    1 clove of garlic, minced
    1 red pepper, chopped
    60g dried green lentils (or 160g tinned green lentils,
        drained)
    400g tin of chopped tomatoes
    250ml vegetable stock
    pinch of chilli powder
    pinch of ground cumin
    a very small pinch of cayenne pepper
    salt and freshly ground black pepper
    160g tinned red kidney beans, washed and drained
    50g uncooked rice
    lemon wedges for garnish

Heat the oil in a pan and fry the onion, carrot, garlic and red pepper gently for about 10 minutes. Add the lentils, tomatoes, stock and all the spices and seasonings. If you are using dried lentils, cover the pan and simmer for about 50 minutes. If you are using tinned lentils, go straight on to the next step.

Add the kidney beans to the mixture, cover the pan, and simmer for 10 minutes while you cook the rice. Garnish with lemon wedges and enjoy!

18. The *Chemical Calorie* Food Guide

I will be quite clear about this – these charts are what losing weight is all about. With this new and totally revolutionary guide to the typical *Chemical Calorie* levels in foods you will be able for the first time ever to get a good idea of which foods are likely to make you fat and which are not – possibly showing many of your favourite foods in a completely new light!

The charts will also enable you to eat lower in *Chemical Calories* without spending a fortune. For example, if money is tight, it would be far better to spend that bit extra on buying an organic lettuce than it would be on buying organic walnuts or an organic cauliflower – as the conventionally grown versions of these tend to be very low in *Chemical Calories* anyway.

Next time you go shopping, make this chart your trusted friend in guiding you to make the right choices and the results will soon become very apparent in the form of a new slimmer you.

HOW THESE CHARTS WERE PRODUCED

To produce these charts, I have used four years' worth of nationally published and publicly available data from the UK Government's Ministry of Agriculture, Fisheries and Food (MAFF; now called DEFRA). They tested for pesticide residues in a whole variety of foods grown in the UK as well as in a very large number of imported foods – particularly from Europe.[1]

For each food I calculated the average number of *Chemical Calories*, using data from over ninety different types of pesticides. Out of interest, the number of different pesticides found on each batch of tested food varied greatly, from 0 to 27, but averaged out at 1.5 for each sample.

If foods were tested more than once, I worked out the average number of *Chemical Calories* for each particular food.

HOW TO USE THE CHARTS

In order to keep things simple, I have created five categories, which will give you an indication of the level of *Chemical Calories* found in each food. These categories are as follows:

- Very low
- Low
- Medium
- High
- Very high

A brief summary of each of these categories will enable you to use them to best effect, as follows.

The foods in the *very low* category are the safest, as they either have no measurable or extremely low levels of *Chemical Calories* detected. Of course, these foods should still be washed thoroughly before eating.

The foods in the *low* category are still relatively safe, as the average level detected in these foods remains reasonably low. But it is still a good idea to wash or peel fruit or vegetables thoroughly just to be on the safe side.

Coming on to the foods with *medium* levels of chemicals, it starts becoming more worthwhile to consider buying the organic version if available, as these foods can contain significant levels of *Chemical Calories*. If no organic alternative is available, it would be worthwhile using the techniques described in Chapter 9 to lower any potential contamination.

When we get to the foods found to have *high* levels of *Chemical Calories*, the problem becomes much more serious, as these levels, over time, could significantly damage your *Slimming System*. So stepping up your efforts to avoid these foods will be definitely worth your while. Again, do look for the organic option or use appropriate methods of preparation to lower potential contamination.

Finally, the foods in the *very high* category should be avoided if possible and the organic alternative substituted wherever appropriate – except for oranges, where peeling will very significantly lower the overall level of *Chemical Calories*.

EXPLAINING THE VARIABILITY BETWEEN DIFFERENT FOODS

One thing to be borne in mind is that these levels are based on the average levels of *pesticides* found in the relatively small samples of foods tested by MAFF. This means that the amounts of *Chemical Calories* will be totally dependent on the farming practices used for those particular foods. As practices can vary greatly, the guide can provide only a rough estimate as to how contaminated the foods you choose to eat might be.

And as you go through the different categories you will find that some foods may be high in *Chemical Calories* in one form but lower in another. This may be because processing often lowers the level of pesticides in the food. This could help explain why many processed foods, such as biscuits, crisps and bread, tend to be relatively low in *Chemical Calories*.

Chemicals tend to be used on foods as a method of preservation, to keep them looking perfect on the supermarket shelf. If you use other forms of food preservation, such as freezing or canning, the need for chemical preservatives (which are also very expensive) tends to diminish. This could explain why items such as frozen and canned raspberries have been found to be very low in *Chemical Calories* while fresh raspberries are high.

In addition, if foods are prepared and cut up before sale, for example the vegetables going into coleslaw, the act of preparation in combination with a reduced need for chemicals to keep the vegetables looking good on the supermarket shelf could explain why some 'processed or pre-prepared' produce tends to be lower in *Chemical Calories*.

Although the *Chemical Calorie* rating of some foods appears to be very high, much of these chemicals tend to be found on the skin of the fruits or vegetables. These levels can be reduced dramatically once the skin has been removed. This would explain why banana chips are lower in *Chemical Calories* than fresh bananas, and orange juice is much lower in *Chemical Calories* than fresh oranges appear to be, because in peeling the fruit you will have removed the main source of chemical contamination.

I also need to mention meat, dairy produce and eggs here. As these charts have been based on the level of pesticides detected in foods, much of this produce appears relatively low in *Chemical Calories*. However, this produce can also contain antibiotics, other growth-promoters, and environmental pollutants, which were not tested for in these MAFF reports. As most of these chemicals also possess weight-promotion abilities, they will also contain a certain amount of *Chemical Calories*. This could result in the meat and products of intensively farmed animals, such as chickens, turkeys and pigs, being much higher in *Chemical Calories* than these initial charts first suggest.

To deal with this I will be re-evaluating all animals and animal produce for these additional added chemicals, and although these results cannot be provided in this book because of time restraints, they will appear on our website, www.chemicalcalories.com, as well as in future publications.

THESE LEVELS ARE NOT CAST IN STONE AND WILL NEED TO BE CONTINUALLY UPDATED

Because the chemicals used on crops keep changing, these charts will need to be renewed every few years to keep up with the changes in agriculture. So as the years go by you should expect changes in the overall level of *Chemical Calories* for different foods. And as more information comes in we will keep updating the information on which foods are high and low in *Chemical Calories* on our website.

Lastly, these charts indicate the levels of *Chemical Calories* from pesticides only, as other *Chemical Calories* from plastics or environmental pollutants are not routinely tested. To ensure that your intake of all sorts of *Chemical Calories* is kept as low as possible, you need to keep in mind the advice in Chapters 7 and 9. As more of this type of information becomes available, I will be able to include the effects of these plastics and environmental pollutants on the overall levels of *Chemical Calories* too.

So good luck, and I hope these exciting new charts will help you not only to lose those excess pounds but also to keep them off for good!

The *Chemical Calorie* Food Guide (All foods listed were produced conventionally, unless marked organic)

POTENTIAL AMOUNT OF *CHEMICAL CALORIES* IN DIFFERENT FOOD TYPES

Dairy and Egg

	Very low	Low	Medium	High	Very high
Butter			*		
Cheese		*			
Cream		*			
Eggs			*		
Ice-cream	*				
Milk	*				
Milk concentrate	*				
Milk powder	*				
Skimmed milk powder	*				
Whey powder	*				
Yoghurt	*				

Fish and Shellfish

	Very low	Low	Medium	High	Very high
Eels				*	
Fish oils				*	
Fish sticks	*				
Jellied eels				*	
Mussels	*				
Oysters	*				

Fruit and Fruit Products

	Very low	Low	Medium	High	Very high
Apples, dessert				*	
Apples, dessert, organic	*				
Apple concentrate		*			
Apple juice concentrate	*				
Apricots				*	
Apricots, dried	*				
Apricot concentrate	*				
Bananas			*		
Banana chips	*				
Blackcurrants, fresh	*				
Blackcurrants, canned				*	
Blueberries			*		
Cherries		*			
Cherry juice concentrate	*				
Clementines	*				
Coconut	*				

continued . . .

	Very low	Low	Medium	High	Very high
Mandarin concentrate		*			
Mandarin juice	*				
Mangoes		*			
Mango concentrate	*				
Melons	*				
Minneolas				*	
Mixed fruit, dried		*			
Navelinas				*	
Nectarines		*			
Oranges					*
Orange concentrate	*				
Orange juice	*				
Orange juice, organic	*				
Ortaniques				*	
Papayas		*			
Peaches		*			
Peach pulp	*				
Pears				*	

Pilchards	*				
Salmon (farmed)					*
Scallops	*				
Tiger prawns	*				
Trout (farmed)				*	
Tuna				*	
White fish	*				
Beverages					
Coffee beans	*				
Tea					*
Wine	*				
Wine, organic	*				
Fats, oils and Shortenings					
Dripping			*		
Lard				*	
Linseed oil				*	
Margarine	*				
Olive oil		*			
Rapeseed oil				*	
Suet			*		
Sunflower oil	*				

Cranberries	*				
Currants		*			
Damsons	*				
Dates, fresh	*				
Dates, dried	*				
Dragon fruit	*				
Figs, fresh	*				
Figs, dried	*				
Fruit salad, fresh				*	
Fruit salad, dried	*				
Gooseberries	*				
Grapefruit			*		
Grapes			*		
Grapes, organic	*				
Infant food, fruit			*		
Infant food, fruit, organic	*				
Kiwi fruit			*		
Kiwi fruit, organic	*				
Lemons				*	
Lemon juice	*				
Lemon peel	*				
Limes	*				
Lime juice	*				
Loganberries	*				
Lychees				*	
Mandarin oranges					*

Pear juice concentrate		*			
Pears, organic	*				
Persimmons		*			
Pineapple		*			
Pineapple, canned	*				
Pineapple, crushed	*				
Pineapple juice	*				
Plums		*			
Plums, organic	*				
Pomegranates	*				
Prunes	*				
Raisins	*				
Raspberries				*	
Raspberries, frozen	*				
Raspberries, canned	*				
Raspberries, organic	*				
Redcurrants			*		
Rhubarb	*				
Satsumas			*		
Star fruit		*			
Strawberries				*	
Sultanas	*				
Tangerines			*		
Tayberries	*				
Whitecurrants	*				

The *Chemical Calorie* Food Guide (All foods listed were produced conventionally, unless marked organic)

POTENTIAL AMOUNT OF CHEMICAL CALORIES IN DIFFERENT FOOD TYPES – *cont.*

Grain Products

	Very low	Low	Medium	High	Very high
Barley	*				
Biscuits, sweet	*				
Biscuits, savoury	*				
Biscuits, crackers	*				
Bread, white	*				
Bread, brown	*				
Bread, wholemeal		*			
Bread, multigrain		*			
Bread, with fruit		*			
Breakfast cereal	*				
Cakes	*				
Cereals, infant food	*				
Corn, cereal grain			*		
Flour, white		*			
Flour, white organic	*				
Flour, brown	*				
Flour, wholemeal	*				
Flour, wholemeal organic	*				
Linseed			*		

continued . . .

	Very low	Low	Medium	High	Very high
Fennel	*				
Garlic	*				
Garlic, chopped dried	*				
Ginger	*				
Mace, ground	*				
Marjoram	*				
Mint					*
Mixed herbs	*				
Mustard seeds	*				
Nutmeg	*				
Oregano	*				
Paprika	*				
Parsley			*		
Parsley root	*				
Pepper, black	*				
Pepper, cayenne	*				
Rosemary			*		
Sage	*				
Tarragon		*			

continued . . .

	Very low	Low	Medium	High	Very high
Turkey	*				
Veal	*				
Venison	*				

Miscellaneous Items

	Very low	Low	Medium	High	Very high
Chocolate, plain		*			
Chocolate, milk		*			
Chocolate, white	*				
Chocolate, continental			*		
Chocolate, cooking		*			
Cider vinegar	*				
Cocoa beans	*				
Cocoa butter			*		
Coleslaw	*				
Honey	*				
Marmalade	*				
Soup, mushroom	*				
Soup, tomato	*				

Section 1

Soup, vegetable *
Sugar *
Tortilla chips *

Nuts, Seeds and Pulses

Almonds *
Beans, baked *
Beans, borlotti *
Beans, butter *
Beans, haricot *
Beans, kidney *
Beans, mung *
Beans, navy *
Brazil nuts *
Cashew nuts *
Chestnuts *
Chickpeas *
Cobnuts *
Coconut *
Hazelnuts *
Lentils, green *
Lentils, red *
Peanuts *
Peas, marrowfat *
Peas, yellow split *
Pecans *
Pistachios *

Section 2

Thyme *
Turmeric *

Meat and Poultry

Bacon *
Beef *
Beef, burgers *
Chicken (see Chapter 7) *
Duck *
Goose *
Guinea fowl *
Kidneys, lamb *
Kidneys, ox *
Kidneys, pig *
Lamb *
Lamb, British *
Liver, lamb *
Liver, ox *
Liver, pig *
Ostrich *
Pâté *
Pheasant *
Pork *
Quail *
Rabbit *
Sausage, beef *
Sausage, pork *

Section 3

Maize *
Maize-based snacks *
Millet *
Muesli, organic *
Oats *
Pasta *
Porridge, infant foods *
Quinoa *
Rice, white *
Rice, brown *
Rye *
Wheat grains *
Wheat grains, organic *

Herbs and Spices

Basil *
Basil, organic *
Bay leaves *
Chillies *
Chives *
Cinnamon *
Coriander *
Coriander, seed *
Cumin, ground *
Dill *

The *Chemical Calorie* Food Guide (All foods listed were produced conventionally, unless marked organic)

POTENTIAL AMOUNT OF *CHEMICAL CALORIES* IN DIFFERENT FOOD TYPES – *cont.*

continued . . .	Very low	Low	Medium	High	Very high
Sesame seeds		*			
Walnuts			*		
Vegetables					
Alfalfa sprouts, organic	*				
Artichoke, globe	*				
Artichoke, Jerusalem			*		
Asparagus	*				
Aubergines	*				
Avocados	*				
Baby vegetables, mixed			*		
Beansprouts	*				
Beans, dwarf	*				
Beans, fine	*				
Beans, flat			*		
Beans, green	*				
Beans, runner		*			

continued . . .	Very low	Low	Medium	High	Very high
Carrots		*			
Cauliflower	*				
Celeriac	*				
Celery				*	
Celery, organic	*				
Chervil	*				
Chicory		*			
Chinese cabbage	*				
Courgettes	*				
Cress	*				
Cucumbers			*		
Greens	*				
Hops					*
Kale			*		
Leeks	*				
Lettuce, varied types				*	
Lettuce, winter					*
Marrow	*				
Mushrooms		*			

continued . . .	Very low	Low	Medium	High	Very high
Parsnips		*			
Peas	*				
Peas, mangetout			*		
Peas, sugar snap					*
Potatoes				*	
Potatoes, baking				*	
Potatoes, new		*			
Potatoes, salad			*		
Potatoes, sweet			*		
Pumpkin	*				
Radishes	*				
Rocket	*				
Spinach			*		
Squash	*				
Squash, patty pan		*			
Swede				*	
Sweet corn	*				
Sweet peppers		*			
Tomatoes			*		

Tomatoes, organic	*		
Tomatoes, cherry	*		
Turnips		*	
Watercress	*		

Okra	*		
Olives		*	
Onions		*	
Onions, red			*
Onions, salad		*	

Beetroot	*	
Beetroot, organic	*	
Broccoli		*
Brussels sprouts		*
Cabbage		*

19. Charting Your Progress on the Detox Diet

Motivation and a sense of achievement are key elements to the success of any diet. It takes so much energy and commitment to achieve our target weight that to succeed we all need to be constantly reassured that our efforts are not in vain – which translates down to having some sort of hard evidence. Therefore having a way of measuring your progress is absolutely crucial to your ultimate dieting success. And once you have attained your wished-for figure, you will be more motivated to keep it.

Fortunately, you can now create your own progress report by recording your exact weight and measurements before you start the programme and taking the same measurements again at regular intervals throughout the rest of your time dieting. You might even want to take pictures or keep a video diary to record your success.

Being able to see how far you've come will really boost your morale when progress appears to slow down or when the going gets tough. Because at these make-or-break moments in time you will be able to look at the real improvement in your photographs, or count the lost pounds and inches in your progress chart. You will find that if anything can, this hard evidence of progress will give you all the encouragement you need to carry on – because you can see for yourself that your efforts are really paying off.

But record-keeping is not just for the long term – a daily record will help you keep track of what you eat and of when you take your supplements. And with the frantic pace at which most of us live, it is easy to forget whether you have taken your supplements or not, even to remember what foods you have just been eating. I know because I have been there too!

To help you keep on top of the situation, at the end of this chapter I have provided some sample daily record sheets which I, and others, have found to be very helpful. You could make photocopies and fill in a record sheet every day – keeping all the sheets in a file. Or you could make a template of it on your computer, or jot it down in your diary or journal, if this is more in keeping with your lifestyle.

But whichever way you do it, it will really help you plan your meals, snacks and supplements so that you can easily keep to the diet guidelines in Chapters 16 and 17. At a glance you will know exactly what supplements you still need to take, and which foods you still have left from your allowance that day.

Although these charts have been designed for those people who are going on the Detox Diet plan, as shown in Chapters 16 and 17, certain parts of it, such as the body measurement section, will also be very relevant for those people who don't wish to diet as such, but who still want to enjoy the longer-term slimming benefits of eliminating *Chemical Calories* from their lives.

So get ready – you will now discover all you need to know about how to acquire all the vital statistics to give you full dieting success!

SETTING UP AND KEEPING YOUR PERSONAL RECORD

You can't see results unless you know where you started from, so this is where you have to be really rigorous with yourself. The importance of getting a true picture of your pre-diet shape and weight can't be emphasized enough. Please believe me when I tell you that the effort you spend in doing this *before* you start the Detox Diet will be paid back many times over the following weeks and months. Just think how disappointed you would be if you put it off for a few weeks – you would never fully know how successful you had been!

Before you start the diet, get a full-length photograph of yourself wearing a swimsuit or some clothing in which your shape is revealed. Now you might find it very difficult to pose for a photograph of yourself in a swimsuit, let alone keep it in a record. So please believe me when I tell you that the harder it is for you now, the greater your commitment and success will be throughout the rest of the diet.

Once you start putting future photographs beside it, you will start glowing with pride at the marked improvement you will see before your very eyes. This growing collection of photographs will be one of the most powerful ways of proving how much your whole body shape has been transformed, and to you it will eventually be worth its weight in gold. All you have to do now is to get busy snapping – so what are you waiting for?

CHARTING WEIGHT LOSS

We can all appreciate that it's difficult to stick to a diet without some regular way of measuring progress. After all, everyone needs some form of continual reassurance or feedback if they put a lot of effort into something.

Although checking our weight is one of the simplest way of seeing results quickly, hence its popularity over the years, it is by no means perfect. In fact there are few, if any, perfect ways of measuring our progress.

To decide which method we should go for – whether it's measuring our weight, or our percentage body fat, measuring our actual body parts such as our chest, hips, waist and thighs, or even a combination of all the above – we need to know a bit more about their individual strengths and weaknesses before we can discover the best way forward.

WEIGHING YOURSELF ON SCALES

Many households own bathroom scales, so the attractions of this method are obvious. Measuring your weight is so quick and easy, and will give you an immediate idea of the size of the problem you are faced with. Despite their ease of use, however, an over-reliance on this way of assessing our weight has brought about major problems – even dictating to some extent the way we now go about dieting.

This is because for many years now most diets have been judged solely on achieving maximum weight loss. The majority of diets have therefore been designed to achieve just this – seemingly without regard as to whether the weight lost is fat, muscle or water. As a result, this type of strict dieting is relatively popular – because it can appear very effective if you go by the measurements you see on the scales alone.

However, it is now well recognized that if you lose more than a kilo or so of weight per week, anything over the kilo will be water, or muscle, which is even worse. The problem is that simple weighing scales cannot distinguish between weight loss from fat and weight loss due to loss of water or muscle. So while you may think you are doing fabulously, in reality you could be wrecking your *Slimming System* by shrinking your muscles.

If this happens, then despite your seemingly stunning weight loss you will be left with proportionately more fat than you had to start with, loose skin, a flabby body, and a much reduced metabolic rate as well. Does the 'yo-yo' diet situation sound familiar? While you are winning on the scales, your figure and your health could actually be the greatest losers!

By contrast, if you step up the amount of exercise you take, your weight may increase slightly, as muscle tends to be relatively heavy. But despite the gain on the scales, your body shape will actually improve, as you will lose inches and look much leaner! So you can see that while the scales are useful, they are definitely not the only way to assess your progress.

While the temptation when you go on a diet is to weigh yourself virtually every day, you must try to break that mentality and limit yourself to once-a-week weigh-ins, if possible. The secret is to use changes in weight as a helpful guide to your progress – but whatever you do, not to let these measurements rule you.

Whether you are keeping a file, journal or computer record, you will find a weekly weight chart like this one very useful. Just fill in the first box before you start and keep a weekly record after that.

Week	0	1	2	3	4
Weight (st/lb/kg)					

Week	5	6	7	8	9
Weight (st/lb/kg)					

ESTIMATING BODY FAT

I think most people now know that excess fat, rather than excess weight, is at the heart of the problem. So the aim of any diet should be to maximize fat loss rather than promote generalized weight loss. Thus, in reality, it would be a great deal better to record fat loss rather than weight loss. Unfortunately this is far less straightforward than you might imagine.

The most accurate methods are only really used for research purposes. These include being weighed in air and then totally immersed in water, drinking radioactive water, getting an electric shock, being exposed to a neutron beam, or X-ray and imaging techniques such as CAT scanning or magnetic resonance imaging. And so long as you are not Superman, you could even use krypton gas![1]

On the more positive side, there are several less accurate but more user-friendly ways to estimate the amount of fat in your body. One involves using callipers to measure the thickness of the fat under the skin, typically over the triceps, the biceps, on the back and just below your waist. This is usually done by doctors, dieticians or health club staff. All they really need are the callipers and the appropriate conversion charts to give you a measurement. As this usually involves the hassle of going somewhere to have the procedure done and returning each time it needs repeating, it can be a bit of a bother. However, it is now possible to buy these callipers, so in fact you could do it all yourself.

Another way is to take your body measurements and to work out a figure using the charts and simple calculations to be found at the back of the book. In reality, it doesn't matter whether or not your estimate is correct down to the last decimal place. What does matter, from the point of view of keeping a record, is to stick to whichever method you start with. Then you will know that the changes are real and in response to your diet.

To give you some guidance on your 'ideal' body fat level, it is about 22 per cent for women and about 15 per cent for men. Athletes tend to have lower levels than this, and the average woman has a much higher level, approximately 32 per cent, with 23 per cent for the average man.

Whichever way you choose to keep your own record, in a journal, scrapbook or file, you will find a weekly measurement chart like the one below very useful to keep you in touch with your progress.

Week	0	1	2	3	4
% Body fat					

Week	5	6	7	8	9
% Body fat					

MEASUREMENTS

As one of the main reasons for going on a diet is to look visibly slimmer, one of the most accurate ways to gauge your success is by taking regular body measurements. As the inches fall off, you will know that you are reaching your goal. If you also put a lot more effort into exercise, it is likely that you will see more rapid progress in your reducing body measurements than you actually achieve in your weight loss – so it is well worth doing!

Now it is one thing to measure different parts of your body, but quite another to measure in exactly the same places a week later! Because it is particularly important to get this right, you should try your best to measure the same part of your body in the same place each and every time.

One way to reduce the margin of error is to take each measurement three times, and record the average value. In addition, stick to either centimetres or inches, and don't swap from one to the other.

Once again, whether you are keeping a journal, scrapbook or file, you will find a weekly measurement chart like the one below very useful. Just fill in the first box before you start, and keep a weekly record after that. Now all you need is a tape-measure!

Week	0	1	2	3	4
Bust/Chest					
Waist					
Hips					
Thighs					

Week	5	6	7	8	9
Bust/Chest					
Waist					
Hips					
Thighs					

KEEPING A FOOD DIARY

It has been found that people who keep some form of food diary while on a diet tend to be much more successful in losing weight. For those of you who think you may need this type of support, I have created the food diary that follows. All you have to do is select the relevant sheet (male or female) and photocopy or reproduce it for your own records so that you have a clean sheet for every day throughout the following weeks and months.

This food diary could really help you if your lifestyle is anything like mine. When I was on the Detox Diet, I personally found it absolutely essential to keep a record of what I had eaten during the day, otherwise it tended to be quickly forgotten in the constant flurry of activities and major demands made on my time.

If you think it could help you, make the diary your constant diet companion, carrying it with you everywhere you go, so that you can jot down whatever you eat or drink. Before long, it will become absolutely invaluable in helping you to stick to the diet and to plan ahead. Then once you begin to lose your excess fat, it will give you great pleasure to go back and read your own personalized record of your progress on the Detox Diet!

The Detox Diet Food Diary

Quantities consumed for a female   Date:

Protein (type and amount, e.g. low-fat plain yoghurt 250g)

1.

2.

Fat

1. Oil, butter or fat spreads (up to 3 teaspoons in total)

   Or nuts and seeds (up to 20g)

2. Milk (up to 200ml)

Complex carbohydrate (type and amount, e.g. potatoes, 100g)

1.   2.

3.   4.

Simple carbohydrate/fruit (type and amount, e.g. apple, 1)

1.   2.

3.   4.

Additional or optional foods

Supplements

Vitamins and minerals

Omega-3 and Omega-6 fat-burning oils

Amino acids

Fibre/detoxing 'drawing powders'

Exercise or activities (type and duration)

NOTES

The Detox Diet Food Diary

Quantities consumed for a male   Date:

Protein (type and amount, e.g. low-fat plain yoghurt 250g)

1.   2.

3.

Fat

1. Oil, butter or fat spreads (up to 3 teaspoons in total)

   Or nuts and seeds (up to 20g)

2. Milk (up to 200ml)

Complex carbohydrate (type and amount, e.g. potatoes, 100g)

1.   2.

3.   4.

5.   6.

Simple carbohydrate/fruit (type and amount, e.g. apple, 1)

1.   2.

3.   4.

Additional or optional foods

Supplements

Vitamins and minerals

Omega-3 and Omega-6 fat-burning oils

Amino acids

Fibre/detoxing 'drawing powders'

Exercise or activities (type and duration)

NOTES

20. Typical Questions and Useful Answers

For all of you who are on, or about to go on, the Detox Diet, this chapter contains a wealth of important and useful information. Don't skip over it, as it could really help you benefit more fully from the programme.

I think by now you will have realized that I like to work on the principle that it is far better to be well-informed than kept in the dark. Consequently the more you understand about a diet, the more you will benefit from it. Although many of your questions will have been answered in the earlier chapters, the answers here will cover a whole range of different issues that will help you achieve and maintain your desired weight. So take a look and see how it could help you.

Q. *Do I need to do everything recommended in this book to lose weight?*
A. No! If you can adopt just a few of the recommendations this will help. Since the vast majority of the most persistent *Chemical Calories* in our bodies come from our food and drink, you can make a huge difference just by buying and eating foods that are low in *Chemical Calories* and taking the appropriate dietary supplements. These are probably the two most important things you can do. If you can adopt any of the other measures recommended, that will be an additional benefit.

Q. *I can't afford to buy organic foods so will this diet still work for me?*
A. Absolutely! If you buy and eat food that is low in *Chemical Calories* and take the required supplements, you should still be able to lose weight permanently.

Q. *I am a confirmed coffee and tea addict and wonder why they are not recommended on the diet?*
A. Coffee and tea interfere with the Detox Diet in two major ways. First, they are nutrient grabbers, so they hijack many of the vitamins and minerals that your *Slimming System* needs to function properly.[1] Second, they contain caffeine, which interferes with and temporarily increases the levels of those powerful fat-burning hormones, catecholamines, in the blood, giving you that extra energy buzz.

However, you will pay for this highly, as caffeine also increases the rate at which these slimming hormones are dispelled from the body. So a few hours later the levels of these hormones can slump to lower than normal body levels, making you feel washed out. In addition the fall in catecholamines may encourage increased food cravings, so you may also end up eating more.[2]

As I do appreciate that it can be very difficult to stop drinking tea and coffee all at once, I have recommended that you make a start by switching to decaffeinated coffee or tea. This alone will make a great difference in boosting the production of many of your most important slimming hormones and keeping them on a steady level – as well as reducing any possible unwanted food cravings.

Q. *I am a heavy smoker and am afraid to quit smoking in case I put on more weight. What should I do?*
A. You are not alone. Many people are afraid to quit smoking in case they gain weight. When you inhale nicotine it artificially alters the levels of certain slimming hormones, so on one level it helps to control your weight in the short term. What you may not realize, though, is that many of the chemicals you inhale in cigarette smoke are very high in *Chemical Calories* and they work to damage your *Slimming System* in the long term.[3]

Quitting smoking may cause a temporary weight gain, but as you rid yourself of *Chemical Calories* you will be able to regain control over your natural *Slimming System*. Don't worry, the Detox Diet will help you lose any initial weight gained, and over

the long term it will be one of the major factors in helping you to
get down to your desired weight.

Q. *We are always being told that a certain amount of alcohol is beneficial
to health, so why do we have to limit our intake of alcohol on the diet?*
A. Normally, drinking moderate amounts of alcohol is not really
a problem, but the situation changes when you embark on a diet.
As well as guzzling up slimming nutrients, alcohol also reduces
our ability to rid our bodies of *Chemical Calories*. The whole point
of the Detox Diet is to mobilize *Chemical Calories* and get rid of
them, so it would be counter-productive to slow down the
process by drinking alcohol while trying to detoxify.

I do understand that for some people cutting out alcohol for
the total period of the diet itself will be very difficult to achieve. If
this is the case, I recommend that you try not to consume any
alcohol for at least the first week, as this is the time the detox
system will be under the greatest pressure, then limit your
consumption to at the very most four drinks a week for women
and eight for men. One drink means a single measure of spirit, a
glass of wine, a small glass of sherry or ½ pint (225ml) of beer or
lager.

Q. *Can I use food that I've not eaten one day in the next day's menu?*
A. I'm afraid it doesn't work like that. Any savings that you make
in your food allowance for one day can't be rolled over to the
next day.

Q. *What if I pig out and break the diet completely?*
A. Don't give up! Most people will have an occasional splurge.
While it is not ideal, breaking your diet from time to time is a
common fact of life. As long as you limit the damage, it will just
slow up weight loss.

However, don't use the odd lapse as an excuse to yourself to
stop dieting. No matter how hard you find it at the beginning, no
situation is irredeemable. The more *Chemical Calories* you shed,
the less you will feel the urge to break the diet. And as you begin

to look and feel better and other people start to notice, the results themselves will be your best motivation.

Finding it hard to stick to the diet is often a sign that your body has very high levels of *Chemical Calories* and is deficient in many essential nutrients. So the best thing to do is to stop actively reducing your food intake for a while and concentrate on cutting down on *Chemical Calories* and taking the right supplements. After a few weeks your body may be better prepared to restart the diet, and you will be one step closer to permanent weight loss.

Q. *From reading your book it seems that many of the persistent* Chemical Calories *tend to be found in animal products, so will it help me to maintain my weight if I become a vegan?*
A. While it is generally a very good idea to eat more fruit, vegetables, pulses, nuts and grains, it is not necessary to cut out meat or dairy products totally, as many of them can be low in *Chemical Calories*.

Q. *How long will it take to remove all the* Chemical Calories *from my body?*
A. Different chemicals are removed from the body at different speeds. It is virtually impossible to remove them all, but so long as you follow the programme and keep current exposure low, many chemicals can be drastically reduced in weeks. Others will take months or even longer to eliminate.

On average, if you follow the programme you should considerably lower your stored levels of *Chemical Calories* within a few months. When you remember that it has taken you a lifetime to build up the levels of many chemicals, clearing the majority in a few months starts to sounds so much more reasonable!

Q. *How are we being damaged by these chemicals, as the actual levels in our bodies are in fact relatively low?*
A. Well, there is a very good explanation. Despite being present at relatively small levels, they bring about many of their toxic effects by damaging our hormones, which are present in even

smaller amounts. These hormones are vital in orchestrating all the reactions taking place in the body.

The consequence of life-long exposure to these chemicals is that the average person is already polluted with chemicals at levels millions of times higher than our natural hormones.[4] Although synthetic chemicals tend to be far less potent than our natural hormones, their presence is very real and can cause real damage.

Q. *Don't we build up a resistance to these toxic chemicals over time?*
A. This is a commonly held belief among many people and needs to be put to rest once and for all. Chemicals are very different beasts from bugs such as viruses and bacteria, which our immune system has been specially developed to fight over many hundreds of thousands of years. Instead of continual exposure resulting in our body's building up a resistance to them, these chemicals actually seem to target and cripple the immune system itself. Consequently, the hard reality is that the more chemicals you are exposed to over time, the more damaged your immune system will tend to become, making you not only increasingly susceptible to a whole range of infections but also more prone to a large number of 'immune-related diseases' such as allergies, eczema, asthma and auto-immune diseases.

Q. *I have just moved into a new house that could be full of* Chemical Calories, *but how am I to find out?*
A. Calling in an environmental house doctor, or leasing equipment to take air and water samples, will help you identify potential problems. The previous owners may be able to tell you whether the house has been treated for wet rot, dry rot or timber infestation, or the guarantees for these treatments may be with the house deeds. You may also be able to find out whether the previous occupants used natural cleaning and building products, or standard commercial products containing chemicals.

Q. *After I went on the programme, I found that my eczema greatly improved. Is this a coincidence or a side-effect of the diet?*

A. Cutting out *Chemical Calories* can greatly improve eczema. Toxic chemicals are thought to be at the heart of many auto-immune disorders, so if you lower their levels and feed the body the nutrients that it needs to repair itself, you will benefit from stronger, healthier skin. You may also find an improvement in other skin disorders, such as acne and dry itchy skin.

Q. *You say that your programme will help people to lose weight. I don't need to lose much weight but I would like to improve my body shape. Will it still help me?*
A. Without doubt. In fact this is one of the major strengths of this programme. As the *Chemical Calories* are removed from the body, the hormones in charge of shaping your body as nature intended will spring into action. As a result, men will find that their muscles increase in size and they lose fat around the middle. Women will tend to lose fat from the waist, hips and thighs, and their muscle tone will also improve.

Q. *Even when I lose weight, I still have cellulite on my thighs and hips. Will your programme reduce cellulite too?*
A. Absolutely. Cellulite is the 'orange-peel' dimpling that we get on our skin, particularly around the thighs, stomach and arms. Reducing our levels of *Chemical Calories* will reduce the size of the fat cells that stretch the skin to cause the dimpling effect. In addition, our skin will become stronger and thicker due to increased production of protein-rich tissues. As a result, the dimples will become less noticeable and start to vanish.

Q. *How can I protect my* Slimming System *if I have to fast for religious purposes?*
A. The sudden release of *Chemical Calories* into the bloodstream during fasting may actually damage the *Slimming System* and the rest of the body. To minimize any damage, you need to take the supplements recommended for the diet for a few days before and after the day of the fast.

In addition, you should take fibre supplements or foods rich in soluble fibre immediately before fasting and for one or two days afterwards. If possible, you should also drink lots of water while you fast and cut down your level of activity.

Q. *What can I do if I am invited out to dinner and am given foods that I know are very high in* Chemical Calories?
A. This can be tricky, but is not an insurmountable problem. When your hosts have gone to great trouble to prepare food it can be rude to refuse it. The easy thing to do is to eat more of the foods that are lower in *Chemical Calories* and less of the rest. If this is not possible, you could eat the food, then when you get back home take an extra dose of fibre and possibly some of the other binding substances mentioned in Chapter 15.

It will take you 6–8 hours to fully digest your food, so the binding substances will still reduce your intake of *Chemical Calories* very significantly. Better still, you could take the binding substances just before you go out.

Q. *I adore eating salmon and can't imagine giving it up. Is there any way of buying or preparing salmon that is low in* Chemical Calories?
A. I'm afraid that will be difficult, as most salmon contains very high levels of *Chemical Calories*. Your best alternative is to choose organic salmon. Organically reared salmon lacks a whole number of chemicals that are added to ordinary farmed salmon, although it may still contain significant amounts of *Chemical Calories* from the fish in its diet.

There is, however, the possibility that in future more vegetable sources of proteins may be used to feed fish, which could potentially significantly cut down on the overall level of *Chemical Calories*.

Otherwise, the best option is to cut off all visible fat while preparing salmon, and to eat the salmon along with foods high in soluble fibre such as pulses or beans. Fibre or charcoal supplements taken before the meal will also help a lot, since they will significantly reduce your uptake of *Chemical Calories* from the fish.

Q. *My job requires me to eat out a lot at places that do not serve organic food. How can I avoid eating too many* Chemical Calories?
A. The good thing about eating out is that you have a choice of foods. Try to order food containing lower levels of *Chemical Calories*. Better still, order dishes that are high in soluble fibre, such as beans or pulses. If you are in any doubt, you could always take a fibre or other *Chemical-Calorie*-binding supplement either before or after your meal.

Q. *It's very difficult to find all the different vitamins and supplements that you recommend, and anyway, it would be extremely expensive to buy them all for a family. Could you offer some advice for families on a budget?*
A. Although it can start to get more expensive as the number of people increases, on the positive side this will allow you to make some savings by buying in bulk. If you shop around you can often pick up special deals on certain supplements such as multivitamins and some of the more commonly used ones such as vitamin C.

Try to get the best multivitamin and mineral tablet you can afford, with levels of nutrient as close as possible to the recommended levels, as this may reduce the need to top up with individual vitamins or minerals. You may have to compromise by buying ordinary flax oil in preference to organic oils (although this is not ideal), as it can be much cheaper. Search around for the cheapest form of binding agent and just stick with that one (probably a soluble fibre). And finally, regarding the amino acids, which are hard to locate anyway, just buy what you can afford.

Q. *I am pregnant, but putting on far too much weight. My doctor says I should try to control my weight but I am finding it almost impossible. What can I do?*
A. The first thing to emphasize is that at no stage of your pregnancy should you actively restrict what you eat. This could harm your unborn baby by mobilizing your stored levels of *Chemical Calories*, and increase the baby's risk for a whole range of illnesses. However, there are many ways to prevent excessive weight gain while still protecting the health of your baby.

The most obvious thing to do is to buy and eat food that is low in *Chemical Calories*. Next, you can take vitamin and mineral supplements specially designed for pregnancy. It is also an excellent idea to take omega-3 supplements in the form of organic flax oil, as this will help your baby's development and boost your own *Slimming System*. These measures, in combination with a diet naturally high in soluble fibre, should help you control your weight.

More and more women are now going on detoxification programmes before they become pregnant. The full programme contained in this book would be ideal for any woman who is considering becoming pregnant in the future but who is not yet actively trying.

Q. *Can I go on the Detox Diet while breastfeeding?*
A. Many people are desperate to lose weight after the birth of a child, something I know from personal experience. However, if you are breastfeeding you should **not** restrict what you eat. If you do, the *Chemical Calories* released as your fat stores break down may accumulate in your breast-milk and be passed on to your baby.[5]

The best option would be to buy and eat food that is low in *Chemical Calories*, take vitamin, mineral, amino acid and essential fat supplements, but avoid going on a food-restrictive diet.

Q. *Despite my best efforts, my five-year-old son seems to be putting on too much weight. What can I do to help him?*
A. More and more children are becoming overweight, but the good news is that there are lots of things you can do to reverse the trend. Young children should not go on a food-restrictive diet, but you should start to encourage your son to eat food that is low in *Chemical Calories*. You should also start him on vitamin and mineral supplements specially formulated for children, and essential fatty acids in the form of organic flax oil.

Children's vitamins often come in fun shapes or fruit flavours, but it is much harder to get children to take flax oil. My own children can taste it no matter how I disguise it, and will spit it out, so occasionally I rub a small amount into their skin after a bath. It may soak into their nightclothes, but it washes off. If your child is not allergic to nuts, you can give him foods rich in essential fatty acids, such as walnuts or pumpkin seeds.

Make sure your child also eats lots of soluble fibre from beans, oats, apples or oranges, and takes more exercise. Together these steps should make a significant improvement in your child's weight problem.

Q. *My teenage daughter has always struggled with her weight, but puberty is making the problem worse. Should she be starting on this programme?*
A. Puberty is a time in which the body's hormones are going through a major upheaval. *Chemical Calories* can interfere with these hormones and have been linked with promoting early puberty in girls.[6] Although this book has been designed for adults, your daughter would definitely benefit from many of its principles.

She should start by changing her diet to include food that is low in *Chemical Calories* and by taking vitamin and mineral, amino acid and fatty acid supplements in doses suitable for her age. This, and an increase in activity, should help her control her weight.

Weight problems can sometimes be exacerbated in puberty, as this life phase increases the need for certain nutrients to fuel adequate growth and sexual development.[7] Most of these nutrients, in particular vitamins A, D and B6, biotin, zinc, calcium, magnesium and essential fatty acids (particularly omega-3 fatty acids), are also used to power the *Slimming System*. They are siphoned off to promote growth, few will be left for weight-control and any shortage will exacerbate the weight gain as well as the other normal problems during puberty, including spots and mood swings.

Q. *I am an athlete, and though I don't want to lose weight I do need to maximize my muscle strength. Could your programme help me to achieve this?*

A. Absolutely. The programme will increase the maximum extent to which your muscles will grow and improve your energy production. In other words your muscle bulk will increase, along with your strength and endurance, which I imagine is just what you will be looking for. If you want to find out more, just turn to the next chapter!

Q. *I have just been through the menopause and want to know if I can lose the excess weight I have gained.*

A. The menopause in women causes a dramatic decline in natural oestrogens and other slimming hormones, so after the menopause the body is naturally 'programmed' to gain a certain amount of weight. *Chemical Calories* accelerate and exacerbate these changes, contributing to 'middle-aged spread'.[8] If you have never detoxed over all these years, the chances are that your build-up of *Chemical Calories* is quite substantial and your *Slimming System* has been under-performing for some time.

This programme is for you, and should help you to lose the weight you have gained by providing your body with the essential nutrients you need in larger amounts around this time, namely vitamins B, D and E, calcium, zinc, magnesium and omega-3 and omega-6 essential fatty acids. Another beneficial side-effect is that your energy levels should greatly improve – which is always very welcome!

Q. *My husband is very overweight and our doctor has put him on a low-fat diet. We'd both like to follow your programme, but most organic dairy foods seem to be full-fat. Is it more beneficial to buy organic products or low-fat products?*

A. Well, the best option is to try to source organic low-fat products. The next best would be to buy a low-fat product as long as it is likely to be low in *Chemical Calories* (see Chapter 18).

Q. *I am getting alarmed at the size of my partner's pot belly, particularly since he has a family history of heart disease. Would he be able to lose his excess fat by going on this diet?*
A. From what you say, your partner would benefit enormously from this programme. It will help to shrink the fat deposits around his abdomen, and lower his risk of future heart disease on a number of different counts.

Q. *I'm confused by all the different labelling systems for meat and poultry. Some are free-range, some are organic, some GM-free, and some are approved by animal welfare organizations. If I can't buy organic chicken, for example, will free-range chicken give me similar benefits?*
A. The short answer is no. Food can be labelled free-range if the animals have a certain amount of living space, but apart from that, their diets are similar to conventionally reared animals, and therefore they are exposed to the same chemicals. However, most organically reared chicken would pass as being free-range, due to generally higher animal rearing standards.

Q. *Do genetically modified foods contain* Chemical Calories?
A. Chemicals only contain *Chemical Calories* by virtue of their ability to damage our *Slimming System*. So the same would hold for genetically modified foods if they too damaged our *Slimming System*. At present, despite the vast amount of research claimed to have been done, very little has been published even about the most basic effects they have on our metabolism. So at present it is impossible to answer this question.

What is interesting is that, in the few studies on animals I have come across, there is a suggestion that there could be some form of damage: for example, ladybirds which ate aphids feeding on genetically modified plants lived approximately half as long as the ladybirds which ate the aphids feeding on ordinary plants.[9] So until more information is published on the effects of GM foods on humans and animals, I choose to avoid them.

21. Maximize Your Fitness

How Exercise Promotes Weight Loss and Detoxification

What you are about to read will help you achieve a level of fitness that you may never have achieved before. Not only will it make you fitter, but it also aims to promote the changes necessary to massively increase the rate at which your muscles burn up fat. As well as making the world of difference to your ability to lose weight, it should help you attain a leaner and better-proportioned body.

Gone will be the fat stores that make you look flabby. In their place will be increased amounts of lean muscle, which will make you look firm and toned. In addition, you will become less fatigued following exercise, your muscles will grow stronger and your energy levels will soar. Even if you are an experienced athlete, you should be able to significantly improve your fitness by following the advice in this chapter.

All I can say is that you will be truly amazed at how much difference it can make to your whole life – to find out how, read on.

EXPOSING THE MYTH

Everywhere we turn, medical experts and politicians alike tell us that we are turning into a nation of slobs. They suggest that overweight people don't take enough exercise, stigmatizing large groups of people who are consequently regarded as plain lazy.[1] This really irritates me, as I don't believe for one second that over half the population who are at any one time putting vast amounts of their energy into trying to lose weight are either lazy or slothful.

So I have great pleasure, once and for all, in exposing the myth that people are overweight simply through their own lack of effort.

In reality, the finger of blame should be pointed at toxic chemicals, which I believe are the true culprits.

To date, I have uncovered an overwhelming amount of evidence showing that *Chemical Calories* damage virtually all the mechanisms that our bodies use to exercise. Chemicals damage the nerves that control exercise,[2] they directly injure and shrink the muscles, they damage the hormones that control the growth of muscles[3] and they reduce our ability to produce energy,[4] so potentially reducing our ability to convert excess energy to heat.[5]

In effect they appear to act like a chemical cosh on our whole ability to exercise, and they even appear to reduce our drive to exercise.[6] An increased sensitivity to being damaged by chemicals could be the reason why when overweight people do exercise, they end up burning fewer calories than their leaner colleagues for the same amount of exercise undertaken.[7]

As you can imagine, any damage to our ability to exercise could massively increase our chances of putting on weight – particularly in those who are less able to defend themselves against the toxic effects of these chemicals. So to anyone in authority – when you next have a go at overweight people, please direct your censure at the right target.

TAKING ACTION TO FIX THE PROBLEM

The good news is that now that the problem has been recognized, we can take the necessary action to put it right. The Detox Diet will help to boost your own desire and ability to exercise by removing *Chemical Calories* from your body, while supplying it with the supplements it needs to repair and strengthen itself.

Gradually, as your levels of natural hormones start to recover, they will start stimulating new muscle growth and your energy levels will start to increase – allowing you to do more for longer. In addition you will regain the motivation to take part in more activities.

However, if you simply diet without taking the recommended supplements, it can actually exacerbate muscle damage.[8] Unfortunately

I have first-hand experience of this debilitating effect, which took months out of my own life, and which I have already briefly touched on in Chapter 14.

THE VITAL NEED FOR SUPPLEMENTS WHEN DETOXING

As previously mentioned, a few years ago I fell ill after dieting hard following the birth of my second son – I did not realize that food-restriction dieting should always now take place with a detox. As I lost weight, I started to experience increasingly severe muscular pains.

Although I stopped dieting the damage appeared to have been done, as for the next six months I suffered from constantly aching muscles which were extremely painful to the touch. I also suffered from constant fatigue; even going up the stairs was very hard work and I seemed to catch one virus after another. Sometimes I was so worn out that I had to go to bed at 7 p.m.

For some reason which I can't recall now, I heard about the potential benefits of taking vitamin C. I was really desperate by that stage and bought some to see if it would help. Up to that point I had the same view of vitamins and minerals as many other doctors and indeed many other people – such as you, perhaps – which is that they are not necessary so long as you have a good diet.

To my complete and utter amazement, about an hour after taking the vitamin C, my muscle aches and cramps totally disappeared for the first time in six months. I probably wouldn't have believed it if I hadn't experienced such a dramatic response first hand. My first thought was to find out if the effect was repeatable, so the next day when my muscle aches came back, I took another vitamin C tablet. The cramps disappeared again within an hour.

At this point, as well as being ecstatic because there now seemed to be a way out of this living nightmare, I also felt driven to find out exactly what had happened to me – not only to discover how to optimize my own recovery but also how to prevent other people from suffering as I did.

ANTIOXIDANTS ARE VITAL PROTECTION

I know now that what I had been experiencing was the poisoning of my muscles by the release of organochlorines from my fat stores into my bloodstream as a direct result of dieting. After entering my muscles they caused a great deal of damage to the muscle structure, which caused the aching, as well as to my ability to exercise by damaging the way the muscle produces energy.[9]

It seems that much of this damage was probably caused by the excessive release of free radicals. And this explained why the powerful antioxidant vitamin C appeared to work so well, because it neutralized and so lowered the levels of these little muscle-wreckers.

But not only will dieting release *Chemical Calories* into the bloodstream, rigorous exercise will also do it. It seems advisable that anyone who exercises intensively now should take antioxidants regularly to prevent any damage from free radicals.

WHICH ANTIOXIDANTS CAN HELP?

Our muscles are largely water and vitamin C is water-soluble, so taking vitamin C is one of the most effective ways of delivering antioxidants directly to the place where they are needed. However, a whole range of other supplements, including vitamin E, are also important to protect the muscles.

Did you know that if trained athletes take vitamin E regularly their muscles recover more quickly after long training sessions? This is because a bout of rigorous training is thought to enhance the release of free radicals, increasing the chances of muscle damage the next day.

Other vital supplements are vitamin A, beta carotene, selenium, zinc, omega-3 oils, glutathione and serotonin, which can all reduce the levels of free radicals.[10] As the supplements recommended on the Detox Diet (see Chapter 15) provide all these nutrients in the levels your muscles need to work fully, they fully cater for those lovers of sport among you all.

In addition to its antioxidant actions, organic flax oil, which is high in omega-3 fatty acids, can also enhance your ability to burn fat. It does this by increasing the sensitivity of muscles to the fat-burning effects of catecholamines.[11] So as well as protecting muscles from toxic damage, flax oil can increase the number of conventional calories that you will burn up exercising – something I imagine most people would like to benefit from.

HOW EXERCISE REVITALIZES YOUR *SLIMMING SYSTEM*

I think deep down most of us already know that exercise has a whole host of benefits for the slimmer. But to be more specific, exercise plays a major role in my programme because it:

- Speeds up detoxification by mobilizing *Chemical Calories* from your fat. So exercise, in conjunction with the right supplement programme, will speed up the rate at which you can detox.
- Increases your level of lean muscle tissue, so you will burn up more of your fat stores throughout the day.
- Boosts the levels of many of the most essential slimming hormones, including thyroid hormones, testosterone and catecholamines.[12] This will increase your desire to exercise, as well as improving the size, strength and ability of your muscles to use up energy.

So it makes sense that if you are planning to start the diet, you will improve your figure much more quickly and effectively if you incorporate exercise as part of your programme. There are many scientific reasons why this is in fact the case.

First, exercise, especially in short bouts, will lower your appetite, helping you to stick to the diet.[13] Second, your mood will improve,[14] because exercise increases the levels of your natural mood-improving hormones. Third, exercise will greatly improve your figure, as it preserves and increases your lean muscle tissue.[15]

In addition, a certain degree of exercise will prevent the fall in metabolic rate that accompanies most food-restriction diets.[16] And finally, an increased level of physical activity will also ensure that your skin keeps firm and toned as you lose weight, so that not only will you look thinner but you will also look fitter and more healthy. So what are you waiting for?

BUT I'M NOT A SPORTY PERSON . . .

Now please believe me: even if you do not consider yourself sporty, you will still be able to exercise enough to reap the full slimming benefits available. Exercise is not just something you do at the gym. For some people, taking a brisk walk will be just as effective as an intensive game of squash is for others.

My husband, Mike, has never been to a gym in his life and does no formal training as such. But while running our estate he is always out and about, climbing up hills, walking across fields, striding through forests, sorting out septic tanks . . . well, who said owning an estate was glamorous! In the course of his normal day he often does the equivalent of an intense workout at the gym.

Of course, you don't need to have an active occupation to keep fit. Anyone can incorporate exercise into their lifestyle by, for example, walking or cycling at least part of the way to work, or using the stairs rather than the lift. Climbing stairs is an excellent way to boost the *Slimming System* and is also highly effective in decreasing appetite and body weight!

Exercise is not necessarily hard work − it can be great fun, very relaxing, extremely sociable and can give you a great feeling of satisfaction after you have finished. The secret is not to think about how strenuous it could be, but just take the plunge and do it!

A REGULAR EXERCISE REGIME

Exercise can be broadly divided into two main types: aerobic exercises such as running or dancing, which improve your stamina and fitness rather than your muscle bulk; and resistance or anaerobic exercise of the kind used by body-builders to build up muscle.

Although both types of exercise are important, resistance exercise has the edge in enhancing your body shape and maintaining your muscle bulk when dieting.[17] Don't worry if you are not keen to go to a gym, as most forms of exercise are actually a mixture of both aerobic and anaerobic types.

To enhance your weight loss for the diet programme, you will need to take active exercise for at least three 30-minute sessions every week, to a level that will leave you out of breath or sweaty. Keep it in your mind that it is also important always to do that little bit extra every time you exercise, whatever you do, so that you stimulate your muscles as well as stimulating the release of your slimming hormones.

There is really no preferred exercise – it could be weight training in the gym, swimming or spring-cleaning the house. These will all help the *Slimming System*, so they are all equally acceptable. The trick is to find some kind of exercise that you really enjoy doing.

Life is full of competing attractions and you will only really stick to something that you enjoy. You should also try to vary your routine every few weeks to avoid getting bored. It is also important not to overdo things or use the gym equipment incorrectly, since that could lead to injury – if you attend a gym, always ask the instructors for advice on how to use the various machines and at what levels of difficulty you should use them.

Personally, I often spend my exercise sessions taking my dog for a brisk walk. It gives me time to think and admire the changes the seasons bring to the beautiful Scottish countryside which surrounds me. These benefits keep enticing me out of doors – all you have to do now is find an activity that inspires and motivates you!

WORKING UP TO NEW LEVELS

To give you some ideas about the level of activity you need, I have divided a variety of activities into 'light', 'moderate' and 'vigorous' categories. Ideally you should be choosing moderate and vigorous activities for your 30-minute sessions.

However, if you have not previously been particularly active, you should start with light activities and work your way up as your fitness improves. One last thing: it is important to exercise for the full 30 minutes (or more) each time to get the maximum benefit from this programme.

LIGHT ACTIVITIES: Table tennis, golf, social dancing and exercises (if not out of breath and sweaty), bowls, fishing, darts, snooker, lighter gardening (weeding), light DIY (for example decorating), long walks at an average or slow pace.

MODERATE ACTIVITIES: Football, swimming, tennis, aerobics, cycling, table tennis, golf, social dancing and moderate exercises, heavy DIY (for example mixing cement), heavy gardening (for example digging), heavy housework (for example spring-cleaning), long walks at a brisk or fast pace.

VIGOROUS ACTIVITIES: Squash, running (all forms), football, swimming, tennis, aerobics, rowing vigorously, energetic social dancing, cycling, energetic exercising, hockey, lacrosse, sawing wood, skiing energetically, skating energetically, some occupations that involve frequent climbing, lifting or carrying heavy loads.
To help prevent injury you should spend a few minutes warming up before you start your activity. After each session you should make a note in your diet diary of what type of activity you participated in, how you felt following each session, and how long you actually spent exercising.

If you ever work out in a gym, as I do, try to go on the running machine when a good song comes on. This way, your mind is occupied listening to the music or watching the video. Dancing is another excellent form of exercise, and has the advantage of being a very social activity. And I always find that time goes much faster if I work out to music.

One more thing: over the years I have also developed a gentle 5-minute body-toning 'work-out' which I do every day – I find it works wonders in keeping my body in shape.

TOP TIPS FOR DETOXIFICATION

Exercise in itself is a wonderful way of detoxifying, but there are a few extra things you can do to maximize the detox benefits from your sessions:

- Have a shower after a workout to wash off any toxic chemicals excreted on to your skin.
- Wipe away sweat during exercise to prevent reabsorption of toxins.
- Drink plenty of water before and after exercising to wash out lots of mobilized toxins.
- Take supplements to ensure you soak up the *Chemical Calories* that you mobilize, and to minimize potential damage from free radicals.

HOW ATHLETES CAN BENEFIT FROM THE PROGRAMME

Finally, it is not only those who want to lose weight and shape up who will benefit from this programme, but also amateur or professional athletes. Ridding yourself of *Chemical Calories* in the ways I have suggested will help everyone to achieve and maintain a new high level of physical fitness. These benefits can include:

- Bigger muscles, as a result of increased hormone production. By changing your hormones you can effectively reprogramme and increase the maximum size to which your muscles can develop.
- Stronger muscles, due to increased muscle size and increased numbers of energy-producing mitochondria – your readily available energy will soar.
- Increased power for short bursts of activity, due to enhanced anaerobic energy metabolism (100-metre sprinting, etc.).
- More energy for sports that use short bursts of power over a medium distance or time (400-metre running, soccer or tennis).
- Greater stamina, due to improved and more efficient aerobic energy metabolism. Important for long-distance events, such as marathon running.

- Less body fat, more efficient fat-burning and so less body weight to carry about.
- Less muscle damage after a training session.

At this point you can see that not only will exercise enhance your *Slimming System*, but keeping your *Slimming System* in shape will enhance your ability to exercise. So to make the most of the slimming benefits now available to you, all you need to do is to get out of your chair and go for it!

PART FOUR

Achieving a Lifestyle Low in *Chemical Calories*

22. Combating Twenty-first-century Illness

Eliminating *Chemical Calories* Can Seriously Improve Your Health

If you value your health, what this chapter has to say could totally revolutionize the rest of your life. For it is not only weight that appears to be affected by toxic chemicals, but a huge spectrum of illnesses – such as hormonal disorders (e.g. diabetes), reproductive problems, heart disease, cancer and a whole range of allergic disorders such as asthma and eczema.[1]

In fact, because of the increasing body of evidence emerging over the last century, a totally new speciality of medicine has evolved to deal with the rising number of people who now suffer from chemical-related damage. But if you are worried about any of these issues, don't panic – help is now at hand.

The real beauty of going on my programme is that by shedding *Chemical Calories* from your body, and increasing the strength of your detoxification systems, not only can you lose weight but you can also actively reduce your risk of developing any one of these chemical-related diseases. This is because many of the chemicals that make you fat are the ones that will make you ill.

And if you already suffer from one of these chemical-related illnesses, the chances are that by dealing with the core of the problem, many of the related symptoms could also improve or, in some cases, even be cured – because similar techniques are used to treat these illnesses in the field of environmental medicine.

To discover more about the immense potential health benefits available to all those of you who adopt a lifestyle low in *Chemical Calories*, read on.

WEIGHT-RELATED ILLNESSES ARE SKY-ROCKETING

Over the last few decades, the relentless rise in the number of people who are overweight has produced another extremely serious trend – a phenomenal rise in the number of people with weight-related illness, resulting in a massive global health crisis.[2] What kind of diseases are we talking about? Well, there are quite a few which are strongly linked to increasing weight, but to keep things simple I have listed only the most common ones:

- **Cardiovascular diseases** (coronary heart disease, heart attacks, strokes, high blood pressure)
- **Metabolic disorders** (diabetes – both insulin and non-insulin dependent – high blood cholesterol, gallstones)
- **Cancer** (in males – cancers of the colon, rectum and prostate; in females – cancers of the breast, ovary, uterus, cervix, gallbladder and bile ducts)
- **Hormonal disorders** (such as sex hormone imbalances)
- **Arthritis** (rheumatoid arthritis, osteoarthritis)
- **Immune system disorders** (allergies, eczema, asthma, increased susceptibility to infections)[3]

Given the overall dramatic increase in weight, it is not too surprising that diabetes, heart disease, cancer and immune system disorders have become the new plagues of our time, especially in the western world. The breakneck speed at which these diseases are spreading is not only causing immeasurable distress at a personal level but is also putting enormous pressure on health-care systems.

Think about it: most people already know someone who is diabetic, has heart disease or is afflicted by cancer. The personal financial costs of these illnesses can be high enough, but the costs at national levels can be horrific. And to get more of a feel for the size of the problem, all you have to do is take a look at the annual US health-care bill for treating weight-related diseases – recently estimated relatively conservatively at a stunning 68 billion dollars.[4]

But it is not just America which is feeling the pinch; many other governments across the world are really struggling to provide the resources necessary to cope with this escalating health crisis.

ARE *CHEMICAL CALORIES* LINKED TO THE INCREASE IN WEIGHT-RELATED ILLNESSES?

This is something which interests me greatly, and although I intend to explore it more fully at some point in the future, I will just briefly touch on it here.

To date, it has been assumed that most weight-related diseases have arisen through the increased strain on the body caused by excess weight alone. This may be true to an extent, but on closer inspection there may be more to it than that.

If you take a closer look at the literature on the subject, you will find that many of these weight-related illnesses are the same as illnesses thought to result from toxic chemical damage. In fact there is quite a marked common ground between weight-linked illnesses and chemical-related illnesses.

This raises the possibility that excess weight may not be the only thing which influences the development of illness, and that chemicals could be exacerbating certain health problems in their own right. And the people most affected by these problems could be those who are particularly vulnerable or sensitive to chemical damage. If that were true, this programme could not only reverse chemical-related weight gain, but might also start turning around much of this chemical-related health damage.

But rather than investigating that intriguing line of inquiry any further, we need to find out a bit more about what these chemical-linked illnesses are – since for most people the idea that toxic chemicals are linked to a wide range of illnesses will be a totally new concept.

SO WHAT ARE THESE CHEMICAL-RELATED ILLNESSES?

To date a very large number of illnesses have been found to be linked to our exposure to toxic chemicals. For example: heart and lung disease, cancers, immunity disorders, auto-immune diseases (such as asthma and allergies), neurological illnesses, mental illnesses, changes in sex drive, hormonal disorders, infertility, birth defects, metabolic disorders (such as diabetes), muscle damage, kidney damage and skin problems such as eczema.[5]

In fact, the more these issues are investigated, the clearer it seems that the real story of how chemicals are damaging our health could be far bigger than we had ever imagined. Almost every other day it seems that another study is published, adding to the growing mountain of studies that appear to connect yet another toxic chemical to another human illness.

Due to the vast amount of information out there, it would take several books to cover this material in the depth it deserves – but for those who are interested, the most detailed book I have found on the subject is vol. 3 of Professor William Rea's textbook on *Chemical Sensitivity*.[6] Although it particularly focuses on people who are extremely sensitive to chemical damage, it describes the different ways in which a whole range of toxic chemicals can damage virtually all our different body systems, and covers in detail how toxic chemicals are linked to all the illnesses up to the year 1995, and since publication, further adverse health effects from exposure to chemicals continue to be discovered. This excellent book is very technical and detailed, containing over 1,000 relevant references, so it is not for the faint-hearted! On the other hand, it could be of immense interest to those who already know they have medical problems and want to learn more about the link between toxic chemicals and their particular illness.

INTRODUCING THE NEW FIELD OF ENVIRONMENTAL MEDICINE

At the beginning of this chapter I mentioned that due to the ever-increasing number of studies revealing the different ways in which toxic chemicals appeared to damage our health, it soon became clear that this area was a significant medical field in its own right and so needed its own particular expertise.

So just as we have cardiologists who deal with heart problems, we now have physicians and scientists who specialize in preventing and treating the health-damaging effects of toxic chemicals. These toxic chemical specialists work in the field which is now commonly known as environmental medicine or environmental health.

Although it is one of the 'new boys' in the medical world, it is of rapidly growing importance, simply because chemicals affect us all to varying degrees. Given that many highly toxic chemicals can last for decades, the problem of toxic chemicals in our food and environment is not going to go away overnight.

The more you understand about these issues, the more able you will be to protect yourself in the future. If you don't, you may even be risking your health.

For more information on how to contact your local specialist in environmental medicine, see page 353.

HOW TOXIC CHEMICALS DAMAGE OUR HEALTH – QUICK OR SLOW POISONINGS

So how exactly do toxic chemicals cause us physical harm? Well, the toxic effects of chemicals can be divided into two main types of damage. The most obvious and best-documented way is 'poisoning' with a relatively large amount of chemicals – inducing almost immediate and often violent symptoms,[7] whereas the second, more subtle way follows long-term exposure to much lower levels of chemicals and usually goes unnoticed by the affected person, so that they do not relate health problems to this toxic build-up.[8]

Not surprisingly, the quicker and more dramatic poisoning episodes are relatively easy to recognize, both by the person affected
and by health professionals. This is because high levels of toxic
chemicals tend to cause rapid and dramatic damage.

Symptoms can range from mild flu-like illnesses to the other
extreme, of convulsions, unconsciousness and death.[9] Since these
symptoms usually follow quickly after the poisoning incident, they
are relatively well documented and on the whole pretty hard to
ignore. And on a wider scale, these high-dose poisoning episodes
account for a staggering 3 million cases of acute severe pesticide
poisonings alone, including 220,000 worldwide fatalities every
year.[10]

SLOW POISONING EFFECTS ARE MORE DIFFICULT
TO DIAGNOSE

However, these figures in all probability vastly underestimate the
true damage that chemicals pose to our health. Because as yet, no
one has found a way to record the number of people suffering from
a whole range of chemical-related illnesses triggered by much lower
levels of chemical exposure.

For instance, exposure to low levels of cancer-inducing chemicals may not make people ill immediately, but it could activate the
development of cancer cells or cause other forms of damage that
may only become apparent many years, even decades, later.

And because of the much longer time factors and the lower levels
of chemicals involved, and the simply massive numbers of toxic
chemicals all around us, it has become far more difficult to draw a
direct link between particular chemicals and particular illnesses.
The other complication here is that since we all have different
genetic make-ups and live in different environments, we may each
react in a slightly different way to a given level of chemical.

One of the real problems preventing a fuller understanding of
the health consequences of this long-term chemical damage stems
from the relatively recent emergence of this speciality, several
decades ago, and the relatively small number of trained specialists

in this field. Environmental medicine – like weight control – is one of the so-called 'Cinderella' medical specialities. And because of this relatively lowly status, very few health professionals learn about this subject during their training – I certainly didn't.

So if the vast majority of health-care professionals have very little knowledge or awareness of the potential health risks involved from our exposure to chemicals, they simply won't be asking the right questions or looking for the relevant signs which would indicate chemical damage. And if you don't look for a problem, the chances are you won't find it. So in this way many potentially soluble problems will be missed.

HOW THIS LACK OF INFORMATION CAN BE TACKLED

Fortunately there is a way round these difficulties. By looking at certain groups of people who are particularly exposed to toxic chemicals at their workplace or in their homes, and by studying their particular health problems, we can start to get a clearer picture of what types of illnesses tend to be related to chemical damage.

For example, there are many studies showing exposure to toxic chemicals resulting in diabetes. G. L. Henriksen and his colleagues looked at the potential health-damaging effects of high levels of the dioxins (a toxic synthetic chemical) in the herbicide 'Agent Orange', which had been widely used in the Vietnam war. He found that the greater the exposure to this substance at that time, the greater the chance that a US veteran would have of developing diabetes in the future.[11]

The same holds for toxic chemicals causing other illnesses such as heart disease and cancer. Another study revealed that workers in a pesticide factory in the Netherlands not only had a higher general mortality (meaning a higher risk of dying prematurely from any cause), but a higher than average chance of getting cancer and ischaemic heart disease.[12]

Disorders of the immune system have also been found to be strongly linked to chemical damage. A recent review has gathered together extensive evidence that pesticides appear to damage both the structure and the functioning of the immune system in both animals and humans.[13]

THE LINK BETWEEN CANCER AND TOXIC CHEMICALS

Although there is not enough time or space here to go into all the different diseases that have been linked to toxic chemicals, I would like to take this opportunity to talk in more detail about the link between sex hormone disrupters (types of synthetic chemicals) and breast cancer. This particular link means a lot to me, for it was largely responsible for triggering my initial interest in this relatively new field.

It all started when I was a medical research fellow at Christ Church, Oxford, working for my scientific doctorate. Part of my initial research then involved investigating a new technique to diagnose recurrent breast cancers, using a type of scanning technique known as magnetic resonance imaging, or MRI for short.

Now although I was mainly interested in the detection of cancer, the question of why the rate of breast cancer was so high had increasingly bugged me during this time. It was already affecting one in eleven women in the UK and had been increasing by around 1 per cent per year since the 1940s.

This rapid rise was happening too quickly to be due only to genetic predisposition, but as no one could explain why this increase was occurring, it remained an unsolved mystery to me – I effectively stored it in the back of my mind. Until quite by chance, many years later, years after I had finished my doctorate and had lived in Scotland for a while, I heard about the existence of a group of artificial chemicals commonly known as xenoestrogens. At this point my memories came flooding back – because in that moment, for me at least, the problem had finally been solved.

HOW XENOESTROGENS ARE LINKED TO
BREAST CANCER

Xenoestrogens are substances that mimic the actions of natural female hormones. They include a large number of man-made chemicals, for instance synthetic oestrogens, or natural substances, for example phytoestrogens in soya. The problem with many of these substances is that at certain doses they can become toxic as they interfere with the functioning of our natural hormones. Unfortunately, in the world we now live in, we are surrounded by ever-increasing amounts of these artificial hormone mimics in a whole range of substances such as plastics, pesticides and detergents. It would seem that these chemicals are causing havoc with our natural hormone systems.[14]

High levels of female hormones are thought to increase the risk of getting breast cancer.[15] Therefore, as xenoestrogens mimic the actions of natural oestrogens, they too could effectively increase the rate at which certain oestrogen-sensitive parts of our body are stimulated. This was shown to be the case in a large number of studies, including one by L. W. Frim-Titulaer *et al.* He demonstrated this process graphically in reports of Puerto Rican children who experienced premature breast growth after eating oestrogen-like compounds in chicken that had been contaminated by hormone-treated feed.[16]

Unlike real female hormones, which are 'switched off' after they produce their desired effect, many xenoestrogens cannot be 'switched off'. They just keep on and on stimulating the cells.[17] As breast cells are highly sensitive to oestrogens, continual stimulation is thought to result in excessive uncontrolled cell division, which could eventually lead to cancer.

This personal realization effectively changed the course of my life, for as soon as I heard about the existence of xenoestrogens, which were already present in our environment at levels which could produce these effects, I realized the huge significance of the link. Although I was by no means the first person to think of this possibility, for me it had finally provided a solid reason for the relentless tide of breast cancer sweeping the developed world.

What this personal discovery really did for me was make me realize that there was a big new world of medicine out there just waiting to be discovered – if these chemicals were already altering one set of hormones so completely they were possibly having further major effects on our other systems. Instinctively I knew that this was the route I now had to take, as this was the direction in which conventional medicine had to turn to survive and be effective in the future.

EVIDENCE SHOWING THAT BREAST CANCER IS LINKED TO TOXIC CHEMICAL EXPOSURE

It is currently thought that a very large number of breast cancers are strongly linked to our exposure to toxic chemicals and other environmental influences. For example, Professor William Rea states in his book that only 5–7 per cent of cases of breast cancer can be fully explained by hereditary predisposition, with the rest possibly due to environmental causes. So in theory, up to 95 per cent of breast cancers could be preventable.[18]

To date, a large number of different studies have taken place looking at the links between chemicals and breast cancer. Falck *et al.* found high levels of certain organochlorines in the breast tissue of women diagnosed with breast cancer,[19] whereas other studies have not found this link. Duell and colleagues found that women who are more exposed to chemicals (farmers for example) are at higher risk.[20] Other researchers have found a link between breast cancer and some chemicals but not with others. So a growing picture is gradually emerging.[21] Moreover, Professor Rea's book shows us that it is not just breast cancer that is linked to exposure to toxic chemicals, a huge range of other cancers are too.

Now that we know a little bit more about how long-term health problems are associated with chemicals, it is time to move on to explore one other way in which the presence of chemicals could be damaging our health. And this is where it gets even scarier.

HOW 'YO-YO' DIETING COULD BE DAMAGING
OUR HEALTH

While it is relatively clear that our daily exposure to chemicals is already damaging our health, it now seems that the way that some of us diet to lose weight could also be exacerbating the degree of damage done. This is because current dieting methods that make our weight fluctuate, or 'yo-yo', don't take into account the arrival of chemicals now present in our bodies.

The link between increased rates of illness and a previous history of major fluctuations in body weight has been found by many researchers, for example L. Lissner *et al.*[22] This study revealed that the more body weight varied the fatter you would become, particularly around the waist, but also the more fat you would tend to eat – signalling damage to the *Slimming System*. But the most serious finding was that weight fluctuation also increased the chances of developing heart disease and diabetes. In fact, the more that weight was found to fluctuate, the greater the risk of getting diabetes.[23] What's more, greater degrees of fluctuation tended to result in higher mortality from all documented types of diseases.[24]

Although this marked rise in illness has hitherto been pretty much of a mystery, an understanding of the role of *Chemical Calories* goes a long way towards explaining it all now. As dieters lose weight, the release of chemicals from the body's fat stores will cause damage to the *Slimming System* and to many other body systems as well. This injury follows direct damage by the chemicals as well as indirect damage from the increased numbers of free radicals released by the higher levels of these chemicals.

It is well known that free radicals increase the chances of getting an extensive range of illnesses.[25] So increased chemical exposure in combination with the rise in free radical production could reasonably explain why so many diseases are linked to 'yo-yo' dieting. Unless these actions are fully anticipated and catered for, as is my aim in this programme, our health and weight are both likely to suffer by 'yo-yo' dieting.

WHAT CAN THE DETOX DIET DO TO HELP?

I hope this chapter has opened your eyes to the possibility that health problems other than excess weight might be caused or exacerbated by *Chemical Calories*. By cutting *Chemical Calories* out of your life and enhancing your *Slimming System*, not only will you be lowering your weight, but your health is also likely to be a major beneficiary.

But the benefits don't stop there: not only are our chances of getting chemical-linked diseases likely to be reduced, but it is also possible that many symptoms of these diseases may be alleviated, even cured – as many people have already discovered to their great delight.

You do need to understand, however, that while it may help considerably with certain problems, this programme is not specifically designed to treat illness. If you have a health problem, you should seek advice from your doctor or environmental health specialist before starting this or indeed any weight-loss programme.

23. Thirty Top Tips to Rid Your Life of *Chemical Calories*

To help you on your way to achieving the body of your dreams, here are thirty excellent ways to help rid your life of *Chemical Calories*. Every single one will help you detoxify and lose weight over the long term. And if you are just about to start the Detox Diet, they will help to make your diet more effective.

The key is to do what you can when you can. While this can look like an awful lot of changes, the more you can cut out *Chemical Calories* the slimmer you will eventually become. Better still, none of these changes require you to give up any food–all they do is cut out the chemicals. This is in effect dieting without food restriction, which for many is a dream come true!

1. Let polluted air escape your home by keeping it well ventilated. Remember that the air indoors tends to be far more polluted than it is outdoors (even in cities). If you live in a really heavily polluted area, you could invest in an air filter.

2. Fill up your rooms with plants that soak up airborne *Chemical Calories*. Spider plants are particularly useful – and can thrive without too much attention!

3. Use organic cosmetics, hair products and toiletries whenever possible. And if you can't find a replacement for a product, just try to use less of it.

4. If you have highlights or other chemical treatments done at the hairdresser, take some extra vitamins C and E and a dose of soluble fibre supplements just before your visit. This will help protect your *Slimming System* from chemical damage – as sometimes a girl's got to do

what a girl's got to do. Better still, see if they have a
chemical-free alternative.

5. Always filter or distil tap water before drinking it.

6. If you use bottled water, buy it in a glass bottle and not a
plastic one. If I can't get glass-bottled water when on the
move, I choose chilled plastic-bottled water over tap water.

7. Install a household water filter to reduce the chemicals
you will absorb from bath or shower water. If you wash
your hair in the bath, don't hang about in the soapy
water, as chemicals from the shampoo and conditioner
will be absorbed straight into your skin.

8. If you have clothes dry-cleaned, let them air outside or
in a well-ventilated place for a day or two before putting
them away in your wardrobe.

9. Transform your bedroom into a *Chemical-Calorie*-free
oasis. Don't forget to keep your bedroom window
slightly open at night if possible, but just to be on the
safe side, make sure it has some sort of security lock.

10. Decorate your home with home-grown flowers rather
than bought ones, which are likely to have been sprayed
with pesticides.

11. If you have new plastic objects or appliances that smell
strongly, keep them in a well-ventilated room, or
outside (if appropriate), until the plastic smell has mostly
gone.

12. Don't store food, particularly fatty foods, in plastic
containers. Fat acts as a 'magnet' for *Chemical Calories*
because of the high fat-solubility of plastics and their
additives.

13. If you do buy fatty foods (such as milk or cheese) in
plastic packaging, either decant them into a glass or
ceramic container, or make sure you keep them at a low
temperature in the fridge or freezer. The higher the
temperature the greater the contamination will be from
the plastic container into the food. As some tins are
lined with plastic, store them in a cool place too. And

one more thing: don't keep tinned foods hanging
around for too long before using them.

14. Try to avoid using those small plastic portions of milk or
cream for your coffee or tea, particularly if they contain
long-life products, since the longer the fatty fluids have
been in contact with the plastic, the greater the potential
contamination.

15. If you buy a new fridge, you can stop the plastic smell
being absorbed into your food by airing it outside with
the door propped open, until the smell subsides.
Alternatively, if you have to use it immediately, you can
make oil traps to soak up the plastic as it off-gasses. Fill a
few small cups with any type of vegetable oil and leave
them inside the fridge. Change the oil every few days
until the plastic smell disappears.

16. Steer clear of fish oils in supplements (unless you are
reasonably sure that their chemical content has been
reliably removed) and in processed foods.

17. On no account microwave or cook food in plastic
containers, as higher temperatures enhance the amount
of chemicals leaching out from plastics.

18. Don't drink boiling hot fluids from polystyrene or
plastic cups. I know it can be tricky to keep to this one
when at work or eating out, but it's worth asking if
there is an alternative container. You never know, the
next time there may well be! At work, you could always
bring in your own cup and supplies of organic coffee,
tea bags, etc.

19. Be ruthless in chucking out all your unwanted plastic
bags or wrappings – this can be hard for natural
hoarders, but do try!

20. When not in use, keep plastic objects packed away in
well-ventilated rooms.

21. Look for toys made from natural materials. They are
safer for your child and they will pollute the air inside
the house less.

22. Make sure that you rinse every trace of washing-up liquid from your cutlery and dishes.

23. Keep paints and solvents in a well-ventilated area, as far away as possible from your living and sleeping space.

24. Safely dispose of all fly sprays, flea powders and other synthetic pesticides. Try to find non-toxic alternatives – there are plenty out there.

25. If you need a spray-on bug repellent, choose a natural remedy such as peppermint oil.

26. Use natural cleaning solutions instead of chemicals to make your home sparkle.

27. Go for the most environmentally friendly option when treating your home for bug infestations.

28. Try to avoid using plastic-coated cooking utensils such as non-stick frying pans.

29. If you eat a meal that is high in *Chemical Calories*, take some soluble fibre and activated charcoal as soon as possible, as this will greatly reduce the amount of *Chemical Calories* you will absorb from the meal. And if you plan to eat out, why not just take the fibre and charcoal in advance, as it will allow you to be more relaxed about what you eat.

30. If you spend a long time in the car, try to get an air filter and keep a good distance away from the car in front. This will let the exhaust fumes disperse before the air gets sucked into your car – as well as reducing your chances of an accident!

24. Slim for Life

Maintaining and Enhancing Your New Slimmer Body

If you have just been on the Detox Diet and lost a significant amount of weight, then you have already accomplished a great deal. Stop for a while and congratulate yourself, as you have made a brilliant start down the path to permanent weight loss.

The real beauty of this programme, unlike other diets, is that once you have lost weight it actually becomes easier to keep it off. This is because the programme tackles the main cause of excess fat, which is the presence of *Chemical Calories*, and not just the symptoms of being overweight. This makes it stand out from every other diet, as its approach is unique.

However, to keep the excess pounds at bay for the rest of your life, you will still need to continue to keep your exposure to *Chemical Calories* as low as possible – the Detox Diet is not a quick-fix gimmick, but the first stage of long-term weight loss.

Stay calm now, because if you have been making the changes in diet and lifestyle advised by this book so far, keeping weight off over the long term should pose no problem to you whatsoever. In fact, as your *Slimming System* regenerates, controlling your weight will get ever easier as your body becomes more able to manage the process all by itself.

In order to ensure this long-term success, you will need to keep to the following guidelines – and if you do, all the benefits of this programme will be yours.

LONG-TERM GUIDELINES — AND WHO THEY ARE FOR

Most of the principles mentioned in the previous chapters still hold true, but here are the most important ones again. They will ensure that you keep that great new body you have worked so hard to get, as well as continually adding to these improvements throughout your life:

- Buy and eat food that is low in *Chemical Calories*.
- Take nutritional supplements to soak up *Chemical Calories* and to keep your *Slimming System* working optimally.
- Eat foods that are high in slimming nutrients and high in soluble fibre.
- Maintain an effective exercise programme.
- Eliminate *Chemical Calories* from your personal environment.

Furthermore, it is not only those people who have been on the diet who can benefit from the long-term programme — the above principles can be used by a whole range of other people who have their own individual needs.

This includes people who want to lose weight more gradually and can't bear the thought of going on a food-restriction diet, or those who are relatively happy with their weight but just want to improve their body shape. It is even ideal for people who are not overweight, but would just like to ensure that they stay that way.

Fortunately these guidelines will give all these people the ability to achieve weight loss or a more natural figure without dieting — which presents for the first time a viable as well as an achievable excellent alternative to the traditional concept of a food-restriction weight-loss diet.

Keeping to these principles will also be vital for those who are particularly overweight when they start the Detox Diet. These people will need to spend a longer time on the diet itself, simply because they have more weight to lose. They should then follow these long-term principles in between each period of active dieting, and of course after they have achieved their ultimate weight-loss goal as well.

KEEPING *CHEMICAL CALORIES* LOW

Keeping your exposure to *Chemical Calories* as low as possible is one of the key ways in which you can prevent future weight gains. By doing this, you will be doing all you can to minimize any future damage to your *Slimming System*. Once you have made the changes suggested for the diet programme, it should take less and less effort to keep your total exposure to *Chemical Calories* as reasonably low as possible.

One more thing: if you plan to have building work done in your house, seize the opportunity to lower your exposure to *Chemical Calories* both now and in the future by using products that are low in artificial chemicals. This can require a bit more effort and planning – try to find a builder who has worked this way before or who is willing to make the relevant inquiries on your behalf.

If you are planning to do the work yourself, a good tip is always to ask for the product data sheet for each type of building material, as this will reveal all the chemicals which have been used in that product. Better still, try to obtain the building materials from a company that supplies organic or naturally sourced products. A good company should also give you advice on how to use the products as well as investigating the available options – if in doubt, just ask.

Sometimes you will have to accept that there will be no natural equivalent, and will have to use chemical-based products. But if you can keep these instances to a minimum, you will have achieved a great deal towards keeping everyone in your home slim and healthy.

WHY YOU NEED TO KEEP TAKING SUPPLEMENTS

You might think that once you have achieved your ideal body weight, you won't need to keep taking all those supplements. Well, while your need for supplements will definitely diminish when you stop dieting, you will still need to keep taking them – they are vital in preventing those pounds from piling on again. There are two reasons for this.

First, although you can remove the majority of *Chemical Calories* from your body, however hard you try you will never be able to remove them all or to prevent some degree of recontamination throughout the rest of your life. You have to be philosophical here and accept that the whole world is so polluted that you cannot realistically prevent yourself from being exposed to any more *Chemical Calories*. By taking the supplements, though, you will be in a far better position to deal with the *Chemical Calories* that sneak past your defences as well as the ones still lurking in your body.

Second, to keep your *Slimming System* in tip-top form, you need to continue giving it all the nutrients it needs, as certain supplements can really make all the difference in helping you to keep slim. It's really worth making the effort, so that your body can continue to do its bit! Therefore, to ensure that your *Slimming System* is in the best possible shape, you need to take the following supplements on a long-term basis. Don't worry if you can't find one single tablet that meets all your needs. The best thing is to buy a good multi-vitamin and then add to it.

Although the need for these supplements can vary greatly between individuals, try to take levels close to the suggested dose.

Essential Supplements	Daily amount
Vitamin A (retinol or betacarotene)	3000–5,000ius*
Vitamin B1 (thiamine)	5–25mg
Vitamin B2 (riboflavin)	5–25mg
Vitamin B3 (niacin)	20–25mg
Vitamin B5	20–25mg
Vitamin B6	10–50mg
Vitamin B12	5–25mcg
Vitamin C	500–2,000mg
Vitamin E	100–200ius
Folic acid	200–400mcg
Choline	25–75mg
Zinc	15–20mg
Magnesium	200–400mg

Iron	10–20mg
Co-enzyme Q10	10–25mg

Essential fats	**Total daily amount**
Omega-3 essential fats, e.g. flax (linseed) oil	5–10g (approx. 1–2 teaspoons)

Detoxers	**Total daily amount**
Soluble fibre (for example grapefruit pectin, psyllium seed husks, or other equivalent)	approx. 3g

* If pregnant or trying to conceive, do not exceed 10,000ius of retinol a day.

You can take all these supplements in the morning, so long as you take the soluble fibre at least half an hour, and preferably an hour, before taking the rest of the supplements. Alternatively, the soluble fibre could be taken last thing at night or before a meal.

Optional Supplements	**Total daily amount**
Omega-6 essential fats, either evening primrose oil or equivalent	250–500mg

Amino acids (protein)*	**Total daily amount**
Tyrosine	100–200mg
L-5 hydroxytryptophan (5HTP, a natural precursor of serotonin)	25–50mg
Methionine	100–200mg
Glutathione	100–200mg

* These may be very hard to locate, so just use what's available.

The omega-6 oils will greatly help you in your efforts to keep your weight steady after dieting, but if you want to minimize the number of tablets you take, these could be cut so long as you are taking the linseed oil, as it contains a certain amount of omega-6 oils anyway.

If, however, you have not been on the Detox Diet and you are following the maintenance plan to lose weight, I would recommend that you take all the supplements. If you need help in discovering where to obtain the most suitable supplements for this programme, visit our website at www.chemicalcalories.com. To get more advice on how to structure taking them into your daily routine, see Chapters 15 and 17.

EATING AND STAYING SLIM FOR EVER

Unlike many weird and wonderful diets, the types of food recommended on the *Slimming System* programme will be the basis for your lifetime's eating habits after you come off the diet. But rather than sticking to the quantities recommended in the diet, the total amount of food can be increased by approximately one third.

Of course, people vary in size and shape, with some taller and more active men needing more food and some shorter and less active women needing less, but this provides an average level to aim for.

EAT MORE *SLIMMING SYSTEM* FRIENDLY FOODS

One of the best ways to keep your *Slimming System* running smoothly is to give it the fuel it needs. I would like to positively encourage people to eat the following two groups of foods – provided of course that they are low in *Chemical Calories*!

- Fresh foods high in slimming nutrients (salads, fruit, vegetables, nuts – if not allergic – and seeds)
- Foods high in soluble fibre (oats, apples, citrus fruit)

By eating a larger proportion of these foods in your diet, you will continue to boost your *Slimming System* and keep its fat-burning ability as high as possible.

Fresh fruit and raw vegetables also contain valuable substances known as phytonutrients ('phyto' means plant). Because of their many recognized benefits, one of the main areas of nutritional research is identifying and isolating phytonutrients so that they can be used as supplements. In the meantime, the simplest option for all of us is to eat them as nature intended.

By eating food high in soluble fibre, you will continue the good work of lowering your levels of *Chemical Calories*. In addition, you will also tend to eat higher levels of the other sort of fibre, roughage. Not only will this help to keep you regular, but it will also leave less room for all the fatty and sugary foods that you should be trying to cut down in your diet. Eating more roughage will also hasten the removal of *Chemical Calories* already bound up with soluble fibre from your diet.

EAT LESS FAT AND SUGAR

Of course, some foods offer little or no benefit and just contain what is commonly described as 'empty calories'. This means that they add conventional calories but give the body or *Slimming System* few nutritional bonuses. In addition, the more of these foods you eat, the more slimming nutrients you will use up in processing them. So they are definitely not *Slimming-System* friendly.

Rather than cutting them out totally, however, you should just cut down on the quantities you eat. This group of foods includes mayonnaise, margarine and spreads, pastries, sweets, chocolates, biscuits, cakes, ice-cream, sugary drinks, crisps and some fatty sauces.

TRY TO MODIFY YOUR EATING HABITS

Initially, it's hard to cut down on the amount of food that you eat, particularly if your *Slimming System* is badly contaminated with *Chemical Calories* – because the hormonal changes caused by chemical damage tend to increase the appetite. However, there are a number of things which you can do to help yourself. For example, an important way of helping yourself to cut down – particularly in the first few days, when these appetite-stimulating effects are at their strongest – is to try to change your eating behaviour.

For instance, if you put a whole pizza on your plate it will be very tempting to gobble the whole thing up – even the strongest-willed person in the world would find it hard not to. But if you cut the pizza into slices, and help yourself to one slice at a time, you may find that you are more likely to stop before it is all gone. More suggestions along the same lines include the following:

- Drink a glass of water a few minutes before a meal, to take the edge off your hunger.
- If hunger pangs strike, eat a piece of fruit or pre-prepared raw vegetable.
- When cooking family meals, try to ensure there are plenty of foods that you can eat too. If you are making a rich sauce, serve it in a separate container so that you can avoid it.
- Eat slowly, giving your body sufficient time to register what you have just eaten.
- Listen to what your body needs and stop when you are just full and not when you couldn't eat another bite.
- Always try to leave a small amount of food on your plate.

Scientists have found that these and many other behavioural techniques are successful, but only in the short term.[1] Interestingly, their lack of success in the long term could be explained by their inability to alter one of the *Slimming System*'s fundamental drives – our appetite.

However, in combination with my programme the techniques can be extremely effective. If you follow my programme, you are likely to find that your need for fatty or sweet foods will diminish naturally over time. This is because there will be fewer *Chemical Calories* to distort your appetite for fats and sugary carbohydrates. In addition your *Slimming System* will have substantially repaired itself and will now be getting all the nutrients it needs to prevent the overwhelming need to eat certain foods, particularly fatty or sweet ones.

I can vouch for this myself, as before I started this programme I was unable to get up from a meal without eating something sweet. Now this is not an issue, and I am rarely driven to seek out sweet things. In fact, now I cannot eat most of the sugary foods I used to adore.

You must accept that this transformation may take some time to happen, depending on the state of your *Slimming System*, but it should happen eventually – making it ever easier to control your weight. In fact, as time goes by, you will find that your ability to reduce the amount of food you eat at any one sitting actually improves.

After a while the ideal situation occurs, as you will find that your *Slimming System* will be able to readjust your appetite to a lower level all by itself – which it was what it was designed to do in the first place!

EXERCISE IS VITAL!

As you can imagine, exercise is extremely important in helping you to lose weight, and essential in maintaining your new slimmer self. Did you know that exercise appears to be one of the few ways in which you can actually lower your body's natural weight?[2]

Once you have achieved your target weight, stepping up your level of activity can lower it even further. The only provision is that to keep your weight at this new lower level you will need to be more active.

The activity recommendations for the diet are found in Chapter 21. To remind you: this involves three activity sessions per week, each lasting at least 30 minutes, and performed at a level where you will become warm or slightly out of breath. The long-term plan is slightly different, as the number of recommended exercise sessions is increased to a total of five 30-minute sessions each week. This will not only ensure that your *Slimming System* is in tiptop form, but also reflects your increased food intake off the diet.

OK, five sessions may seem daunting at first, but it really could be much easier than you think. The way to do it is to think of them as activity sessions and not exercise sessions. Whereas exercise sessions imply a workout at the gym, activity sessions also extend to digging the garden, doing housework or even taking the dog for a brisk walk. While it is ideal to have a formal workout, how you take your exercise will be totally up to you.

Start by looking at your daily routine to see where activity sessions could fit in. For instance, rather than jumping in a car to drive a short distance, walk or cycle there instead. That could easily make up two or three of your sessions every week.

The bottom line is that people who keep exercising after they have lost weight are far more successful in keeping it off than people who fail to keep up their activity levels. If you want to keep your new-found body, you have got to keep working on it!

HOW TO AVOID RELAPSES

After you have achieved your ideal weight, you should be feeling very pleased with yourself. Your great new looks are probably receiving a lot of positive attention. You will almost certainly be on a high, and why not? You have changed your life in an extremely positive way. At this point you really do need to be careful. It's one thing to lose weight on a diet, but quite another to keep weight off when you are not giving it your full attention.

As time goes on, maintaining your weight may become less and less of a priority. The activity sessions, which you used to complete so easily, go by the board. You find that you have run out of supplements and forget to reorder them. The care you took in choosing and preparing food low in *Chemical Calories* is forgotten and you go back to eating convenience foods. The several glasses of water you used to drink every day have been replaced by sugary drinks or coffee. And finally you find that the clothes you bought just after you lost weight seem to be getting tighter. Panic sets in: after losing all that weight, things seem to be going pear-shaped.

At this point, or, better still, before this point, you need to stop and reconsider your situation. If you don't keep your exposure to *Chemical Calories* down, and continue to take your supplements, your *Slimming System* will go on being damaged and you will start to put on weight again.

The best thing to do is to start keeping a daily diary again. As well as acting as a memory aid, it will help you to see whether your food intake has risen too high and your intake of essential supplements has fallen or even stopped.

If you have regained more than just a couple of pounds, you could re-start the Detox Diet. It may be the case that you are still relatively contaminated with *Chemical Calories* and that further efforts are needed to get rid of them. Don't forget that it has taken you a lifetime to build up your personal toxic store, so it may take more than a few weeks to shift!

But if you are still unable to maintain your weight despite following all the instructions as closely as possible, there are two possibilities. The first is that, unknown to you, you may be being continually exposed to chemicals, say at your office or in your house. So you could make further inquiries at work or call in a building specialist to help you isolate and identify the problem in your home.

Secondly, there might be a problem with your ability to detoxify. It takes a whole range of different reactions to metabolize *Chemical Calories*, and if one of these is faulty, your ability to detoxify will plummet. To find out if you have a problem, you will need to see a specialized nutritionist or, better still, a medical practitioner trained in environmental medicine. They can test your system for a variety of detoxification disorders, which can then be treated accordingly.

ONE LAST THING

For all you who have struggled with your weight day in and day out for years, this programme could be the answer to your prayers. Actually tackling the cause of excess weight has now made it possible to believe that permanent weight loss is no longer just a faraway myth.

The long-term programme set out in this chapter will not only help you to maintain your weight, but can also help you to keep losing weight after you have finished the diet – the more your inner levels of *Chemical Calories* drop, the more your *Slimming System* is then able to regenerate itself. And a more efficient *Slimming System* will be reflected by continued gradual weight loss until it reaches the point where your body-weight set-point gets as low as it possibly can. Don't forget, your *Slimming System* is the most valuable weapon you have in the battle against weight gain, so give it all the attention it deserves!

I do hope that you now understand more fully why you need to make the lifestyle alterations to achieve your long-term weight-loss goals. At the end of the day, whether you do or don't is in your hands and your hands alone – all I have done is provide you with a workable structure for how best to achieve it – it's now up to you to fully realize your dreams. So go on, you can do it!

Finally, it is time to start asking questions about how to deal with and lower the levels of pollution throughout the world. For until these vital issues are tackled, the levels of *Chemical Calories* in every aspect of our lives will continue to rise, making it constantly harder for us to keep our weight down and our bodies in good health.

25. Where Do We Go from Here?

The conclusions from my own personal search into what makes us fatter, and what we can do about it, can be found in this book, which is the culmination of years of painstaking research. Personally I have reaped a great deal of benefit from the research, since my weight now controls itself with little effort from me. In addition, my energy levels have shot up and I am no longer plagued with coughs and colds. I hope that the same information about combating the fattening effects of toxic chemicals will now also revolutionize the lives of others.

I think by now you will have realized that my approach differs fundamentally from the old methods of dieting, which use simple food-restriction alone. Dieting just by drastically cutting down what you eat is now in my belief virtually obsolete, and could be downright dangerous in the twenty-first century. The evidence stacked up over the past fifty years shows this approach to be not only ineffective but actually fattening over the long term, in addition to being a potentially significant cause of ill-health.

For most of us, recognizing that we are contaminated with *Chemical Calories* will be the biggest step forward we can make. Once we accept this, it becomes much easier to understand why we gain weight and therefore why we need to protect ourselves against the re-release of chemicals as we lose weight.

The guidelines set out in these chapters describe a safe way in which we should now lose weight in our increasingly contaminated environment. For the first time ever you have the power to control your own weight – by actively reversing the damage done by many years of chemical injury.

BLAME TOXIC CHEMICALS, NOT OVERWEIGHT PEOPLE

What has motivated me all along this major journey of discovery has been a burning desire to help others control their weight. I know it sounds corny, but I get really upset by people suffering unnecessarily. It's probably what got me into medicine in the first place.

I don't for one minute underestimate how much overweight people really can suffer. There's a powerful social stigma associated with being overweight, because it is widely assumed that it is the person's own fault. I hope that the information I've gathered about toxic chemicals will help to get rid of that stigma.

In addition, there are a whole range of other disadvantages that come with being overweight, such as the relative lack of medical support. The medical establishment currently offers relatively little active help and encouragement towards solving weight problems. I don't think this is malicious, though, just a lack of understanding and minimal or no training in how to deal with the problem.

Happily I have been able to move the finger of blame away from the individual and point it at our increasing exposure to toxic chemicals. In the future, I hope that being overweight will be seen as a medical problem arising from the person's sensitivity to chemicals and specific nutritional deficiencies, rather than as a condition that is their own fault. If I accomplish this, then all the hard work and effort I have put into researching and writing this book over the last few years will be completely worthwhile.

IMPROVING THE FUTURE FOR EVERYONE

Although we can't remove much of the pollution that already afflicts our planet, we can all influence the production of less toxic and fattening substances in the future. By buying organic foods and environmentally friendly products we will be sending an extremely powerful message to big business and industry.

Consumer power is by no means something to underestimate.

Since commercial companies are in the business of making money, if the products they produce aren't popular it won't take long before they come up with alternative products that are lower in *Chemical Calories*. If the demand grows, I predict that these types of goods will become ever easier to get hold of.

By choosing products low in *Chemical Calories*, not only will you be making a real difference to your own weight, body shape and health, but also, at the same time, you will be helping to reduce the overall use of toxic chemicals.

And the more people start to make these changes, the greater the overall chemical-lowering effect will be. So in addition to losing weight and getting fitter, you will also be doing your bit to help save the planet!

THE HEADLINES ONCE AGAIN

Since my findings are so topical and ground-breaking, I expect them to trigger a much wider debate about chemicals and their many toxic effects. In my view, though, the more debate and research on this subject, the better. In order to bring things together, let's take a final look at the key issues raised throughout the book:

- *The current fat epidemic is being caused mainly by the presence of toxic chemicals*. Why? Because these toxic chemicals interfere with and damage the body's *Slimming System*, which humans have developed over millions of years in order to control their body weight. Damage to this system can result in an increased appetite, slower metabolism, a reduced ability to burn off fat stores and a reduced ability to exercise. All these changes can actively promote weight gain.
- *The way to lose weight permanently is by restoring and rejuvenating your* **Slimming System**. You already have a highly developed system in place designed to promote weight loss. If you give your *Slimming System* what it needs to work properly and protect it from further damage, your body will become able to shift excess weight and keep it off by regulating your appetite, metabolism and level of activity accordingly.

- ***What are* Chemical Calories *and why are they so important?* I** have created a new unit known as a *Chemical Calorie* in order to estimate the fattening ability of all the different toxic chemicals we are now surrounded by. They are important because, by knowing which foods and non-food products are low in *Chemical Calories*, we can be more selective in targeting the removal of those products which chemically appear to be the most fattening.

- ***A diet of processed foods has increased the severity of the fat epidemic.*** Processed foods tend to lack many of the vitamins, minerals and essential fats that are essential in powering the *Slimming System* and in ridding our bodies of toxic chemicals. So a diet of highly processed foods will result in higher body levels of *Chemical Calories* and therefore excess fat.

  The foods recommended on my programme are *Slimming-System-*friendly. In other words, they are high in slimming nutrients and low in *Chemical Calories*. They make all the difference when it comes to keeping your *Slimming System* in excellent shape.

- ***Pesticides and other synthetic chemicals increase vitamin and mineral deficiencies.*** The presence of *Chemical Calories* in every aspect of our lives has permanently increased our body's needs for certain nutrients. As a result, however good we may consider our diet to be, we all need to take nutritional supplements to ensure that our *Slimming System* is in full working order.

- ***Traditional dieting methods can make us fatter and damage our health.*** The way we need to diet has been permanently changed by the presence of toxic chemicals. Simple food-restriction, without considering the presence of *Chemical Calories*, releases high levels of toxins into the blood-stream from the body's fat stores. The resulting damage to the *Slimming System* and the rest of the body reduces our ability to lose weight and greatly increases our chance of developing a serious illness.

  However, given the right conditions, food-restriction dieting can be a great way to mobilize and rid our bodies of even the most persistent and hard-to-shift *Chemical Calories* that we are now plagued with.

- ***To maximize our ability to lose weight we need to cut down our total exposure to* Chemical Calories**. Eating organic foods or foods low in *Chemical Calories*, in combination with lowering exposure to *Chemical*

Calories in our personal environment, will significantly reduce the harm done to our *Slimming System*. As a result, our natural ability to burn up excess fat stores will be enhanced as our body's load of *Chemical Calories* falls.

- **Your body's store of Chemical Calories *must be safely removed to achieve maximum weight loss***. The only effective way in which to remove many of the most highly fattening and persistent toxins is to take substances that bind to the chemicals, such as soluble fibre. This should take place alongside adequate nutrient supplementation, in order to enhance the body's natural detoxification system and protect the *Slimming System* from damage. Together, this will result in the safe removal of your lifetime's build-up of *Chemical Calories*, while minimizing any damage as a result of toxin mobilization.

- **By optimizing your Slimming System *you will be enhancing the quality of your life***. When you enhance your *Slimming System*, you will not just reduce your body fat, you will effectively be reprogramming your body shape (by reducing the amount of fat and increasing the proportion of lean muscle), improving your health and greatly enhancing your physical performance. In other words, by preventing the damage from toxic chemicals you will be allowing your body to achieve its full potential.

THE EFFORT BRINGS RICH REWARDS

As we all know from experience, in order to achieve anything worthwhile in life you have to make a concerted effort. The same is true here. In order to gain these benefits you will have to accept that you must make certain changes in how you shop for food, how you eat and in your lifestyle. In addition, you will need to take quite a few supplements.

I admit this can't all be done overnight – it will take some time to achieve all the necessary changes. For instance, depending on where you live, it may be either very easy or quite difficult to source organic produce or to get used to shopping with the benefit of the new *Chemical Calorie* charts. But as demand rises, these less polluted products will become more widely available, making it easier to keep your exposure to *Chemical Calories* as low as you can reasonably manage.

The beauty of this programme is that you can actually lose weight by simple lifestyle changes that don't require any form of food deprivation at all. For example, just by filtering your household water or by using natural household cleaners you can still lose weight. That realization is a true breakthrough.

And the more you achieve, the more you will find that your efforts are having a significant effect on your weight. This continual positive reinforcement will provide you with the encouragement you need to continue making lifestyle changes. I have seen the greatest sceptics totally converted into the greatest followers of this programme because of the amazing results they have experienced.

One such sceptic, Jonathan Gold, started making various comments to his wife Fiona just after she had begun the programme. When she started to cut down on certain foods which are potentially high in *Chemical Calories*, such as salmon, he began to comment on changes in her shopping habits, since salmon was one of his favourite foods. After complaining greatly about how he would never stop eating salmon and how she was so stupid in following these 'cranky' ideas, to prove his point he then went out and bought an extremely large quantity of it and then proceeded to wolf it down during the Christmas and New Year holidays.

By chance, just as he finished the last mouthful, he found himself listening to a news item about how extremely polluted our salmon now is with highly toxic chemicals which have been strongly linked to cancer. She said that after a couple of days of similar stories in the press, he turned positively green and began to take a bit more of an interest in what my programme was actually all about.

Not long after that he started on the programme himself. And although he never actively cut down on his food, after just a couple of months of cutting out *Chemical Calories* and taking the supplements, he discovered to his great delight that he had lost 4.5 kilos in weight, totally effortlessly! His old suits began to fit again and more and more people started commenting on his sleeker and healthier form. And to top it all, the severe symptoms of hay-fever which had bothered him greatly for all his adult life virtually disappeared. For the first time in all their years together, he didn't have to take any medication for it!

Well, now he is totally over the moon with his new self and is a total convert to my programme. And to his wife's constant amusement – because of his initial strongly negative attitude, arising from just a lack of information – he now takes the lead in ensuring that the food he eats and the environment that surrounds him are kept as free from *Chemical Calories* as possible. This just shows there is nothing quite like experiencing these great benefits first hand to provide a powerful motivating force!

On a final note, I feel extremely privileged to be able to present you with the means to achieve something that other weight-loss programmes have failed to achieve – permanent weight loss. I know from personal experience how much it has helped me, and I hope it will help you too. So with all my heart, I wish you good health and a very long and happy life.

Appendix A: Common Toxic Chemicals

We are exposed to vast numbers of chemicals containing high levels of *Chemical Calories* in a huge number of everyday products. Although it would be impractical to go through all of them individually, I have picked out some of the most common chemicals, just to highlight some of the places in which they can now be found.

The more you appreciate how widely these chemicals are used, and their individual longevity, the more clearly you will understand why we are now so contaminated with them.

ORGANOCHLORINES (AND OTHER ORGANOHALIDES)

What are they? Synthetically manufactured chemicals.
Examples: Organochlorine pesticides such as DDT, chlordecone, aldrin, dieldrin, endrin, toxaphene, heptachlor, lindane and its isomers, HCB (hexachlorobenzene); organochlorine pollutants such as dioxin, PCBs (polychlorinated biphenyls); organobromine fire-retardants such as the PBBs (polybrominated biphenyls – used mainly in the USA) and PBDEs (polybrominated diphenyl ethers – used mainly in northern Europe).
Background information: Most developed countries have banned many types of organochlorine pesticides now, but owing to their previous extensive use, and their long-lasting effects, their production is thought to have resulted in the permanent pollution of the entire planet.

Moreover, these pesticides continue to be produced and used in developing countries, largely because of their relatively low cost, even though many of their dangers are well-known. As contaminants, they accumulate up the food chain, and because of their high fat solubility and stability they tend to concentrate in fatty tissues.

Compounds very similar to the organochlorine industrial chemicals (PCBs) and pesticides (DDT) are used as fire-retardants. These substances, known as PBDEs and PBBs, are extensively used in developed and developing countries alike. These are also stable fat-loving chemicals which accumulate in fatty tissues and are nearly as toxic as their organochlorine counterparts.

Intended uses: General pesticides, common herbicides, insecticides and fungicides; wood preservatives and treatment for termite protection; anti-malaria spray; electrical conductors, fire-retardants; paints and dyes, medicines.

Where they are found: In food, as deliberately applied pesticide residues (in chocolate, for example); as environmental contaminants in carnivorous fish, fatty meats, dairy products, human tissue, soil, water and air adjacent to pollution sources; as contaminants in combusted leaded petrol; as contaminants in pesticides; as fire-retardants on fabrics, clothes, curtains, furniture coverings, plastics and wood; in electrical sealants, small capacitors, old refrigeration units, starter motors for fluorescent light switches; in carpets, carbonless duplicating paper, surface coatings, inks, and adhesives; in medicines such as nit shampoo and treatments for head and crab lice.

Estimated fattening ability: Extremely powerful, due to their extreme stability, our inability to expel them and their widespread toxicity to the body's natural *Slimming System*.

ORGANOPHOSPHATES

What are they? Synthetically manufactured chemicals.

Examples: Organophosphate insecticides.

Background information: Organophosphates were originally created in 1845. Later they were developed as a nerve gas and used in the Second World War. Since then they have been used very extensively in many different areas of manufacturing, food production and even medicine. They are now some of the commonest pesticides detected on our foods.

Intended uses: Nerve gas in human warfare; pesticides for crops; sheep dips, cattle treatments, flea treatments for pets; wood infestation treatments; animal growth-promoters; medicines, particularly treatment for lice, crabs and nits; widespread industrial uses such as petrol additives, stabilizers in lubricating and hydraulic oils, plastic additives, rubber additives and flame-retardants.

Where they are found: In food as pesticide residues, particularly on soft fruit, vegetables and grain products; as pesticides used in agriculture; in household and garden pesticides such as fly spray; in pet treatments; on treated wood; as medicines; in car oil, petrol fumes, plastics and rubber.

Estimated fattening ability: Organophosphates were previously used as animal growth-promoters. Although not as fat-soluble and persistent as the organochlorine pesticides, they have different toxicities. They appear to be particularly damaging to the ability to exercise.

CARBAMATES

What are they? Synthetically manufactured chemicals.

Examples: Carbamate insecticides, dithiocarbamate fungicides, ETU (ethylenetiourea).

Background information: Action thought to be similar to that of organophosphates, but generally considered to be less toxic. Some effects last for a shorter period than those of organophosphates, but other toxic actions can last for much longer periods and result in permanent damage.

Intended uses: In pesticides such as insecticide, herbicide, fungicide and anti-microbials; preventing potatoes from sprouting; ridding livestock and chicken of parasites; in flea treatments for pets; in forestry and wood infestation treatments; as animal growth-promoters; in manufacturing synthetic rubber; in plastics; as metal chelating agents.

Where they are found: In a wide range of foods and drinks including potatoes, soya beans, citrus fruits, peanuts, tomatoes, beer and wine; in cigarettes and cigars; in cotton; in household and garden pesticides including pet treatments, fly sprays and mothballs; in treated wood; in water as contaminants; in medicines (see below).

Estimated fattening ability: Very powerful. Carbamates have been used as growth promoters in battery farm situations because of their ability to slow down the overall metabolic rate. They are used in medicine for their anti-thyroid hormone actions.

PLASTICS AND PLASTICIZERS

What are they? Synthetically manufactured chemicals.

Examples: Common plastic additives known as phenols (e.g. bisphenol A), phthalates and phthalate esters.

Background information: The main function of phenols and phthalates is to give flexibility to plastic. Bisphenol A was originally created as an oestrogen mimic in the 1930s, but is now extremely commonly used as a plasticizer in food packaging: for example, it is used in the lining of metallic food containers.

Intended uses: Phthalates, phthalate esters and phenols are used as additives in PVC and in virtually all other types of plastics; as a pesticide dilutant; as surface active agents (cleaning compounds commonly derived from petroleum); in industry they are widely used in rubber and plastic manufacturing, as industrial cleaning agents, lubricants and corrosion inhibitors.

Where they are found: In plastic wrappings for food, in food containers, in plastic bottles for baby milk, in the lining of cardboard and aluminium food containers, in the lining of metal food cans; in food and water as contaminants; in some types of fish; in fatty foods such as eggs, dairy and breast milk; as human tissue contaminants; in household pesticides and insect-repellents; in cosmetics, perfumes, shampoo, hair products and nail polish; in inks, synthetic leather, vinyl floors, carpet backing, water pipes, adhesives and glues and waterproof clothing; in medical devices such as catheter bags and blood storage bags; in all kinds of tubing; in dental sealant and dental impression material; in detergents and paints.

Estimated fattening ability: Strong. Particularly damaging to the slimming hormones.

HEAVY METALS

What are they? Naturally occurring toxic metals.

Examples: cadmium, lead, mercury, methyl mercury and tributyl tin (TBT).

Background information: These toxic substances occur naturally. However, due to their extensive industrial use, we are now being exposed to them in levels many times greater than are usually found in nature.

Intended uses: Industrial uses include use in pesticide formulations, electroplating, nickel plating, for soldering, in alloys, in photoelectric cells and in storage batteries. Released in mining practices. Household uses include plumbing, building materials, cable covering and paints; also used in dentistry, as petrol additives and in insecticides.

Where they are found: As contaminants in drinking water and in food grown near roadsides. Found as human contaminants and in effluent in heavily polluted areas; used in amalgam fillings, crystal glass, petrol, batteries, roofing.

Estimated fattening ability: Moderate, but their tendency to accumulate in the body over a number of years makes them very important.

SOLVENTS

What are they? Synthetically manufactured chemicals.

Examples: Organic solvents (styrene and polystyrene), chlorinated solvents (trichloroethylene), industrial solvents.

Background information: These chemicals are very widely used in a whole range of products. Certain liquid solvents, such as styrene, can be converted into polystyrene.

Intended uses: Solvents are used extensively throughout industry to dissolve or dilute oils and fats; as a petrol additive; as a plastic strengthener and major component of packaging and household materials; a major substance used in the dry-cleaning industry; used in manufacturing plastics, synthetic rubbers, latex and resins.

Where they are found: As synthetic fragrances in toiletries, detergents, skincare products, perfumes and aftershaves; in plastics and
synthetic rubbers; as a heat seal coating on metal foils (on yogurt and
cream containers, etc.); as polystyrene cups and plates or polystyrene
packaging; as a solvent for paints, in turpentine substitute, in shoe
creams, floor waxes or dyes; in household pesticides and medicines;
as an environmental contaminant found in water, in the urban
atmosphere and in wildlife; in foods packaged in polystyrene; as a
human contaminant; in glass fibre, petrol vapour and exhaust fumes.

Estimated fattening ability: Moderate, but still significant because
of their very extensive presence in the environment. In particular
they appear to damage our slimming hormones.

Appendix B: Your Ideal Weight and Body Fat Percentage Charts

THE IDEAL WEIGHT FOR YOUR HEIGHT
(SEE NOTE ON PAGE VII)

The following tables give you an idea of what your ideal weight should be, for a person of average build, depending on your height and sex.

Men aged 25 and over		Women aged 25 and over	
Height	Weight (lb)	Height	Weight (lb)
5'1"	112–129	4'8"	92–107
5'2"	115–133	4'9"	94–110
5'3"	118–136	4'10"	96–113
5'4"	121–139	4'11"	99–116
5'5"	124–143	5'0"	102–119
5'6"	128–147	5'1"	105–122
5'7"	132–152	5'2"	108–126
5'8"	136–156	5'3"	111–130
5'9"	140–160	5'4"	114–135
5'10"	144–165	5'5"	118–139
5'11"	148–170	5'6"	122–143
6'0"	152–175	5'7"	126–147
6'1"	156–180	5'8"	130–151
6'2"	160–185	5'9"	134–155
6'3"	164–190	5'10"	138–159

BODY FAT PERCENTAGE

Your body fat percentage is actually a more important statistic than your ideal body weight, since it gives you an indication of how much excess fat you are carrying around. It also provides a very useful tool in enabling you to see the real progress made on the diet.

This is particularly useful in the situation when your body is using up fat and converting it to muscle, but the reduction in the overall body weight appears to be slowing down. By working out the percentage body fat you can actually see progress which is not readily apparent on the scales.

If you don't have access to somewhere where your percentage body fat can be estimated, such as a gym, the following equation allows you to work out an approximation of your body fat percentage in the comfort of your own home. An ideal body fat percentage for a man is around 15 per cent and for a woman around 22 per cent.

STEP 1:   Find your Body Weight (BW) on the charts on pages 345–7 and write down the corresponding Conversion Factor. For weights which are not multiples of 5lb, take the figure below your weight and add 1.08 to the Conversion Factor for every pound over it. For example:

If you weigh 175lb, your Conversion Factor is 189.36.

If you weigh 132lb, your Conversion Factor is 142.83 (140.67 + [2 + 1.08])

STEP 2:   Find your Waist Girth on the chart and write down the corresponding Conversion Factor. For example:

If you have a 35-inch waist, your Conversion Factor is 145.26.

STEP 3:   Subtract the Waist Conversion Factor from the Body Weight Conversion Factor. For example:

189.36 − 145.26 = 44.10

STEP 4: Men add 98.42 to the result. Women add 76.76. This gives your Lean Body Weight (LBW). For example:

44.10 + 98.42 = 142.52

STEP 5: To calculate your Fat Weight (FW), subtract the LBW from the BW. For example:

175 − 142.52 = 32.48

STEP 6: To determine your Body Fat percentage, divide FW by BW and multiply by 100. For example:

(FW/BW) x 100 = %BF.

(32.48/175) x 100 = 19%

Body fat percentage calculation chart

Body weight (lb)	Conversion factor	Waist girth (inches)	Conversion factor
100	108.21	25	103.75
105	113.62	25.5	105.83
110	119.03	26	107.9
115	124.44	26.5	109.98
120	129.85	27	112.05
125	135.26	27.5	114.13
130	140.67	28	116.2
135	146.08	28.5	118.28
140	151.49	29	120.35
145	156.9	29.5	122.43
150	162.31	30	124.51

Body weight (lb)	Conversion factor	Waist girth (inches)	Conversion factor
155	167.72	30.5	126.58
160	173.13	31	128.66
165	178.54	31.5	130.73
170	183.95	32	132.81
175	189.36	32.5	134.88
180	194.77	33	136.96
185	200.18	33.5	139.03
190	205.59	34	141.11
195	211	34.5	143.18
200	216.41	35	145.26
205	221.82	35.5	147.33
210	227.23	36	149.41
215	232.64	36.5	151.48
220	238.05	37	153.56
225	243.46	37.5	155.63
230	248.87	38	157.71
235	254.28	38.5	159.78
240	259.69	39	161.86
245	265.1	39.5	163.93
250	270.51	40	166.01
255	275.92	40.5	167.08
260	281.33	41	170.16

Body weight (lb)	Conversion factor	Waist girth (inches)	Conversion factor
265	286.74	41.5	172.23
270	292.15	42	174.31
275	297.56	42.5	176.38
280	302.97	43	178.46
285	308.38	43.5	180.53
290	313.79	44	182.61

Appendix C: Glossary of Terms

Adrenaline (epinephrine) Functions to stimulate heart rate, respiration rate and metabolism. One of the most important slimming hormones we possess. It plays an important role in burning up excess fat and carbohydrates. Unfortunately, it is very easily damaged by toxic chemicals.

Amino acids These are the basic building blocks from which proteins are made up.

Antioxidants Substances which are able to effectively neutralize and soak up harmful free radicals. Examples include vitamin A and beta-carotene, vitamins C and E, zinc, selenium, Co-enzyme Q10 and the amino acid glutathione.

Bioaccumulation A build-up of chemicals which the body is unable to remove, so they end up being stored.

Body-weight set-point The body weight (different for each individual) which the body tries to maintain through feast and famine.

Calorie The energy needed to raise the temperature of 1 gram of water through 1 degree Centigrade (now usually defined as 4.1868 joules).

Calorific value The amount of energy which the body can extract from a food.

Carbamates A class of very widely used pesticides, added to food because of an ability to kill fungus. They are used on a vast scale in agriculture and are commonly used in veterinary practice, in medicine and as wood preservers.

Chemical Calories^{TM} A *Chemical Calorie* is a measure of how damaging a toxic chemical is to the body's natural *Slimming System*. Foods high in *Chemical Calories* will be more chemically 'fattening' than those low in *Chemical Calories*.

Chemical Calories™ **rating** A score allocated to particular chemicals indicating how toxic and damaging they are to the *Slimming System*. In practical terms, the higher the score a chemical possesses the more fattening it will be.

Co-enzyme Q10 This is a semi-essential nutrient which plays a central role in boosting our energy levels. Like vitamins and minerals, it can be taken as a supplement.

Detoxification The removal of toxic substances from the body by the body's waste-disposal systems.

Free radicals These are highly damaging particles which are produced in cells in the normal process of energy creation or from the detoxification of certain toxins. They are harmful because they damage and age all the tissues they are created in. Certain things increase the number of free radicals produced and they are as follows: pesticides, smoking, exhaust fumes, pollution, infections, burnt foods, fried foods and sunburn.

Fungicide A chemical that destroys fungus.

Glutathione An amino acid that is essential in breaking down toxic chemicals.

Growth-promoter A chemical or substance that encourages growth in animals.

Herbicide A chemical that is toxic to plants and is commonly used as a weedkiller.

Hormones These are natural substances which act as natural internal chemical messengers in our bodies. They are released from one part of our bodies (glands) and are then carried around in the bloodstream to a tissue or organ which they then stimulate.

Insecticide A substance used to kill insects.

Insulin A hormone, the main role of which is to control our blood sugar levels. It also has a role in controlling our fat metabolism.

Metabolic rate The rate at which heat and other energy is produced and released from our bodies as a result of all the individual chemical reactions taking place.

Metabolism All the chemical reactions that occur within a living organism in order to maintain life.

Mineral An inorganic substance which occurs naturally and is needed by the human body in small quantities, for good health.

Noradrenaline (norepinephrine) One of the most important slimming hormones we possess – for as well as its role in powerfully suppressing our appetite, it is also absolutely essential in order to burn up excess body fat. Unfortunately it is also exquisitely vulnerable to chemical damage.

Nutrient A substance that provides nourishment essential for the maintenance of life and growth.

Oestrogens A group of female hormones (but also found in low levels in men) that promote female physical characteristics. Their decrease in women after the menopause reduces the effectiveness of the *Slimming System*.

Organic The term organic has three popular definitions that can result in a certain amount of confusion. In the first popular definition, organic means natural plants and animals, or made from natural substances, or allowed to grow naturally. People even talk about companies having organic growth, meaning gradual growth resulting from the hiring of employees as the company gains more business, as opposed to sudden growth resulting from the takeover of another company.

The second popular definition is in using the term to describe food legally certified as organic. This means that organic food is supposed to have few added manufactured pesticides, antibiotics, hormones, and other additives – that is, meat, eggs, vegetables and fruit produced without the use of artificial synthetic chemicals. These first two different meanings can result in confusion, as the ambiguity allows manufacturers to say that shampoo or other cosmetics are made from organic ingredients when they can actually just mean that they contain plant extracts that have been grown in a conventional way.

And in the chemistry world, organic simply refers to any chemical with carbon and hydrogen in it. The study of organic chemistry is the study of compounds with carbon and hydrogen in them. Most pesticides and synthetic chemicals contain carbon, as they are often synthesized from petroleum or oil. So strictly speaking they are organic compounds but unlike the substances they are derived from they do not exist in nature.

Organic chemicals Substances derived from living organisms containing carbon and hydrogen.

Organic foods Food and other products grown, stored, preserved, and transported with a minimal use of chemicals – so they tend to be less chemically contaminated than those produced using conventional means.

Organochlorines A number of organic chemicals which contain the element chlorine. These types of compounds are not found to occur naturally. And due to our inability to remove them from our bodies – and their ability to accumulate in fatty tissues – they tend to be extremely persistent in the body, as well as toxic. This varied group includes chemicals known as DDT, PCBs and lindane.

Organobromides A number of artificial and toxic compounds, which include the PBB and PBDE fire-retardants. They are particularly persistent, fat-soluble and toxic. These substances tend not to be found in nature. And since they possess such a difficult molecular shape (because of the bromine component), our bodies' waste-disposal systems can find it very difficult to get rid of them.

Organophosphates Synthetic organic compounds containing phosphorus, which include highly toxic pesticides and nerve gases.

PBBs (polybrominated biphenyls) and PBDEs (polybrominated diphenyl ethers) These are organic compounds which contain the element known as bromine. These substances are not usually found in nature and include a number of highly stable compounds which are particularly heat-resistant – and because of these qualities they are commonly used as fire-retardants. However, due to our relative inability to remove them from our bodies, our bodily levels of these chemicals tend to accumulate throughout our lives.

PCBs (polychlorinated biphenyls) Although the manufacture of these types of organochlorines is now banned, these very stable organochlorines are still found in our environment as they are extremely persistent. They are also extremely persistent in our bodies.

Pesticide A substance used for destroying insects or other organisms harmful to cultivated plants or to animals and humans.

Plasticizers Chemicals added to plastics (synthetic resins) to produce or promote flexibility and to reduce brittleness.

Pollutants Substances that pollute or contaminate the environment, especially harmful chemical or waste material discharged into the atmosphere and water, including gases, particulate matter, pesticides, radioactive isotopes, sewage, organic chemicals and phosphates, solid wastes and many others.

Slimming System™ A set of highly evolved body functions that work together to bring about weight loss.

Supplement A substance taken to remedy the deficiencies in a person's diet.

Sympathetic nervous system (SNS) This is a specialized part of the body's nervous system which plays a key role in controlling our body weight.

Synthetic chemical A man-made substance made by chemical synthesis, especially to imitate a natural product. These synthetic chemicals or substances do not exist in nature.

Testosterone A hormone that controls the development of male sexual characteristics. It is also very vulnerable to chemical damage.

Thermogenesis The production of heat in an animal or human. Many chemicals are able to reduce the body's ability to convert body fat stores into heat energy. So their net effect is to lower the body's temperature.

Thyroid hormones A group of hormones that regulate growth and development through altering the body's metabolic rate.

Vitamin Any of a group of compounds which are essential for normal growth and nutrition and are required in small quantities in a person's diet because they cannot be created by the body.

Xenobiotics Foreign or unnatural compounds or chemicals (i.e. those that do not exist in nature).

Xenoestrogen A synthetic or phyto (plant) chemical not naturally found in the body, that mimics the actions of natural oestrogens (female hormones).

'Yo-yo' dieting (or weight cycling) This is when people lose weight on a diet, then regain it when they have stopped dieting. They may repeat this pattern many times.

Appendix D: Useful Contacts

Slimming Systems Ltd: To help make it easier for people to follow the Detox Diet, Dr Paula Baillie-Hamilton has founded the company Slimming Systems Ltd. Contact us at Slimming Systems Ltd for the latest information on *Chemical Calories*, to be put on a mailing list, to find out more about our products and services, or to comment on your own experiences with the Detox Diet. Please visit our Internet address **www.slimmingsystems.com** or send your mail to:

Dr Paula Baillie-Hamilton
Slimming Systems Limited
PO Box 14
Callander
FK17 8WA

ENVIRONMENTAL MEDICINE

To see a local specialist in environmental medicine, contact one of the following organizations:

British Society for Allergy, Environmental and Nutritional Medicine (BSAENM)
PO Box 7
Knighton LD7 1WT
UK
Tel: +44 (0) 1547 550378
Fax: +44 (0) 1547 550339
www.jnem.demon.co.uk

American Academy of Environmental Medicine
7701 East Kellogg, Suite 625
Wichita
KS 67207
USA
Tel: +1 316 684 5500
Fax: +1 316 684 5709
www.aaem.com

Australasian College of Nutritional and Environmental Medicine
13 Hilton Street,
Beaumaris
Victoria 3193
Australia
Tel: +61 3 9589 6088
Tel: +61 3 9589 5158

Australian Society for Environmental Medicine Inc.
2/11 Howell Close
Doncaster East
Victoria 3109
Australia
Tel: +61 3 9842 1886
Fax: +61 3 9841 4336

ORGANIC LIVING

To dig deeper into organic issues, check out the following contacts:

International Federation of Organic Agriculture Movements (IFOAM)
Okozentrum Imsbach
D-66636
Tholey-Theley
Germany
Tel: +49 6853 5190
www.ifoam.org
IFOAM's website has comprehensive links to organic organizations around the world.

The Soil Association
Bristol House
40–56 Victoria Street
Bristol BS1 6BY
UK
Tel: +44 (0) 117 929 0661
Fax: +44 (0) 117 925 2504
www.soilassociation.org
Another very helpful website.

Henry Doubleday Research Association (HDRA)
Ryton Organic Gardens
Coventry CV8 3LG
UK
Tel: +44 (0) 24 7630 3517
Fax: +44 (0) 24 7663 9229
www.hdra.org.uk
For gardening products and information.

Pesticide Action Network UK (formerly the Pesticides Trust)
Eurolink Centre
49 Effra Road
London SW2 1BZ
UK
Tel: +44 (0) 20 7274 8895
www.pan-uk.org
e-mail: admin@pan-uk.org
For information on the effect of pesticides as well as finding alternatives.

Association for Environmentally-Conscious Building
PO Box 32
Llandysul SA44 5ZA
UK
Tel/fax: +44 (0) 1559 370 908
www.aecb.net
e-mail: admin@aecb.net
They advise on natural and organic materials in new buildings, extensions etc.

Construction Resources
16 Great Guildford St
London SE1 0HS
UK
Tel: +44 (0) 207 4502211
Fax: +44 (0) 207 450 2212
www.ecoconstruct.com
Ecological builders' merchant and building centre who also provide useful advice.

Building Investigations Ltd (Environmental House Doctor)
Peter Broach
The Cartshed
Church Lane
Osmington
Dorset DT3 6EW
UK
Tel: +44 (0) 1305 837223
www.building-investigations.co.uk
e-mail: mail@building-investigations.co.uk
Detects pesticides and pollutants in houses.

The range of organic products on the market is currently increasing at a tremendous pace. To find out how to source these products, there are many books available which contain this information for an ever-expanding number of countries. In addition, the internet is a very good source of information.

Notes

Introduction: Making the Discovery

1. G. Gardner and B. Halweil, 'Overfed and Underfed: The Global Epidemic of Malnutrition', *World Watch Paper* (2000), 150, pp. 7–11.

Chapter 1: The Fat Epidemic

1. G. Critser, 'Let them eat fat: The heavy truths about American obesity', *Harpers, USA* (2000), April.
2. ibid.
3. ibid.
4. M. S. Tremblay *et al.*, 'Secular trends in the body mass index of Canadian children', *Canadian Medical Association Journal* (2000), 163 (11), pp. 1429–33.
5. R. J. Kuczmarski *et al.*, 'Increasing prevalence of overweight among US adults', *Journal of the American Medical Association* (1994), 272 (3), pp. 205–11.
6. D. Collcutt and C. Evans, 'Yes girls, it's true. You really are bigger these days', *Daily Mail*, London, 2 February 2000.
7. B. Marsh, 'A two-inch pinch as men lose war of the waistline', *Daily Mail*, London, 15 June 2000.
8. K. D. Brownell and C. G. Fairburn (eds.), *Eating disorders and obesity: A comprehensive handbook*, Guilford Press, New York, 1995, p. 56.
9. S. N. Steen *et al.*, 'Are obese adolescent boys ignoring an important health risk?', *International Journal of Eating Disorders* (1996) 20 (3), pp. 281–6.
10. A. G. Dulloo, 'Regulation of body composition during weight

recovery and thermogenesis', *Clinical Nutrition* (1997), 16 (1), pp. 25–35.

11. ibid.

12. G. A. Colditz, 'Economic costs of obesity', *American Journal of Clinical Nutrition* (1992), 55, pp. 503s–7s.

13. L. Lissner *et al.*, 'Body weight variability in men: Metabolic rate, health and longevity', *International Journal of Obesity* (1990), 14 (4), pp. 373–83.

14. J. Baxter, 'Obesity surgery – another unmet need', *British Medical Journal* (2000), 321 (2), pp. 523–3.

15. K. M. Flegal, 'Overweight and obesity in the United States: prevalence and trends, 1960–1994', *International Journal of Obesity and Related Metabolic Disorders* (1998), 22 (1), pp. 39–47.

16. C. A. Dell *et al.*, 'Lipid and fatty acid profiles in rats consuming different high-fat ketogenic diets', *Lipids* (2001), 36 (4), pp. 373–8.

17. H. Tarnower and S. S. Baker, *The Complete Scarsdale Medical Diet*, Bantam Books, London, 1993.

18. B. Sears and B. Lawren, *Enter the zone: A dietary road map*, Regan Books, New York, 1995.

19. R. Atkins, *Dr Atkins' New Diet Revolution*, Avon Books, New York, 1999.

20. A. M. Prentice, and S. A. Jebb, 'Obesity in Britain: gluttony or sloth?', *British Medical Journal* (1995), 311 (12), pp. 437–9.

21. HMGO (Her Majesty's Government Offices), 'Health of the Nation; Obesity results', *Health Survey of England* (1998), pp. 282–303.

22. E. Ravussin, 'Rising trend may be due to "pathoenvironment"', *British Medical Journal* (1995), 311, p. 1569.

23. ibid.

24. *Allied Dunbar National Fitness Survey*, Sports Council, London, 1992.

25. R. B. Harris, 'Role of set-point theory in regulation of body weight', *FASEB Journal* (1990), 415, pp. 3310–18.

26. E. Alleva *et al.*, 'Statement from the work session on environmental endocrine-disrupting chemicals: neural, endocrine and behavioural effects', *Toxicology and Industrial Health* (1998), 14 (1–2), pp. 1–7.

27. United States Tariff Commission, 'Synthetic Organic Chemicals', US Government Printing Office, Washington, 1918–94.

Chapter 2: The Synthetic Revolution

1. T. Colborn *et al.*, 'Environmental neurotoxic effects: the search for new protocols in functional teratology', *Toxicology and Industrial Health* (1998), 14 (1/2), pp. 9–23.

2. B. Holdsworth *et al.*, *New Civil Engineer Supplement*, 25 September 2000.

3. D. V. Bailey, 'Vyvyan Howard in bullet points', *Living Earth* (2001), 211 (July-Sept.).

4. Health and Safety Executive, *Annual Report of the Working Party on Pesticide Residues*, Ministry of Agriculture, Fisheries and Food, HMSO, London, 1996, pp. 97 and 129–34.

5. J. L. Jacobson and S.W. Jacobson, 'Dose-response in perinatal exposure to polychlorinated biphenyls (PCBs): The Michigan and North Carolina cohort studies', *Toxicology and Industrial Health* (1996), 12 (3/4), pp. 435–45.

6. L. S. Birnbaum, 'Endocrine effects of prenatal exposure to PCBs, dioxins, and other xenobiotics: implications for policy and future', *Environmental Health Perspectives* (1994), 102 (August), pp. 676–9.

7. F. Bordet *et al.*, 'Organochlorine pesticide and PCB congener content of French human milk', *Bulletin of Environmental Contamination and Toxicology* (1993), 50, pp. 425–32.

8. J. L. Jacobson and S. W. Jacobson, 'Sources and implications of interstudy and interindividual variability in the developmental neurotoxicity of PCBs', *Neurology and Teratology* (1996), 18 (3), pp. 257–64.

9. Health and Safety Executive, *Annual Report of the Working Party on Pesticide Residues*, Ministry of Agriculture, Fisheries and Food, HMSO, London, 1997, pp. 157–9 and 55.

10. Bordet *et al.*, 'Organochlorine pesticide and PCB congener content'.

11. P. Beaumont, 'The chronic effects of pesticides', in *Pesticides, Policies and People; a guide to the issues*, Pesticides Trust, London, 1993, pp. 83–92.

12. L. R. Goldman, 'Children – Unique and vulnerable. Environmental risks facing children and recommendations for response', *Environmental Health Perspectives* (1995), 103 (suppl. 6), pp. 13–18.

13. W. Rea, *Chemical Sensitivity*, vol. 2, Lewis Publishers, Boca Raton, Florida, 1994, pp. 1935–2006.

14. A. L. Rodrigues *et al.*, 'Effect of perinatal lead exposure on rat behaviour in open-field and two-way avoidance tasks', *Pharmacology and Toxicology* (1996), 79 (3), pp. 50–56.

15. United States Tariff Commission, 'Synthetic Organic Chemicals'.

16. S. Steingraber, *Living Downstream*, Virago Press, London, 1998, pp. 90–93.

17. ibid.

18. J. A. Thomas and H. D. Colby (eds.), *Endocrine Toxicology*, Taylor & Francis, Washington, DC, 1996, p. 190.

19. L. E. Sever *et al.*, 'Reproductive and developmental effects of occupational pesticide exposure: the epidemiologic evidence', *Occupational Medicine* (1997), 12 (2), pp. 305–25.

20. K. Rozman *et al.*, 'Histopathology of interscapular brown adipose tissue, thyroid, and pancreas in 2,3,7,8-tetrachlorodibenzo-p-dioxin', *Toxicology and Applied Pharmacology* (1986), 82 (3), pp. 551–9.

21. J. R. Brown, 'The effect of environmental and dietary stress on the concentration of 1,1-bis(4-chlorophenyl)-2,2,2,-trichloroethane', *Toxicology and Applied Pharmacology* (1970), 17, pp. 504–10.

22. D. W. Nebert, *Human genetic variation in the enzymes of detoxification. Enzymatic Basis of Detoxification*, 1, ed. W. B. Jakoby, Academic Press, Orlando, 1980, p. 32.

23. O. A. Iakovleva *et al.*, '[Vitamin A and E allowance of the body in xenobiotic exposure]', *Voprosy Pitaniia* (1987), 3, pp. 27–9.

24. R. W. Chadwick *et al.*, 'Effects of age and obesity on the metabolism of lindane by black a/a, yellow Avy/a, and pseudoagouti Λvy/a phenotypes of (ys xvy) F1 hybrid mice', *Journal of Toxicology and Environmental Health* (1985), 16, pp. 771–96.

25. C. Denzlinger *et al.*, 'Modulation of the endogenous leukotriene production by fish oil and vitamin E', *Journal of Lipid Mediators and Cell Signalling* (1995), 11 (2), pp. 119–32.

26. P. Beaumont, *Pesticides, Policies and People; a guide to the issues*, Pesticides Trust, London, 1993, p. 121.

27. Health and Safety Executive, *Annual Report of the Working Party on Pesticide Residues*, 1997, p. 49.

Chapter 3: Chemicals Make You Fat

1. J. Turner, 'The welfare of broiler chickens – an analysis of the European Scientific Committee report of March 2000', Compassion in World Farming Trust, 2000.

2. J. F. Hancock, 'Effects of Estrogens and Androgens on Animal growth', in A. M. Pearson (ed.), *Growth regulation in farm animals*, Elsevier Applied Science, London, 1991, p. 267.

3. T. Baptista *et al.*, 'Mechanism of the neuroleptic-induced obesity in female rats', *Progress in Neuro-Psychopharmacology and Biological Psychiatry* (1998), 22, pp. 187–98.

4. J. Gawecki *et al.*, 'The effect of poisoning with dithane M-45 on oxygen uptake and energy balance in adult rats', *Acta Physiologica Polonica* (1976), 27 (2), pp. 169–74.

5. M. L. Trankina *et al.*, 'Effects of in vitro Ronnel on metabolic activity in subcutaneous adipose tissue and skeletal muscle from steers', *Journal of Animal Science* (1985) 60 (3), pp. 652–8.

6. United States Tariff Commission, 'Synthetic Organic Chemicals'; K. M. Flegal, 'Overweight and obesity in the United States'.

7. G. Critser, 'Let them eat fat: The heavy truths about American obesity', *Harpers, USA* (2000), April.

8. S. D. Stellman *et al.*, 'Adipose and serum levels of organochlorinated pesticides and PCB residues in Long Island women: Association with age and body mass', *American Journal of Epidemiology* (1997), SER Abstract S21, p. 81.

9. J. Ashby *et al.*, 'Lack of effects for low dose levels of bisphenol A and diethylstilbestrol on the prostate gland of CFI mice exposed in utero', *Regulatory Toxicology and Pharmacology* (1999), 30 (2, pt 1), pp. 156–66.

10. B. D. Hardin *et al.*, 'Evaluation of 60 chemicals in a preliminary developmental toxicity test', *Carcinogens, Mutagens and Teratogens* (1987), 7, pp. 29–48.

11. D. R. Clark, 'Bats and environmental contaminants: A review', US Department of the Interior: Fish and Wildlife Service, Special Scientific Report, Washington, DC, *Wildlife* No. 235 (1981), pp. 1–29.

12. K. Takahama *et al.*, 'Toxicological studies on organochlorine pesticides. 1. Effect of long term administration of organochlorine pesticides on rabbit weight and organ weight', *Nippon Hoigaku Zasshi* (1972), 26 (1), pp. 5–10.

13. J. C. Lamb *et al.*, 'Reproductive effects of four phthalic acid esters in the mouse', *Toxicology and Applied Pharmacology* (1987), 88 (2), pp. 255–69.

14. Ashby *et al.*, 'Lack of effects for low dose levels of bisphenol A and diethylstilbestrol'.

15. Trankina *et al.*, 'Effects of in vitro Ronnel'.

16. J. E. Morley, 'Anorexia in older persons', *Epidemiology* (1996), 8 (2), pp. 134–55.

17. P. B. Kaplowitz and S. Jennings, 'Enhancement of linear growth and weight gain by cyproheptadine in children with hypopituitarism receiving growth hormone therapy', *Journal of Pediatrics* (1987), 110 (1), pp. 140–43.

18. M. T. Antonio *et al.*, 'Neurochemical changes in newborn rat's brain after gestational cadmium and lead exposure', *Toxicology Letters* (1999), 104 (1–2), pp. 1–9.

19. E. A. Field *et al.*, 'Developmental toxicology evaluation of diethyl and dimethyl phthalate in rats', *Teratology* (1993), 48 (1), pp. 33–44.

20. B. N. Gupta *et al.*, 'Effects of a polybrominated biphenyl mixture in the rat and mouse. I. Six-month exposure', *Toxicology and Applied Pharmacology* (1983), 68 (1), pp. 1–18.

21. Trankina *et al.*, 'Effects of in vitro Ronnel'.

22. J. L. De Bleecker *et al.*, 'Neurological aspects of organophosphate poisoning', *Clinical Neurology and Neurosurgery* (1992), 94, pp. 93–103.

23. S. F. Ali *et al.*, 'Effect of an organophosphate (Dichlorvos) on open field behaviour and locomotor activity: correlation with regional brain monoamine levels', *Psychopharmacology* (1980), 68 (1), pp. 37–42.

24. J. T. Yen *et al.*, 'Effect of carbadox on growth, fasting metabolism, thyroid function and gastrointestinal tract in young pigs', *American Institute of Nutrition* (1984), 115, pp. 970–79.

25. T. Tanaka, 'Reproductive and neurobehavioural effects of chloropham administered to mice in the diet', *Toxicology and Industrial Health* (1997), 13 (6), pp. 715–26.

26. A. Heeremans *et al.*, 'Elimination profile of methylthiouracil in cows after oral administration', *Analyst* (1998), 123, pp. 2625–8.

27. A. L. Sawaya and P. G. Lunn, 'Lowering of plasma triiodothyronine level and sympathetic activity does not alter hypoalbuminaemiain rats fed a low protein diet', *British Journal of Nutrition* (1998), 79 (5), pp. 455–62.

28. K. J. Van den Berg *et al.*, 'Interactions of halogenated industrial chemicals with transthyretin and effects of thyroid hormone levels in vivo', *Archives of Toxicology* (1991), 65, pp. 15–19.

29. A. Vigano *et al.*, 'Anorexia and cachexia in advanced cancer patients', *Cancer Surveys* (1994), 21, pp. 99–115.

30. M. C. Nesheim, 'Some observations on the effectiveness of anabolic agents in increasing the growth rate of poultry', *Environmental Quality and Safety. Supplement* (1976), 5, pp. 110–14.

31. J. S. Cranmer and D. L. Avery, 'Postnatal endocrine dysfunction resulting from prenatal exposure to carbofuran, diazinon or chlordane', *Journal of Environmental Pathology and Toxicology* (1978), 2, pp. 375–67.

32. J. F. Hancock, 'Effects of estrogens and androgens on animal growth', p. 271.

33. V. W. Hays, 'Effect of antibiotics', in Pearson (ed.), *Growth regulation in farm animals*, pp. 299–320.

34. ibid.

35. Vigano *et al.*, 'Anorexia and cachexia'.

36. S. H. Kennedy and D. S. Goldbloom, 'Current perspectives on drug therapies for anorexia nervosa and bulimia nervosa', *Practical Therapeutics* (1991), 41 (3), pp. 367–77.

37. ibid.

38. Morley, 'Anorexia in older persons'.

39. E. M. Walker Jr *et al.*, 'Prevention of cisplatin-induced toxicology by selected dithiocarbamates', *Annals of Clinical and Laboratory Science* (1994), 24 (2), pp. 121–33.

40. E. Van Ganse *et al.*, 'Effects of antihistamines in adult asthma: a meta-analysis of clinical trials', *European Respiratory Journal* (1997), 10 (10), pp. 2216–24.

41. Bailey, 'Vyvyan Howard in bullet points'.

42. Alleva *et al.*, 'Statement from the work session on environmental endocrine-disrupting chemicals'.

43. Nebert, *Human genetic variation*, p. 32.

44. W. B. Deichmann *et al.*, 'Effects of starvation in rats with elevated DDT and dieldrin tissue levels', *Internationales Archiv für Arbeitsmedizin* (1972), 29, pp. 233–52.

45. R. W. Chadwick *et al.*, 'Possible antiestrogenic activity of lindane in female rats', *Journal of Biochemical Toxicology* (1988), 3, pp. 147–58.

46. D. C. Villeneuve *et al.*, 'Effect of food deprivation on low level hexachlorobenzene exposure in rats', *Science of the Total Environment* (1977), 8 (2), pp. 179–86.

47. Stellman *et al.*, 'Adipose and serum levels'.

48. M. E. Hovinga, *et al.*, 'Environmental exposure and lifestyle predictors of lead, cadmium, PCB, and DDT levels in Great Lakes fish eaters', *Archives of Environmental Health* (1993), 48, pp. 98–104.

49. E. Dar *et al.*, 'Fish consumption and reproductive outcomes in Green Bay, Wisconsin', *Environmental Research* (1992), 59 (1), pp. 189–201.

50. E. Lonky *et al.*, 'Neonatal behavioural assessment scale performance in humans influenced by maternal consumption of environmentally contaminated Lake Ontario fish', *Journal of Great Lakes Research* (1996) 22 (2), pp. 198–212.

51. A. Bernhoft *et al.*, 'Effects of pre- and postnatal exposure to 3, 3', 4, 4', 5-pentachlorobiphenyl on physical development, neurobehaviour and xenobiotic metabolising enzymes in rats', *Environmental Toxicology and Chemistry* (1994), 13 (10), pp. 1589–97.

Chapter 4: Your Natural Slimming System

1. Harris, 'Role of set-point theory'.

2. C. Michel and M. Cabanac, 'Effects of dexamethasone on the body weight set point of rats', *Physiology and Behavior* (1999), 68 (1–2), pp. 145–50.

3. R. E. Keesey and M. D. Hirvonen, 'Body weight set-points: determination and adjustment', *Journal of Nutrition* (1997), 127 (9), pp. 1875s–1883s.

4. M. E. Hadley, *Endocrinology*, Prentice-Hall International (Publishers), New Jersey, 3rd edn, 1992, pp. 19–21.

5. ibid., pp. 362–90.

6. Brownell and Fairburn (eds.), *Eating disorders and obesity*, pp. 3–7.

7. J. Clarke, *Body foods for life*, Weidenfeld & Nicolson, London, 1998, p. 200.

8. Harris, 'Role of set-point theory'.

9. P. Bjorntorp, 'Endocrine abnormalities of obesity', *Metabolism* (1995), 44: 9 (suppl. 3), pp. 21–3.

10. P. T. Williams, 'Weight set-point theory predicts HDL-cholesterol levels in previously obese long-distance runners', *International Journal of Obesity* (1990), 14 (5), pp. 421–7.

11. Y. Hu *et al.*, 'Comparisons of serum testosterone and corticosterone between exercise training during normoxia and hypobaric hypoxia in rats', *European Journal of Applied Physiology* (1998), 78, pp. 417–21.

12. S. V. Roberts *et al.*, 'Energy expenditure and intake in infants born to lean and overweight mothers', *New England Journal of Medicine* (1988), 318, p. 461.

13. T. Archer and A. Fredriksson, 'Functional changes implicating dopaminergic systems following perinatal treatments', *Developmental Pharmacology and Therapeutics* (1992), 18 (3–4), pp. 201–2.

14. J. A. Levine *et al.*, 'Role of nonexercise activity thermogenesis in resistance to fat gain in humans', *Science* (1999), 283 (5399), pp. 212–14.

15. D. S. Miller and P. Mumford, 'Obesity: physical activity and nutrition', *Proceedings of the Nutritional Society* (1966), 25 (2), pp. 100–107.

16. R. Scott Van Zant, 'Influence of diet and exercise on energy expenditure – a review', *International Journal of Sport Nutrition* (1992), 2, pp. 1–19.

17. C. Bouchard *et al.*, 'Genetic effect in resting and exercise metabolic rates', *Metabolism* (1989), 38, p. 364.

18. L. Landsberg *et al.*, 'Sympathoadrenal system and regulation of thermogenesis', *American Journal of Physiology* (1984), 247 (2, pt 1), E181–9.

19. G. R. Goldberg *et al.*, 'Longitudinal assessment of the components

of energy balance in well-nourished lactating women', *American Journal of Clinical Nutrition* (1991), 54, pp. 788–98.

20. A.G. Dulloo and D.S. Miller, 'The effect of parasympathetic drugs on energy expenditure: Relevance to the autonomic hypothesis', *Canadian Journal of Physiology and Pharmacology* (1986), 64, pp. 586–91.

21. R.T. Jung *et al.*, 'Reduced thermogenesis in obesity', *Nature* (1979), 279, pp. 322–3.

22. B. Zahorska-Markiewicz, 'Thermic effect of food and exercise in obesity', *European Journal of Applied Physiology* (1980), 44, pp. 231–5.

23. Ali *et al.*, 'Effect of an organophosphate (Dichlorvos)'.

24. A. Moor de Burgos *et al.*, 'Blood vitamin and lipid levels in overweight and obese women', *European Journal of Clinical Nutrition* (1992), 46, pp. 803–8.

25. S. Klaus, 'Functional differentiation of white and brown adiposities', *Bioessays* (1997), 19 (3), pp. 215–23.

26. Moor de Burgos *et al.*, 'Blood vitamin and lipid levels'.

27. T. Decsi *et al.*, 'Reduced plasma concentrations of alpha-tocopherol and beta-carotene in obese boys', *Journal of Pediatrics* (1997), 130 (4), pp. 653–5.

28. G.J. Naylor *et al.*, 'A double blind placebo controlled trial of ascorbic acid in obesity', *Nutrition and Health* (1985), 4 (1), pp. 25–8.

29. Gardner and Halweil, 'Overfed and Underfed'.

30. M. Ohrvall *et al.*, 'Lower tocopherol serum levels in subjects with abdominal adiposity', *Journal of Internal Medicine* (1993), 234 (1), pp. 53–60.

31. R.B. Singh *et al.*, 'Association of low plasma concentrations of antioxidant vitamins, magnesium and zinc with high body fat per cent measured by bioelectrical impedance analysis in Indian men', *Magnesium Research* (1998), 11 (1), pp. 3–10.

Chapter 5: How Chemicals Make You Fat

1. H.D. Colby *et al.*, 'Toxicology of the adrenal cortex: Role of metabolic activation', *Endocrine toxicology*, 2nd edn., eds. J.A. Thomas and H.D. Colby, Taylor and Francis, Washington, DC, 1997, pp. 81–131.

2. W. Rea, 'Nervous system', *in Chemical Sensitivity*, vol. 3, Lewis Publishers, Boca Raton, Florida, 1995, pp. 1727–885.

3. M.B. Abou-Donia and D.M. Lapadula, 'Mechanisms of organo-phosphorus ester-induced delayed neurotoxicity: Type I and type II', *Annual Review of Pharmacology and Toxicology* (1990), 30, pp. 405–40.

4. N.C. Rawlings *et al.*, 'Effects of the pesticides carbofuran, chlor-pyrifos, dimethoate, lindane, triallate, trifluralin, 2,4-D, and penta-chlorophenol on the metabolic endocrine and reproductive endocrine system in ewes', *Journal of Toxicology and Environmental Health* (1998), 54 (Part A), pp. 21–36.

5. M.J. DeVito and L.S. Birnbaum, 'Dioxins: Model chemicals for assessing receptor-mediated toxicity', *Toxicology* (1995) 102, pp. 115–23; G. Cehovic *et al.*, 'Paraxon: Effects on rat brain cholinesterase and on growth hormone and prolactin of pituitary', *Science* (1972), 175, pp. 1256–8.

6. J.A. Richardson *et al.*, 'Catecholamine metabolism in humans exposed to pesticides', *Environmental Research* (1975), 3 (9 June), pp. 290–94.

7. Colby *et al.*, 'Toxicology of the adrenal cortex'.

8. J.R. Beach *et al.*, 'Abnormalities on neurological examination among sheep farmers exposed to organophosphorous pesticides', *Occupational and Environmental Medicine* (1996), 53, pp. 520–25.

9. T. Namba *et al.*, 'Poisoning due to organophosphate insecticides', *American Journal of Medicine* (1971), 50, pp. 475–92.

10. R.J. Zwiener and C.M. Ginsburg, 'Organophosphate and carbamate poisoning in infants and children', *Pediatrics* (1988), 81 (5), p. 683.

11. Iakovleva *et al.*, '[Vitamin A and E allowance]'.

12. E.J. Cheraskin, 'Antioxidants in health and disease', *Journal of the Optometric Association* (1996), 67 (1), pp. 50–57.

13. P. Holford, 'The myth of the well balanced diet', *The Optimum Nutrition Bible*, Piatkus, London, 1999, pp. 27–33.

14. Field *et al.*, 'Developmental toxicology evaluation'.

15. Vigano *et al.*, 'Anorexia and cachexia'.

16. R. Husain *et al.*, 'Differential responses of regional brain polyamines following in utero exposure to synthetic pyrethroid insecticides:

a preliminary report', *Bulletin of Environmental Contamination and Toxicology* (1992), 49 (3), pp. 402–9.

17. Gawecki *et al.*, 'The effect of poisoning with dithane M-45'.

18. F.P. Guengerich, 'Influence of nutrients and other dietary materials on cytochrome P-450 enzymes', *American Journal of Clinical Nutrition* (1995), 61 (3), pp. 651s–658s.

19. Cehovic *et al.*, 'Paraxon'.

20. Guengerich, 'Influence of nutrients'.

21. W.B. Deichmann *et al.*, 'Dieldrin and DDT in the tissues of mice fed aldrin and DDT for seven generations', *Archives of Toxicology* (1975), 34 (3), pp. 173–82.

22. P.D. Hrdina *et al.*, 'Role of noradrenaline, 5-hydroxytryptamine and acetylcholine in the hypothermic and convulsive effects of alpha-chlordane in rats', *European Journal of Pharmacology* (1974), 26 (2), pp. 306–12.

23. Richardson *et al.*, 'Catecholamine metabolism'.

24. W. Rea, 'Nutritional status and pollutant overload', *Chemical Sensitivity*, vol. 1, Lewis Publishers, Boca Raton, Florida, 1992, pp. 395–6.

25. Deichmann *et al.*, 'Dieldrin and DDT'.

26. Nebert, *Human genetic variation*, p. 32.

27. J.L. Jacobson and S.W. Jacobson, 'Intellectual impairment in children exposed to polychlorinated biphenyls in utero', *New England Journal of Medicine* (1996), 355 (11), pp. 783–9.

28. Hancock, 'Effects of estrogens and androgens'.

29. E. Showalter and A. Griffin, 'Commentary: all women should have a choice', *British Medical Journal* (1999), 335(7222), p. 1401.

30. P. Bundred *et al.*, 'Prevalence of overweight and obese children between 1989 and 1998: population based series of cross sectional studies', *British Medical Journal* (2001) 322 (7282), pp. 326–8.

31. Chadwick *et al.*, 'Effects of age and obesity'.

32. Holford, 'The myth of the well-balanced diet'.

33. J. To-Figueras *et al.*, 'Mobilization of stored hexachlorobenzene and p,p-dichlorodiphenyldichloroethylene during partial starvation in rats', *Toxicology Letters* (1988), 42 (1), pp. 79–86.

34. S. N. Blair *et al.*, 'Body weight change, all-cause mortality, and cause-

specific mortality in the multiple risk factor intervention trial', *Annals of Internal Medicine* (1993), 119, 7 (part 2), pp. 749–57.

Chapter 6: *All about* Chemical Calories

1. Harris, 'Role of set-point theory'.
2. A. C. Casey *et al.*, 'Aroclor 1242 inhalation and ingestion by Sprague-Dawley rats', *Journal of Toxicology and Environmental Health* (1999), 56 (5), pp. 311–42.
3. Gupta *et al.*, 'Effects of a polybrominated biphenyl mixture in the rat and mouse'.
4. K. N. Chetty *et al.*, 'Effect of cadmium on ATPase activities in rats fed on iron-deficient and sufficient diets', *Journal of Environmental Science and Health* (1980), 15 (4); pp. 379–93.
5. I. Chu *et al.*, 'Long term toxicity of octachlorostyrene in the rat', *Fundamental and Applied Toxicology* (1986), 6 (1), pp. 69–77.
6. V. C. Moser *et al.*, 'A multidisciplinary approach to toxicological screening: III. Neurobehavioural toxicology', *Journal of Toxicology and Environmental Health* (1995) 45 (2), pp. 173–210.
7. Health and Safety Executive, *Annual Report of the Working Party on Pesticide Residues*, Ministry of Agriculture, Fisheries and Food, HMSO, London, 1995–8.

Chapter 7: *What Makes Lettuce More 'Fattening' Than Avocado?*

1. Health and Safety Executive, *Annual Report of the Working Party on Pesticide Residues*, 1995–8.
2. J. E. Bjerk and E. M. Brevik, 'Organochlorine compounds in aquatic environments', *Archives of Environmental Contamination and Toxicology* (1980), 9 (6), pp. 743–50.
3. J. Leake, 'How farming turned salmon into a high fat food', *Sunday Times*, London, 22 July 2001.
4. R. Young and A. Craig, 'Too hard to swallow', *Soil Association*, Bristol, 4 June 2001.
5. P. M. Friar and S. L. Reynolds, 'The effect of home processing

on post-harvest fungicide residues in citrus fruit', *Food Additives and Contaminants* (1994), 11 (1), pp. 57–70.

6. ibid.

7. Trankina *et al.*, 'Effects of in vitro Ronnel'.

8. A. Watterson, *Pesticides and Your Food*, Greenprint, Merlin Press, London, 1991.

9. B. J. Liska and W. J. Stadelman, 'Effects of processing on pesticides in foods', *Residue Reviews* (1969), 29, pp. 61–72.

Chapter 8: Don't Panic, Go Organic

1. V. Worthington, 'Effect of agricultural methods on nutritional quality: A comparison of organic with conventional crops', *Alternative Therapies* (1998), 4 (1), pp. 58–69.

2. S. S. Schiffman *et al.*, 'Environmental pollutants alter taste responses in the gerbil', *Pharmacology, Biochemistry and Behavior* (1994), 52 (1), pp. 189–94.

3. P. Kendall, 'Why eating fruit and vegetables was better for us 50 years ago', *Daily Mail*, London, 5 March 2001.

4. V. Worthington, 'Nutritional quality of organic versus conventional fruits, vegetables, and grains', *Journal of Alternative and Complementary Medicine* (2001), 7 (2), pp 161–73.

5. J. B. Pangborn and B. Smith, 'Elemental content of some organic foods vs. commercial foods', presented at the 13th Annual International Symposium on Man and his Environment in Health and Disease, Dallas, Texas, 1995.

6. ibid.

7. Soil Association, 'Standards for organic food and farming', Bristol (1999), September, pp. 52–5.

8. ibid., pp. 57–9.

Chapter 9: *Eating Low in* Chemical Calories

1. M. N. Jacobs, 'Organochlorine residues in fish oil dietary supplements: Comparison with industrial grade oils', *Chemosphere* (1998), 37 (9–12), pp. 1709–21.

2. M. E. Zabik and R. Schemmel, 'Influence of diet on hexachlorobenzene accumulation in Osborne Mendel rats', *Journal of Environmental Pathology and Toxicology* (1980), 4 (5–6), pp. 97–103.

3. S. S. Rizvi, 'Requirements for food packaged in polymeric films', *Critical Reviews in Food Science and Nutrition* (1981), 14 (2), pp. 111–34.

4. F. A. Arcadi *et al.*, 'Oral toxicity of bis(2-ethylhexyl) phthalate during pregnancy and suckling in the Long-Evans rat', *Food and Chemical Toxicology* (1998), 36 (11), pp. 963–70.

5. L. Castle *et al.*, 'Migration of plasticizers from printing inks into foods', *Food Additives and Contaminants* (1989), 6 (4), pp. 437–43.

6. M. Karstadt, 'PVC: health implications and production trends', *Environmental Health Perspectives* (1976), 17, pp. 107–15.

7. L. Fishbein, 'Toxicity of the components of poly (vinylchloride) polymers additives', *Progress in Clinical and Biological Research* (1984), 141, pp. 113–36.

8. M. S. Tawfik and A. Huyghebaert, 'Polystyrene cups and containers: styrene migration', *Food Additives and Contaminants* (1998), 15 (5), pp. 592–9.

9. F. Farabollini *et al.*, 'Perinatal exposure to the estrogenic pollutant bisphenol A affects behaviour in male and female rats', *Pharmacology, Biochemistry, and Behavior* (1999), 64 (4) pp. 687–94.

10. Castle *et al.*, 'Migration of plasticizers from printing inks into foods'.

11. Fishbein, 'Toxicity of the components of poly (vinylchloride) polymers additives'.

12. Y. Okai and K. Higashiokai, 'A simple estimation method for the embryonic toxicity of plastic wrapping sheets using an egg shell free culture system of chick embryos', *Sangyo Ika Daigaku Zasshi* (1999), 21 (3), pp. 191–8.

13. A. B. Badeka and M. G. Kontominas, 'Effect of microwave heating

on the migration of dioctyladipate and acetyltributylcitrate plasticizers from food-grade PVC and PVDC/PVC films into olive oil and water', *Zeitschrift für Lebensmittel-Untersuchung und -Forschung* (1996), 202 (4), pp. 313–17.

14. B. Aurela *et al.*, 'Phthalates in paper and board packaging and their migration into Tenax and sugar', *Food Additives and Contaminants* (1999), 16 (12), pp. 571–7.

15. L. Castle *et al.*, 'Migration from plasticized films into food. 2. Migration of di-(2-ethylhexyl) adipate from PVC films used for retail food packaging', *Food Additives and Contaminants* (1987), 4 (4), pp. 399–406.

16. ibid.

17. ibid.

18. J. H. Petersen *et al.*, 'PVC cling film in contact with cheese: health aspects related to global migration and specific migration of DEHA', *Food Additives and Contaminants* (1995), 12 (2), pp. 245–53.

19. Aurela *et al.*, 'Phthalates in paper and board packaging'.

20. L. Gramiccioni *et al.*, 'Aluminium levels in Italian diets and in selected foods from aluminium utensils', *Food Additives and Contaminants* (1996), 13 (7), pp. 767–74.

21. P. Rajwanshi *et al.*, 'Aluminium leaching from surrogate aluminium food containers under different pH and fluoride concentration', *Bulletin of Environmental Contamination and Toxicology* (1999), 63 (2), pp. 271–6.

22. Aurela *et al.*, 'Phthalates in paper and board packaging'.

23. Castle *et al.*, 'Migration of plasticizers from printing inks'.

24. Farabollini *et al.*, 'Perinatal exposure to the estrogenic pollutant bisphenol A'.

25. H. J. Schattenberg, 3rd *et al.*, 'Effect of household preparation on levels of pesticide residues in produce', *Journal of AOAC International* (1996), 79 (6), pp. 1447–53.

26. Friar and Reynolds, 'The effect of home processing'.

27. J. C. Street, 'Methods of removal of pesticide residues', *Canadian Medical Association Journal* (1969), 100, pp. 154–60.

28. ibid.

29. Liska and Stadelman, 'Effects of processing'.

30. Friar and Reynolds, 'The effect of home processing'.

31. D. D. Hemphill *et al.*, 'Effect of washing, trimming and cooking on levels of DDT and derivatives in green beans', *Journal of Agricultural and Food Chemistry* (1967), 15, p. 290.

32. Parents for Safe Food and Friends of the Earth, 'Dangerous Agrochemicals in Supermarket foods', Parents for Safe Food and Friends of the Earth press release, UK, 14 February 1990.

33. A. Schecter *et al.*, 'A comparison of dioxins, dibenzofurans and coplanar PCBs in uncooked and broiled ground beef, catfish, and bacon', *Chemosphere* (1998), 37 (9–12), pp. 1723–30.

34. M. D. Rose *et al.*, 'The effect of cooking on veterinary drug residues in food: 7. Ivermectin', *Food Additives and Contaminants* (1998), 15 (2), pp. 157–61.

35. Tawfik and Huyghebaert, 'Polystyrene cups and containers'.

Chapter 10: Pure Water, the Slimmer's Friend

1. L. McTaggart, 'Assault on a generation', *What Your Doctor Doesn't Tell You* (2000), 11 (6), p. 5.

2. G. Lean and F. Pearce, 'Your tap water – Pure or poisoned', *Observer*, London, 8 August 1989.

3. J. M. Esch, 'Hydrological Investigation, Nottawa Sepee Site, Village of Napoleon, Jackson County', Michigan Department of Natural Resources, 1995.

4. M. A. Medinsky *et al.*, 'Effects of a thirteen-week inhalation exposure to ethyl tertiary butyl ether on Fischer-344 rats and CD-1 mice', *Toxicological Science* (1999), 51 (1), pp. 108–18.

5. K. Cooke and M. H. Gould, 'The health effects of aluminium – a review', *Journal of the Royal Society of Health* (1991), 111 (5), pp. 163–8.

6. C. F. Mello *et al.*, 'Effect of lead acetate on neurobehavioural development of rats', *Brazilian Journal of Medical and Biological Research* (1998), 31 (7), pp. 943–50.

7. W. Rea, 'Avoidance-Water', in *Chemical Sensitivity*, vol. 4, Lewis Publishers, Boca Raton, Florida, 1996, pp. 2359–82.

8. Lean and Pearce, 'Your tap-water – Pure or poisoned'.

9. F. Craig and P. Craig, 'The poison in the pipes', in *Britain's Poisoned Water*, Penguin Books, London, 1989, pp. 31–44.

10. A. L. Gittleman, 'Water: The Chlorine Connection', *The Living Beauty Detox Program*, HarperCollins, San Francisco, 2000.

11. S. Clark, 'Water, the drink of life', *The Times 2 Alternative Health*, London, 21 March 2000.

12. S. Welle *et al.*, 'Increased plasma norepinephrine concentrations and metabolic rates following glucose ingestion in man', *Metabolism* (1980), 29 (9), pp. 806–9.

Chapter 11: Chemical Calories *Lurk All around You*

1. E. J. Routledge *et al.*, 'Some alkyl hydroxy benzoate preservatives (parabens) are estrogenic', *Toxicology and Applied Pharmacology* (1998), 153 (1), pp. 12–19.

2. G. M. Currado, and S. Harrad, 'The significance of indoor air inhalation as a pathway of human exposure to PCBs', *Organohalogen Compounds* (1997), 33, pp. 377–81.

3. R. P. Benedetti, 'Understanding fire retardant and flame resistant materials', *Journal of the American College Health Association* (1979), 27 (6), pp. 311–41.

4. K. Nesaretnam *et al.*, '3,4,3',4'-Tetrachlorobiphenyl acts as an estrogen in vitro and in vivo', *Molecular Endocrinology* (1996), 10, pp. 912–36.

5. H. M. Haynes *et al.*, 'Case control study of canine malignant lymphoma: Positive association with dog owners use of 2,4-D', *Journal of the National Cancer Institute* (1991), 83, pp. 1226–31.

6. M. Levy, 'Dental Amalgam: toxicological evaluation and health risk assessment', *Journal of the Canadian Dental Association* (1995), 61 (8), pp. 667–8 and 671–4.

7. A. Boehncke and A. Curtis, 'Volatilisation of selected pesticides from glass, leaf, and soil surfaces', *Proceedings of IUPAC Congress*, Hamburg, 1990.

Chapter 12: *Beating the* Chemical Calorie

1. P. Dingle *et al.*, 'Reducing formaldehyde exposure in office environments using plants', *Bulletin of Environmental Contamination and Toxicology* (2000), 64 (2), pp. 302–8.
2. A. R. Seyal, 'A relationship of quality of garments to blood pressure in young school children', *Clinical Ecology* (1986/7), 4 (3), pp. 115–19; A. R. Seyal *et al.*, 'Systolic blood pressure, heart rate, and premature ventricular contractions in a population sample: Relationship to cotton and synthetic clothing', *Clinical Ecology* (1986/7), 4 (2), pp. 69–74.
3. A. Clarke *et al.*, 'Organic home', in *Living Organic: Easy steps to an organic family lifestyle*, Time-Life Books, London, 2001, p. 98.

Chapter 13: *Repair and Revitalize Your Natural Slimming System*

1. C. S. Hun *et al.*, 'Increased uncoupling protein2 mRNA in white adipose tissue, and decrease in leptin, visceral fat, blood glucose, and cholesterol in KK-Ay mice fed with eicosapentaenoic and docosahexaenoic acids in addition to linolenic acid', *Biochemical and Biophysical Research Communications* (1999), 259 (1), pp. 85–90.
2. G. V. Skuladottir and M. Johannsson, 'Inotropic response of rat heart papillary muscle to alpha 1- and beta-adrenoceptor stimulation in relation to dietary n-6 and n-3 polyunsaturated fatty acids (PUFA) and age', *Pharmacology and Toxicology* (1997), 80 (2), pp. 85–90.
3. T. Horie *et al.*, 'Docosahexaenoic acid exhibits a potent protection of small intestine from methotrexate-induced damage in mice', *Life Science* (1998), 62 (15), pp. 1333–8.
4. S. M. Watkins *et al.*, 'DHA reduces free radicals generation in the fetal rat brain', *Journal of Lipid Research* (1998), 39 (8), pp. 1583–8.
5. A. P. Simopoulous, 'Omega-3 fatty acids in health and disease and in growth and development', *American Journal of Clinical Nutrition* (1991), 54 (3), pp. 438–63.
6. Jacobs, 'Organochlorine residues in fish oil dietary supplements'.
7. L. H. Garthoff *et al.*, 'Blood chemistry alterations in rats after single

and multiple gavage administration of polychlorinated biphenyl', *Toxicology and Applied Pharmacology* (1981), 60 (1), pp. 33–44.

8. ibid.

9. P. Pittet *et al.*, 'Thermic effect of glucose in obese subjects studied by direct and indirect calorimetry', *British Journal of Nutrition* (1976), 35, p. 281.

10. ibid.

11. Zabik and Schemmel, 'Influence of diet on hexachlorobenzene accumulation'.

12. Guengerich, 'Influence of nutrients'.

13. W. Rea, 'Nutritional status and pollutant overload', in *Chemical Sensitivity*, vol. 1, Lewis Publishers, Boca Raton, Florida, 1992, pp. 345–93.

14. ibid.

15. G. Y. Nicolau, 'Circadian rhythms of RNA, DNA and protein in the rat thyroid, adrenal and testis in chronic pesticide exposure. II. Effect of the herbicides, aminotriazole and alachlor', *Endocrinologie* (1983), 21 (2), pp. 105–12.

16. Rea, 'Nutritional status and pollutant overload'.

17. J. C. Street and R. W. Chadwick, 'Ascorbic acid requirements and metabolism in relation to organochlorine pesticides', *Annals of the New York Academy of Sciences* (1975), 258 (30 September), pp. 132–43.

18. 'A square meal for Britain?' Research by the Bateman Catering Organization, 1981.

Chapter 14: Shed Your Body Stores of Chemical Calories

1. Street and Chadwick, 'Ascorbic acid requirements and metabolism'.

2. P. J. Korytko *et al.*, 'Induction of hepatic cytochromes P450 in dogs exposed to a chronic low dose of polychlorinated biphenyls', *Toxicological Sciences* (1999), 47 (1), pp. 52–61.

3. W. Rea, 'Thermal chamber depuration and physical therapy', in *Chemical Sensitivity*, vol. 4, Lewis Publishers, Boca Raton, Florida, 1996, pp. 2433–79.

4. R. M. Cook and K. A. Wilson, 'Removal of pesticide residues from dairy cattle', *Journal of Dairy Science* (1971), 54 (5), pp. 712–18.

5. R. M. Cook, 'Metabolism of xenobiotics in ruminants. Dieldrin

recycling from the blood to the gastro-intestinal tract', *Journal of Agricultural and Food Chemistry* (1970), 18 (3), pp. 434–6.

6. G. F. Fries *et al.*, 'Effect of activated carbon on elimination of organochlorine pesticides from rats and cows', *Journal of Dairy Science* (1970), 53 (11), pp. 1632–7.

7. ibid.

8. W. Rea, 'Nutrient replacement: Alkalization', in *Chemical Sensitivity*, vol. 4, Lewis Publishers, Boca Raton, Florida, 1996, pp. 2563–7.

9. Goldman, 'Children – Unique and vulnerable'.

10. Chadwick *et al.*, 'The effects of age and obesity'.

11. L. E. Holt and P. H. Holz, 'The black bottle', *Journal of Pediatrics* (1963), 63 (2), pp.306–14.

12. ibid.

13. S. J. Stohs, 'The role of free radicals in toxicity and disease', *Journal of Basic and Clinical Physiology and Pharmacology* (1995), 6 (3–4), pp. 205–28.

14. M. S. Desole *et al.*, 'Neuronal antioxidant system and MPTP induced oxidative stress in the striatum and brain stem of the rat', *Pharmacology, Biochemistry, and Behavior* (1995), 51 (4), pp. 581–92.

15. Cheraskin, 'Antioxidants in health and disease'.

16. Moor de Burgos *et al.*, 'Blood vitamin and lipid levels'.

17. Rea, 'Nutritional status and pollutant overload'.

18. ibid.

19. Guengerich, 'Influence of nutrients'.

20. S. D. Phinney *et al.*, 'Reduced adipose 18:3 omega 3 with weight loss by very low calorie dieting', *Lipids* (1990), 25 (12), pp. 798–806.

21. Department of Health, 'Dietary Reference Values for Food Energy and Nutrients for the United Kingdom (41): Report on Health and Social Subjects, 1997', Stationery Office, London, pp. 61–71.

22. T. J. Meredith and J. A. Vale, 'Treatment of paraquat poisoning in man: Methods to prevent absorption', *Human Toxicology* (1987), 6, pp.49–55.

23. M. von Ardenne, 'Oxygen multistep therapy: Physiological and technical foundations', George Thieme Verlag, Stuttgart/New York, 1990.

24. Rea, 'Thermal chamber depuration'.

Chapter 15: Guide to the Detox Diet

1. Jacobson and Jacobson, 'Dose-response in perinatal exposure'.
2. M. Schlaud *et al.*, 'Organochlorine residues in human breast milk: Analysis through a sentinel practice network', *Journal of Epidemiology and Community Health* (1995), 49 (suppl. 1), pp. 17–21.
3. Cheraskin, 'Antioxidants in health and disease'.
4. W. Rea, 'Nutritional Replacement', in *Chemical Sensitivity*, vol. 4, Lewis Publishers, Boca Raton, Florida, 1996, pp. 2541–684.
5. Department of Health, 'Dietary Reference Values'.

Chapter 18: The Chemical Calorie *Food Guide*

1. Health and Safety Executive, *Annual Report of the Working Party on Pesticide Residues*, 1995–8.

Chapter 19: Charting Your Progress on the Detox Diet

1. E. Bender and A. Bender, 'Body Composition', in *Nutrition: a reference handbook*, Oxford University Press, Oxford, 1997, pp. 11–17.

Chapter 20: Typical Questions and Useful Answers

1. Moor de Burgos *et al.*, 'Blood vitamin and lipid levels'.
2. R. V. Patwardhan *et al.*, 'Effects of caffeine on plasma free fatty acids, urinary catecholamines, and drug binding', *Clinical Pharmacology and Therapeutics* (1980), 28 (3), pp. 398–403.
3. Hovinga *et al.*, 'Environmental exposure and lifestyle predictors'.
4. Alleva *et al.*, 'Statement from the work session on environmental endocrine-disrupting chemicals'.
5. Schlaud *et al.*, 'Organochlorine residues in human breast milk'.
6. Birnbaum, 'Endocrine effects of prenatal exposure to PCBs, dioxins, and other xenobiotics'.
7. L. Brabin and B. J. Brabin, 'The cost of successful adolescent growth

and development in girls in relation to iron and vitamin A status', *American Journal of Clinical Nutrition* (1992), 55 (5), pp. 955–8.

8. T. Baptista *et al.*, 'Antipsychotic drugs and reproductive hormones: Relationship to body weight regulation', *Pharmacology, Biochemistry, and Behavior* (1999), 62 (3), pp. 409–17.

9. A. N. E. Birch *et al.*, 'Tri-trophic interactions involving pest aphids, predatory 2-spot ladybirds and transgenic potatoes expressing snowdrop lectin for aphid resistance', *Molecular Breeding* (1999), 5, pp. 75–83.

Chapter 21: Maximize Your Fitness

1. Prentice and Jebb, 'Obesity in Britain'.

2. Namba *et al.*, 'Poisoning due to organophosphate insecticides'.

3. R. A. Cassidy *et al.*, 'The effects of chlordane exposure during pre- and postnatal periods at environmentally relevant levels on sex steroid mediated behaviours and functions in the rat', *Toxicology and Applied Pharmacology* (1994), 126 (2), pp. 326–37.

4. F. Janik and H. U. Wolf, 'The Ca2+-transport-ATPase of human erythrocytes as an in vitro toxicity test system – Acute effects of some chlorinated compounds', *Journal of Applied Toxicology* (1992), 12 (5), pp. 351–8.

5. P. Schrauwen *et al.*, 'Human uncoupling proteins and obesity', *Obesity Research* (1999), 7 (1), pp. 97–105.

6. Ali *et al.*, 'Effect of an organophosphate (Dichlorvos)'.

7. Zahovska-Mankiewicz, 'Thermic effect of food and exercise'.

8. H. Itoh *et al.*, 'Vitamin E supplementation attenuates leakage of enzymes following 6 successive days of running training', *International Journal of Sports Medicine* (2000), 21 (5), pp. 369–74.

9. Namba *et al.*, 'Poisoning due to . . .'

10. M. Battino *et al.*, 'Oxidative injury and inflammatory periodontal diseases: the challenge of anti-oxidants to free radicals and reactive oxygen species', *Critical Reviews in Oral Biology and Medicine* (1999), 10 (4), pp. 458–76.

11. Y. Mori *et al.*, 'Influence of highly purified eicosapentaenoic acid

ethyl ester on insulin resistance in the Otsuka Long-Evans Tokushima Fatty rat, a model of spontaneous non-insulin-dependent diabetes mellitus', *Metabolism* (1997), 46 (12), pp. 1458–64.

12. Hu *et al.*, 'Comparisons of serum testosterone and corticosterone'; M. Lafontan and M. Berlan, 'Fat cell adrenergic receptors and the control of white and brown cell function', *Journal of Lipid Research* (1993), 34 (7), pp. 1057–91.

13. Miller and Mumford, 'Obesity'.

14. N. L. Keim *et al.*, 'Effect of exercise and dietary restraint on energy intake of reduced obese women', *Appetite* (1996), 26, pp. 55–70.

15. J. L. Thompson *et al.*, 'Effects of diet and diet-plus-exercise programs on resting metabolic rate: a meta-analysis', *International Journal of Sport Nutrition* (1996), 6, pp. 41–61.

16. ibid.

17. D. L. Ballor *et al.*, 'Resistance weight training during caloric restriction enhances lean body weight maintenance', *American Journal of Clinical Nutrition* (1988), 47, pp. 19–25.

Chapter 22: Combating Twenty-first-century Illness

1. Beaumont, 'The chronic effects of pesticides'.

2. Gardner and Halweil, 'Overweight and Underfed'.

3. S. Y. Young *et al.*, 'Body mass index and asthma in the military population of the northwestern United States', *Archives of Internal Medicine* (2001), 161 (13), pp. 1605–11.

4. Baxter, 'Obesity surgery'.

5. W. J. Rea, *Chemical Sensitivity*, vol. 3, Lewis Publishers, Boca Raton, Florida, 1995.

6. ibid.

7. P. Beaumont, 'Acute pesticide poisoning', in *Pesticides, Policies and People; a guide to the issues*, Pesticides Trust, London, 1993, pp. 62–82.

8. Beaumont, 'The chronic effects of pesticides'.

9. Beaumont, 'Acute pesticide poisoning'.

10. World Health Organization, *Public health impact of pesticides used in agriculture*, WHO/UNEP, Geneva, 1990.

11. G. L. Henriksen *et al.*, 'Serum dioxin and diabetes mellitus in veterans

of Operation Ranch Hand', *Epidemiology* (1997), 8 (3), pp. 252–8.

12. M. Hooiveld *et al.*, 'Second follow-up of a Dutch cohort occupationally exposed to phenoxy herbicides, chlorophenols, and contaminants', *American Journal of Epidemiology* (1998), 147 (9), pp. 891–901.

13. I. Voccia *et al.*, 'Immunotoxicity of pesticides: a review', *Toxicology and Industrial Health* (1999), 15 (1–2), pp. 119–32.

14. K. S. Korach *et al.*, 'Xenoestrogens and estrogen receptor action', in J. A. Thomas and H. D. Colby (eds.), *Endocrine Toxicology*, Taylor & Francis, Washington, DC, 1996, pp. 181–211; E. C. Dodds and W. Lawson, 'Synthetic oestrogenic agents without the phenanthrene nucleus', *Nature* (1936), 13 June, p. 996.

15. G. B. Phillips, 'Hyperestrogenemia, diet, and disorders of western societies', *American Journal of Medicine* (1985), 78, pp. 363–6.

16. L. W. Frim-Titulaer *et al.*, 'Premature thelarche in Puerto Rico: a search for environmental factors', *American Journal of Diseases of Children* (1986), 140, pp. 1263–7.

17. Korach *et al.*, 'Xenoestrogens and estrogen receptor action'.

18. Rea, *Chemical Sensitivity*, vol. 3.

19. F. Falck Jr. *et al.*, 'Pesticides and polychlorinated biphenyl residues in human breast lipids and their relation to breast cancer', *Environmental Health* (1993), 5 (5), pp. 143–6.

20. E. J. Duell, *et al.*, 'A population-based case-control study of farming and breast cancer in North Carolina', *Epidemiology* (2000), 11 (5), pp. 523–31.

21. J. F. Dorgan *et al.*, 'Serum organochlorine pesticides and PCBs and breast cancer risk: results from a prospective analysis (USA)', *Cancer Causes and Control* (1999), 10, pp. 1–11.

22. Lissner *et al.*, 'Body weight variability in men'.

23. A. Vidal-Puig and S. O'Rahilly, 'Resistin: a new link between obesity and insulin resistance?', *Clinical Endocrinology* (2001), 55 (4), pp. 437–8.

24. L. Lissner, *et al.*, 'Variability of body weight and health outcomes in the Framingham population', *The New England Journal of Medicine* (1991), 324 (26), pp. 1839–44.

25. Stohs, 'The role of free radicals'.

Chapter 24: Slim for Life

1. K. D. Brownell and F. M. Kramer, 'Behavioural Management of Obesity', *Medical Clinics of North America* (1989), 73 (1), pp. 185–201.
2. Williams, 'Weight set-point theory'.

Recommended Reading

Allied Dunbar Fitness Survey, Sports Council, London, 1992.

P. Beaumont, *Pesticides, Policies and People; a guide to the issues*, Pesticides Trust, London, 1993.

K. D. Brownell and C. G. Fairburn (eds.), *Eating Disorders and Obesity: A Comprehensive Handbook*, Guilford Press, New York, 1995.

A. Clarke *et al.*, *Living Organic: Easy steps to an organic family lifestyle*, Time-Life Books, London, 2001.

F. Craig and P. Craig, *Britain's poisoned water*, Penguin, London, 1989.

Dr U. Erasmus, *Fats That Heal, Fats That Kill*, Alive Books, 1987/94.

S. Heaton, *Organic Farming, Food Quality and Human Health*, Soil Association, Bristol, 2001.

P. Holford, *The Optimum Nutrition Bible*, Piatkus, London, 1997.

J. Humphrys, *The Great Food Gamble*, Hodder & Stoughton, London, 2001.

A. M. Pearson (ed.), *Growth regulation in farm animals*, Elsevier Applied Science, London, 1991.

W. Rea, *Chemical Sensitivity*, Vols. 1–4, Lewis Publishers, Boca Raton, Florida, 1992–6.

S. Steingraber, *Living Downstream*, Virago Press, London, 1998.

A. Watterson, *Pesticides and your food*, Greenprint, Merlin Press, London, 1991.

Index

References to charts and tables are given in italics.